STUDENT WORKBOOK

Clinical Medical Assisting

Foundations and Practice

MARGARET SCHELL FRAZIER, RN, CMA, BS

DEBORAH J. BEDFORD, CMA, AAS
North Seattle Community College
Seattle, Washington

KRISTIANA SUE ROUTH, RMA
Certfied Healthcare Instructor

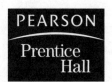
PEARSON

Prentice
Hall

Upper Saddle River, New Jersey 07458

Pearson Prentice Hall™ is a trademark of Pearson Education, Inc.
Pearson® is a registered trademark of Pearson plc.
Prentice Hall® is a registered trademark of Pearson Education, Inc.

Pearson Education Ltd., *London*
Pearson Education Australia Pty. Limited, *Sydney*
Pearson Education Singapore, Pte. Ltd.
Pearson Education North Asia Ltd., *Hong Kong*
Pearson Education Canada, Ltd., *Toronto*
Pearson Education de Mexico, S.A. de C.V.
Pearson Education—Japan, *Tokyo*
Pearson Education Malaysia, Pte. Ltd.
Pearson Education, Upper Saddle River, New Jersey

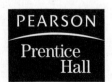

10 9 8 7 6 5 4
ISBN-10 0-13-089339-0
ISBN-13 978-0-13-089339-0

Contents

INTRODUCTION

This student workbook is designed as a study guide and practice tool to accompany the student text, *Clinical Medical Assisting: Foundations and Practice*. Read the Chapter Outlines and Chapter Reviews to reinforce what you have learned. Test your knowledge of medical terminology by defining the terms listed in the Medical Terminology Review section. Measure whether you have achieved the learning objectives in each chapter by answering the short answer questions in the Learning Activities sections of the workbook. Apply your knowledge to real-life situations by answering the Critical Thinking Questions. Take the Chapter Review Tests for each chapter to test your knowledge of key concepts.

Each chapter of this student workbook includes the following:

Chapter Outline: A list of the major content areas in the chapter. Review each of the topics and refer back to your textbook for any topics that remain unclear to you.

Chapter Review: A short summary of the chapter content. If any of the material presented in the review is unclear to you, refer back to your student text.

Learning Activities/Study Aids: Short answer questions/tasks allow you to measure whether or not you have achieved the learning objectives for the chapter.

Medical Terminology Review: A list of the medical terms and abbreviations presented in the chapter. Use a dictionary and the highlighted terms in the chapter to prepare the definitions.

Critical Thinking Questions: Challenging questions that allow you to apply your knowledge to real-life situations.

Chapter Review Test: Multiple choice, true/false, and short answer questions that test your knowledge of key concepts.

Procedure Skill Sheets: These boxed procedures correspond to those in the student textbook and allow students to demonstrate the skills needed to become a medical assistant. A space is included for your instructor to document that you have successfully completed the skill. Each step is weighted to better indicate proficiency of the skill.

LIST OF REVIEWERS

Kristen Anderson, RN, BSN
Medical Assisting Instructor
Wisconsin Technical College
Evansville, WI

Minda Brown, RMA
Pima Medical Institute
Colorado Springs, CO

Lisa M. Schoestek, BA, MLT(ASCP), RMA, CPC, CMBS, AHI
Lakeland Community College
Kirtland, OH

CHAPTER 1
The Medical Assistant Profession and Healthcare

CHAPTER OUTLINE

Review the Chapter Outline. If any content area is unclear, review that area before beginning workbook exercises.

- A. The Medical Assistant's Role in Health Care
- B. The History of Medicine
- C. Ethics and Patient Rights
- D. Professionalism
- E. Health-Care Team Members
- F. Job Opportunities
- G. Medical Assistant Educational Programs

CHAPTER REVIEW

The following is a summary of the chapter. If any of this material is unclear, review it in the textbook.

The medical assistant's role on the healthcare team has become increasingly more important, and assistants are now considered important multiskilled members for their vital support to the physician. The medical assistant must be well-trained and professional. Knowing the history of the evolution of modern medicine is the start of a medical assistant's education and includes such things as the Hippocratic Oath, the ethics set forth by the American Medical Association (AMA), and the Patient Bill of Rights, all of which affect the medical assisting profession. It is also very important that medical assistants know and understand their scope of practice and their own credentialing from their specific organizations: the American Association of Medical Assistants (AAMA) and the American Medical Technologists (AMT).

LEARNING ACTIVITIES AND STUDY AIDS

Review the following study aids and/or complete the activities to ensure that you have achieved the learning objectives for this chapter.

1. Terminology and abbreviations are absolutely critical and will be used daily. Always study both the terms and abbreviations in each chapter. For this chapter, list and define the terminology words and abbreviations in this chapter from memory. Then look at the terminology list in the text to determine any you forgot and add those words along with their definitions to this list. Those that need more study should be highlighted in a different color or underlined.

cadaver, dead body used for studying; prognosis - prediction of outcome of illness; indigestion - inability to digest; empathy - understanding of peoples thoughts, emotions; practitioner - person who practices in a profession.

epidemiology - branch of science that studies diseases.
RMA - Registered medical assistant, AAMA - American Association
of Medical Assistants, PCP - primary care physician, NCCA -
National Commission for Certifying Agents, HMO - health
maintenance org - CMA certified medical assistant - ABHES
Accreation bureau of Health Education schools

2. Review the material in the textbook specifically for the role of the medical assistant on the healthcare team. Explain this role. Also list at least six other professions that are included under the allied healthcare umbrella.

medical assistants are trained to perform many administrative
tasks, including, but no limited to, scheduling appointments & procedure
processing insurance claims & bookkeeping. Clinical includes
understanding & preforming procedures, specimen collection, diagnostic
testing & patient care.
1. OT - work with people who are physically, emotionally, developmentally
disabled. 2. nuclear med. technologist - despensing radioactive substances 3. Ultra
sound tech - Fetal/cardiac ultrasounds 4. Radiology tech - takes X rays 5 Phlet
mist - take blood specimens 6. Clinical dietitian - coordinates patients diet/meals.

3. After reading about Hippocrates and the classical and the modern versions of the Oath in the textbook, you will likely find the modern version to be clearer than the original Hippocratic Oath as it was first written. Review both Oaths and review the material on the history of medical assisting. Consider if any of the Oath would be relevant to medical assisting in the past and in the present. Find at least one statement or portion of a statement in the modern version that would apply to a modern medical assistant.

_____
_____
_____
_____
_____
_____
_____

4. Review the American Medical Association's Principles of Medical Ethics in your textbook. Then write an explanation in your own words of those Principles of Medical Ethics.

_____
_____
_____
_____
_____
_____
_____
_____

5. Using your textbook and the website of the American Hospital Association, search for the intent of the Patient Bill of Rights. What is its purpose? Explain both in your own words.

_____

_____

_____

_____

_____

_____

_____

6. In reading this chapter and browsing the two professional associations' websites (in question 1 above), you likely located information on:

   a. the professional characteristics expected of the medical assistant
   b. the typical job responsibilities of a medical assistant
   c. the medical assistant's place on the healthcare team

   For each of the three items above, provide the following information in your own words:

   For **a,** list the characteristics a medical assistant must possess to be professional, effective in patient care, and efficient for the physician.

   _____

   _____

   For **b,** list the responsibilities of a medical assistant when working in a clinic, physician's office, or other facility. Then choose any three and give a scenario-type example of the MA's performing that responsibility or the situation in which it could arise.

   _____

   _____

   For **c,** list four or five of the other various members of the healthcare team and state their primary jobs or expertise. Make a list of those members (no explanation needed) who may work daily or often in the clinic or office with an MA.

   _____

   _____

7. Check your local newspaper classified ads for open positions for medical assistants to determine the number and type of jobs available. If any ad states a starting pay or a pay range, write it down with the name of the facility. If any ad states a few of the duties of that position, write them down and the name of the facility. Finally, check the ads for jobs listed by other names that would be appropriate for a medical assistant (i.e., clinic assistant, assistant to physician, back office assistant, etc.). As above, list them along with the facility's name. After reading these ads, briefly summarize the job opportunities for MAs in your area.

   _____

   _____

   _____

   _____

   _____

   _____

8. What are the two professional associations for medical assistants? Provide their abbreviations and the full names. Explain the main purpose(s) for the existence of such organizations and list three or four reasons why it is beneficial to join the organization.

CMA-Certified medical Assistant

9. In your textbook, the section Medical Assistant Educational Programs contains critical information regarding the credentials available to the medical assistant. Review this information carefully and then list the requirements for eligibility to take the CMA and RMA examinations.

MEDICAL TERMINOLOGY REVIEW

Use a dictionary and highlighted terms in the textbook to define the following terms.

Terms

cadaver a dead body used for dissection, study, and tissue examples

empathy understanding of and sensitivity of feelings, thoughts and experiences of others

epidemiology branch of science that studies the incidence, spread and control of disease in a population

indigestion inability to digest, often with pain in the gastro-intestinal (GI) tract

practitioner a person who practices in a profession, such as medicine

prognosis an outcome prediction for the course of a disease and patient recovery (literal meaning: knowledge before)

Abbreviations

AAMA American Association of Medical Assistants

ABHES Accrediting Bureau of Health Education Schools

AMT American Medical Technologists

CMA Certified Medical Assistant

HMO Health Maintaince Organization

NCCA National Commission for Certifying Agencies

PCP Primary Care Physician

RMA Registered Medical Assistant

CRITICAL THINKING

1. Read the Case Study at the beginning of the textbook chapter. First, explain what Janet is worried about and why she is so worried.

   Janet is worried because she was told that the office manager is updating files & having everyone needs to be certified by taking & passing the AAMA exam within 12 months. Janet confessed she never took the exam because she was "grandfathered" in & didn't have to take an exam.

2. Annette, the office manager, will implement several changes, including the requirement that all medical assistants will become certified. Name three ways this may emotionally affect the non-certified medical assistants who have already been working for some time without certification.

3. How has the increasing focus on credentials and certification for medical assistants improved medical assisting? Improved patient care? How do you think patients feel about their healthcare workers being certified or not certified?

4. Why do you feel the medical assistant should know something about the history of medicine? The Code of Ethics for physicians? The Hippocratic Oath?

_____

_____

_____

5. Explain why introducing yourself as a "nurse" is not acceptable.

Introducing myself as a "nurse" is not acceptable because M.A's are not nurses. M.A.'s and nurses have different training, schooling and different things that they specialize in.

CHAPTER REVIEW TEST

MULTIPLE CHOICE

Circle the letter of the correct answer.

1. Which credential is offered by the AAMA?
   a. RMA
   b. CMA
   c. AAMA
   d. healthcare team member

2. Medical assistant education does not include
   a. the historical evolution of medical science.
   b. the ages of those training for medical assisting.
   c. phlebotomy.
   d. respect for individuals and cultural differences.

3. Medical terms are comprised of word parts including
   a. verbs.
   b. prefixes.
   c. nouns.
   d. vowels.

4. Medical assistants are trained in administrative tasks, which include
   a. pharmacology.
   b. lab tests.
   c. appointment scheduling.
   d. patient care.

5. One duty of the medical assistant in the area of communication is
   a. to calm the patient as much as possible.
   b. to avoid therapeutic touch to avoid a charge of sexual harassment.
   c. recommend diagnoses to assist the physician.
   d. avoid medical terminology so as not to confuse patients.

6. A reason that the medical assistant needs flexibility and strength is
   a. that only administrative medical assistants' duties require a lot of sitting.
   b. to work effectively with the other medical team members.
   c. to hear the telephone.
   d. to transfer a patient from the wheelchair to the exam table.

7. The professional performance of a medical assistant
   a. must follow a specific list of skills that covers all aspects.
   b. includes the requirement to act independently.
   c. depends on the needs of the physician.
   d. includes performing both administrative and clinical tasks.

8. The job outlook for medical assistants
   a. is moving away from clinics and group practices.
   b. always requires previous experience in the field.
   c. is promising.
   d. will legally require certification by ABHES and/or CAAHEP.

9. The scope of practice for the medical assistant is
   a. strictly limited to a specific list of skills.
   b. either for administrative or clinical duties.
   c. restricted to only certified medical assistants.
   d. what is delegated within the physician's scope of practice and the medical assistant's training, education, and experience.

10. To qualify for the CMA examination requires
   a. graduation from a CAAHEP- or ABHES-accredited program.
   b. recertification every year.
   c. preparing to take the exam in October.
   d. formal medical services training by the U.S. Armed Forces.

TRUE/FALSE

Indicate whether the statement is true (T) or false (F).

F   1. The Hippocratic Oath is no longer used, but it was around for nearly 2,000 years.

F   2. The American Medical Association wrote a code of ethics for physicians in 1846.

F   3. A medical assistant can only call him- or herself a nurse if certified by either an ABHES- or a CAAHEP-accredited medical assisting program.

T   4. Many early and historic plant remedies are still used today for heart conditions, indigestion, bleeding, and urinary tract infections.

T   5. The term *trepanning* means to bore a hole in the patient's skull to release evil spirits.

F   6. Galen (A.D. 129–199) is known as the Father of Medicine.

T   7. Ethics has been a part of medical practice since ancient times.

T   8. The medical assistant should understand the *Principles of Medical Ethics* as explained by the AMA's Council on Ethical and Judicial Affairs.

F   9. The AAMA does not have a Code of Ethics for medical assistants.

F   10. Medical assistants are licensed, not certified.

FILL IN THE BLANK

Using words from the list below fill in the blanks to complete the following statements.

continuing education	networking
flexibility and strength	physician's assistant
Hippocratic Oath	scope of practice
managed care	supernatural origin
multiskilled	therapeutic touch

1. Both AAMA and AMT offer *networking* possibilities at different levels within the organization and professional information through various publications.

2. Diseases were often believed to be of *supernatural origin* caused by evil spirits and angry gods.

3. *Flexibility & strength* is/are required for both clinical and administrative tasks.

4. To keep CMA status, you must recertify by testing on a five-year cycle or by fulfilling *continuing education* requirements.

5. The *Hippocratic Oath* was the first physician's code of ethics.

6. To protect the public welfare and the right of the medical assistant to practice and to provide a basis for legislation with the documents mentioned in the chapter, the AAMA has developed the *scope of practice* for medical assistants.

7. *Therapeutic touch* and an assuring manner help to lessen a patient's fear or anxiety by showing empathy and caring.

8. Health maintenance organizations (HMOs), *managed care*, and preferred providers have created another title for physicians: primary care physician (PCP), also called the gatekeeper.

9. A *physician's assistant* provides patient care under the supervision of a physician.

10. No longer just the physician's general helper, the medical assistant is now considered a *multiskilled* healthcare professional.

CHAPTER 2
Interpersonal Communication

CHAPTER OUTLINE

Review the Chapter Outline. If any content area is unclear, review that area before beginning workbook exercises.

    A.   The Medical Assistant's Role in Communication

    B.   Verbal Communication

    C.   Nonverbal Communication

    D.   Listening

    E.   Developmental Stages of the Life Cycle

    F.   Barriers to Communication

    G.   The Grieving Process

CHAPTER REVIEW

The following is a summary of the chapter. If any of this material is unclear, review it in the textbook.

Communication is one of the most important skills in any workplace and particularly in the medical field. The medical assistant must be well aware of the various components of good communication, whether verbal or written. Many patients also have special needs in communication, and there are various ways to ensure information is conveyed correctly. The ability to send and receive messages accurately to all patients is vital and avoids errors that can be dangerous to patients, as well as a legal liability. The art of listening is a first step in good communication, as well as being knowledgeable in many aspects that affect a patient's ability to communicate, such as Maslow's hierarchy of needs, a patient's age, cultural background, and state of illness.

Patients often use defense mechanisms to cope; this is particularly true of patients who have been diagnosed with serious or terminal illness. The medical assistant will also deal with terminally ill patients and those who experience other types of serious loss. The medical assistant should be aware of the various stages of grief as well as the effects on the patient's family and make the communication techniques appropriate for the individual patient.

LEARNING ACTIVITIES AND STUDY AIDS

Review the following study aids and/or complete the activities to ensure that you have achieved the learning objectives for this chapter.

1. Give some general information about the medical assistant's role in the communication process.

    medical assistants role in the communication process is very important and there are a variety of ways to communicate. There is verbal communication, written communication & nonverbal communication. Verbal Communication is the most commonly used

2. Explain in your own words what comprises verbal and nonverbal communication.

3. State three examples of both oral and written communication in the medical office or clinic.

4. What is symbolic language? Review this information in the text and give two examples of the most common types of symbolic communication.

Symbolic language is an alternative way of communicating

5. What is meant by "personal space"? Which is the space where most communication takes place: the personal distance or the public distance?

_____

_____

_____

6. Give an example of each of the four types of body language (such as one emotion you can convey with eye contact).

_____

_____

_____

_____

_____

_____

_____

7. Describe why listening is such an important part of communication.

_____

_____

_____

_____

_____

_____

_____

8. Read the information on Maslow's Hierarchy of Needs in the textbook. Then research the Hierarchy on the Internet and explain why a medical assistant needs to be familiar with this.

_____

_____

_____

_____

_____

_____

_____

_____

9. There are many barriers to communication. Name four barriers and explain them.

_____

_____

_____

_____

_____

_____

10. Culture and age are factors that can affect a person's communication. Review the material in your textbook and state in your own words how those two factors play a role in communication.

_____

_____

_____

_____

_____

_____

11. List any five common defense mechanisms and briefly describe each one.

_____

_____

_____

_____

_____

_____

12. A grieving patient, as well as those who are sharing the grief with that patient, is a person in need of special understanding. Review the section on the grieving process and Kübler-Ross's stages of grief. While a medical assistant cannot counsel or advise patients or their families, there are some things that the MA can do. List the three basic tasks stated in your textbook that the MA can do without going beyond his or her scope of practice.

_____

_____

_____

_____

_____

_____

MEDICAL TEMINOLOGY REVIEW

Use a dictionary and highlighted terms in the textbook to define the following terms.

Terms

anxiety fear of the unknown; a feeling of worry or fear about the future

hearing impaired unable to hear, or having a diminished sense of hearing

vocally impaired unable to speak, or having a diminished ability to speak

Abbreviations

ASL American Sign Language

CRITICAL THINKING

1. There are twelve common defense mechanisms listed and defined in the textbook. Write a scenario (either real or imagined) in which a patient or healthcare worker used one of the twelve defense mechanisms and how another person replied or reacted. If you choose to describe a real-life situation, you do not have to use real names or any personal information.

2. If a patient stands very close to you and invades your personal space, how would you handle that? What would you do or say?

   Personally, I do not think that I would say anything. I think I would just back away from the patient until I no longer felt like they were in my personal space.

3. In the Case Study at the beginning of the textbook chapter, imagine that the office manager does not come in to see the patient's look of frustration and how Oksana was acting. What would you say or do as the patient? How do you think Oksana would react, given her actions so far, if the patient became very angry?

4. What are two or three ways that you could help a 74-year-old patient when he confides in you that his wife and many friends have died, that he is quite sad and seems to have given up on his own care? Consider the various aspects of communication as well as the stages of life for the age brackets.

_____

_____

_____

_____

5. At a well-baby checkup, you notice that the 3 1/2-year-old patient could not speak well and could not make a sentence. The child's measurements on the growth charts are normal. How would you alert the physician to a possible problem?

_____

_____

_____

_____

CHAPTER REVIEW TEST

MULTIPLE CHOICE

Circle the letter of the correct answer.

1. An MA could do all of the following by email or the Internet, except

   a. obtain diagnostic test results.
   b. access patient records from other medical facilities.
   c. research information.
   d. complete a transmission log.

2. A patient who is 8 to 13 years old is considered to be

   a. school age.
   b. a young adult.
   c. a teenager.
   d. an adolescent.

3. Effective listening includes all except which one of the following techniques?

   a. maintaining eye contact
   b. watching body language and behavior
   c. interrupting the patient tactfully to ask questions
   d. asking relevant questions to keep the patient on track

4. Folding your arms over your chest is

   a. a posture that says "I am ready to give you the time you need."
   b. a closed position that separates you from the patient.
   c. a professional way to tell the patient he or she is annoying.
   d. simply your most comfortable posture when standing a lot all day.

5. An individual's ability to understand communication depends on
    a. his or her developmental stage in life.
    b. whether he or she is 12 or not and maturing.
    c. whether he or she speaks English as well as he or she understands it.
    d. whether you speak in medical or layman's terms.

6. The medical assistant's roles in communications include all of the following except
    a. charting as an essential form of communication in the medical office.
    b. paying attention to how and why to send messages to communicate accurately.
    c. being well-versed in the physician's practice and procedures in order to tell
    every patient the same thing the same way.
    d. using a warm, casual approach with patients, combined with empathy for the patient.

7. Body language includes all of the following except
    a. facial expressions.
    b. eye contact.
    c. what you wear.
    d. gestures.

8. A common mistake that people make when communicating with the elderly is
    a. talking too loud.
    b. reacting with sympathy.
    c. speaking the same way as with any patient.
    d. talking as if the patient were a baby or child.

9. Communication may be influenced by people's needs. Which of the following individuals created principles for these needs at various levels of development to ensure better understanding and therefore better communication?
    a. Antoine Braille
    b. William C. Stokoe
    c. Erik Erickson
    d. Abraham Maslow

10. Which *two* of the following statements are true in relation to listening?
    a. Make eye contact with the patient.
    b. Do not paraphrase the patient's words or he or she might feel you are mocking him or her.
    c. Tell the patient your own story or experience to let him or her know you
    really understand what he or she is saying.
    d. Allow the person to finish what he or she is saying without interrupting.

TRUE/FALSE

Indicate whether the statement is true (T) or false (F).

T 1. An entry into a patient's chart is considered written communication.

F 2. It is best to write emails in all capital letters for emphasis.

T 3. Symbolic language refers to such alternative ways of communicating as sign language or Braille.

_____ 4. Speak to hearing-challenged persons in a louder than usual voice.

_____ 5. Body language shows emotion and feeling and is a type of nonverbal communication.

_____ 6. The medical assistant must know how to project appropriate nonverbal and body language as well as how to read it as patients convey it.

_____ 7. Personal space only relates to strangers, not to those close to you or to healthcare workers.

_____ 8. It is important to communicate with each individual at his or her developmental level.

_____ 9. Two negative coping characteristics are insecurity and dependency.

_____ 10. Only approximately half of the people have mental and emotional defenses to deal with stress and anxiety.

FILL IN THE BLANK

Using words from the list below fill in the blanks to complete the following statements.

birth	heartbeat	~~sending~~
~~communicating~~	legal	stare
conflict	nonverbal	symbolic
English	office procedures	telephone procedures
express	save face	verbally
~~face him or her~~	selective forgetting	~~words~~
fetus	self-esteem	written

1. When __communicating__ with a hearing-challenged person, __face him/her__ at all times.

2. Nonverbal communication is __sending__ a message without __words__.

3. The three types of oral communication are _____, _____, and _____.

4. Medical charts are _____ documents and are a form of _____ communication.

5. Some individuals believe that communication begins before _____ with the _____ hearing the voice and _____ of the mother among other things.

6. Some foreign-born persons may understand the _____ language very well but may not _____ their responses and thoughts _____ in English.

7. Make eye contact with the patient or person, but do not _____.

8. Defense mechanisms protect a person's _____ but do not effectively deal with _____.

9. Repression is sometimes referred to as _____.

10. Rationalization helps to "_____" in embarrassing and anxiety-producing situations.

CHAPTER 3
Patient-Centered Care

CHAPTER OUTLINE

Review the Chapter Outline. If any content area is unclear, review that area before beginning workbook exercises.

A. The Medical Assistant's Role in Patient-Centered Care
B. Wellness
C. A Holistic Approach to Health Care
D. Pain
E. Patients with Special Needs

CHAPTER REVIEW

The following is a summary of the chapter. If any of this material is unclear, review it in the textbook.

The goal of patient care is to encourage and promote wellness in patients. There are various methods for this, and holistic medicine can be an alternative if conventional medicine does not help the patient. Pain is a common problem for patients for many reasons, and pain assessment and management are vital to help patients manage pain, especially when chronic. The medical assistant will deal with many patients with many types of pain and reasons for it, and patient teaching is a very important part of assisting patients to cope with their pain. The medical assistant must also recognize and respond appropriately to patients with special needs to ensure they can get the appropriate care.

LEARNING ACTIVITIES AND STUDY AIDS

Review the following study aids and/or complete the activities to ensure that you have achieved the learning objectives for this chapter.

1. There are ten terminology words and three abbreviations listed at the beginning of the textbook chapter. Review the list and then close the textbook and take a few minutes to recall them. Then list and define all words and abbreviations you can from memory and look up the rest to ensure extra study of those not remembered easily.

   [handwritten answers]

   cerebral - forepart of brain
   controlled sub - narcotics, stimulants
   BMI - body mass index
   PSA - prostate-specific antigen
   JCAHCO - Joint Commission on Accrediation of Health Care Org.
   acute - sharp, severe, short period of time
   chronic - long period of time, slow progression
   afferent nerves - sensory nerves → to cns
   efferent nerves - motor nerves → from cns to peripheral nervous system
   analgesic - pain reducing
   risk factor - factor making person vulnerable to disease/disorder
   referred pain - pain in different areas from injured area
   endorphins - proteins in brain

2. State the four roles of the medical assistant in patient-centered care.

_____

_____

_____

_____

_____

_____

_____

3. Wellness is the state that results from a healthy lifestyle, although there are some risk factors that are beyond a person's control. Using Table 3-1 in the textbook, list each common risk factor and give one example of how to change the factor. Note the one that is not changeable.

_____

_____

_____

_____

_____

_____

_____

_____

4. Discuss holistic medicine and the mind–body connection.

_____

_____

_____

_____

_____

_____

5. Briefly describe the three types of pain and give two examples of each type.

_____

_____

_____

_____

_____

_____

6. State how pain is assessed. Review the information in your textbook about pain. List three things that can heighten pain. Give an example of chronic pain.

_____

_____

_____

_____

_____

_____

_____

7. List the six methods of treating pain found in the Pain Management section of your book.

_____

_____

_____

_____

_____

_____

_____

8. There are patients with various special needs, both physical and emotional. For the following list of special needs, state two things (equipment, supplies, certain types of communication) about each need that is required or helpful to the MA when assisting these patients.

physical challenge:

_____

_____

hearing impairment:

_____

_____

speech impairment:

_____

_____

emotional challenge:

_____

_____

visual impairment:

_____

_____

cultural diversity:

_____

_____

geriatic:

_____

_____

MEDICAL TERMINOLOGY REVIEW

Use a dictionary and highlighted terms in the textbook to define the following terms.

Terms

acute sharp, severe, sudden; having a sudden onset & usually of short duration

afferent nerves sensory nerves that carry impulses to the central nervous system

analgesic pain reducing

cerebral pertaining to the cerebrum, forepart of the brain

chronic long duration, often slow progression

controlled substances narcotics, stimulants & certain sedatives

efferent nerves motor nerves that carry impulses from the central nervous system to the peripheral nervous system

endorphins proteins in the brain that have analgestric properties

referred pain pain that is felt in a different area from the injuried or diseased part of the body

risk factor factor that makes a person particularly vulnerable to certain diseases & disorders

Abbreviations

BMI body mass index

JCAHCO Joint Commission on Accreditation of Health Care Organizations

PSA prostate-specific antigen

CRITICAL THINKING

1. In the Case Study at the beginning of this chapter, Marina is smoking outside of the clinic. How might this make a patient feel about Marina? About the practice?

   If a patient walks into a doctors office who studies naturopathic medicine, one might feel very upset with *marina & not believe what she says. They will also think that she's a hypocrit and/or think they can smoke & be healthy because marina seems to be.*

2. What would you recommend that Marina say to the patient after noticing his reaction? If the patient tells the physician, what do you feel the physician should do or say about the incident with Marina?

I would recommend that Marina apologizes to the patient and tells him that she is trying her best to break the habit. If news gets to the physician, I am sure she would get in trouble because there must be a designated smoking place for workers.

3. a. Consider that you are a family member of a patient with chronic pain going with him or her to a clinic visit. You know that the patient is truly in pain and is not a drug seeker. What do you think you would say or do if the MA or any staff gave the impression, through body language only, of not believing the patient had as much pain as the patient indicated?

_____

_____

b. What do you think you would say or do if the MA did not make eye contact, was not warm and caring, and didn't chat at all except to ask the required questions then hurried out when the patient started to ask a question?

I would think that the M.A. did not really care about me and/or didn't like his job.

c. What do you think you would say or do if the MA would not talk over the medication treatment with you, only the patient, stating that the patient needs to be able to handle their medications themselves?

_____

_____

4. You are a new medical assistant and the physician has asked you to go into the exam room and give patient teaching to Mrs. McCarty about her rheumatoid arthritis pain management plan. The physician has written in the chart what the plan is but you are not very familiar with rheumatoid arthritis. Would you (a) try to do the best you can? (b) ask another MA to tell you what to do or how to do it? (c) ask the patient to wait while you research by office policy manuals and the Internet to figure it out? Choose one of the options and then explain your reasoning.

_____

_____

_____

_____

5. Again read over the Case Study for this chapter and answer the following: How do you feel about Marina's being a smoker yet teaching patients about a healthy lifestyle? What would it convey to patients if they knew she smoked?

_____

_____

_____

_____

CHAPTER REVIEW TEST

MULTIPLE CHOICE

Circle the letter of the correct answer.

1. Which of the following is an open-ended question?
   a. Do you feel nauseated?
   b. Does the pain feel severe and sharp?
   c. Where is the pain located?
   d. Did the pain start yesterday?

2. Which of the following are common methods to rate pain? (circle all that apply).
   a. face scale
   b. continuous scale based on a daily diary
   c. numerical scale or also known as the symbolic scale
   d. patient indicates on a full body picture where the pain is and what type of pain

3. An amputation often causes
   a. phantom pain.
   b. emotional pain.
   c. psychological pain.
   d. physical pain.

4. In the list of common words that can be used to describe pain, *intermittent* means
   a. deep inside.
   b. the very worst pain imaginable.
   c. comes and goes.
   d. pain in children.

5. Which of the following is *not* a treatment goal for patients with pain?
   a. lessen the pain
   b. reduce stress that makes pain worse
   c. keep the pain tolerable
   d. promote physical functioning

6. Which of the following are reasons that a patient may choose not to manage his or her pain with medications?
   a. A neighbor told them about an herbal remedy that would work better.
   b. Potential side effects of the medications prescribed.
   c. The amount and schedule of taking will be too difficult.
   d. Potential drug dependence.

7. Quality care involves (circle all that apply)
   a. focusing on the patient.
   b. patient-centered care.
   c. charting a patient's pain levels.
   d. assisting patients with special needs.

8. Which of the following is not a good role model for a child in developing a healthy lifestyle?
   a. eating healthy food
   b. taking lots of vitamins and herbal supplements
   c. exercising
   d. not smoking

9. Which of the following is *not* one of the three types of physical pain?
   a. superficial
   b. deep
   c. visceral
   d. organic

10. Which of the following statements about nerve impulses is true?
   a. Afferent nerves send impulses to the spinal cord and brain.
   b. The brain signals efferent nerves to send impulses to the spinal cord and brain.
   c. Referred nerves send impulses from the brain to various areas in the body.
   d. Response nerves send impulses to the spinal cord and brain.

TRUE/FALSE

Indicate whether the statement is true (T) or false (F).

_____ 1. The average life span in the United States is 72 years.

_____ 2. To maintain a healthy mind and body, a person needs 60 minutes of exercise per day.

_____ 3. Magnet therapy is one of the alternative methods of treating pain.

_____ 4. A patient with a broken bone would experience phantom pain.

_____ 5. Chronic pain lasts longer than acute pain.

_____ 6. Comfort measures are a way of treating pain.

_____ 7. Physical pain is a symptom of a disease process, inflammation, or trauma.

_____ 8. Patient teaching by the medical assistant is not done for pain management; that is left to RNs.

__F__ 9. Acute pain often lasts for a lifetime.

__T__ 10. In some cultures, people learn to hide pain.

FILL IN THE BLANK

Using words from the list below, fill in the blanks to complete the following statements. Note: Some words may be used more than once.

analgesic

chronic

complete

debilitating or weakening
    conditions

emotional

exercising

games

healthy lifestyle

holistic

lifestyle

medical data

more energy

negative

ongoing

threshold

pain

pain levels

positive

protein

relaxation

sensory

special needs

tolerance

1. Each person responds differently to _____, depending on his or her _____ and pain _____.

2. A person who starts _____ three times a week often has _____ for daily tasks.

3. Wellness is the _____ process of practicing a healthy _____.

4. Pain is an unpleasant _____ and _____ experience.

5. A medical assistant in the role of patient-centered care may do the following:

   Chart a patient's _____, obtain the patient's _____, and assist patients with _____.

6. Endorphins are a group of _____ in the brain with _____ properties.

7. Ignoring a healthy _____ puts people puts people at risk for developing _____ illnesses and/or _____.

8. A _____ approach to healthcare recognizes and addresses the _____ care of the patient.

9. Laughter, _____, and _____ have been effective treatment for chronic and terminal pain.

10. Finding ways to release _____ emotions and replace them with _____ experiences is an excellent way to start the steps toward a _____.

CHAPTER 4
Considerations of Extended Life

CHAPTER OUTLINE

Review the Chapter Outline. If any content area is unclear, review that area before beginning workbook exercises.

    A. The Medical Assistant's Role in Extended Life Care

    B. Organ and Tissue Donations

    C. Transplant Costs

    D. Organ and Tissue Donation Rules and Regulations

    E. Advance Medical Directives

    F. Hospice

CHAPTER REVIEW

The following is a summary of the chapter. If any of this material is unclear, review it in the textbook.

The incredible strides made in the medical field in the last fifty years alone have allowed people to live much longer lives. Along with this, however, come many issues concerning the quality of life. Among the beneficial advances that extend life are organ and tissue donations and transplants. Various agencies and organizations have enacted laws, rules, and regulations to ensure that donations and transplants are handled in the best interest of the patient and offer resources for patients, donors, and families alike.

Living wills, durable powers of attorney for healthcare, and advance directives are all examples of legal documents that came into being for the good of the patient.

Hospice care has also evolved along with the rapid medical advances. Terminally ill patients used to be cared for until their death in hospitals. Now hospice provides an option where patients can either be cared for at home with assistance to the family or cared for in an atmosphere that is more like home. Either option allows patients to pass away with dignity, without life-saving measures (or with whatever measures they wish) except medications for comfort. These issues—organ donation/transplantation, living wills and advance directives, and hospice—are all for the best interest of patients and their quality of life.

LEARNING ACTIVITIES AND STUDY AIDS

Review the following study aids and/or complete the activities to ensure that you have achieved the learning objectives for this chapter.

1. Explain the medical assistant's role in extended life care.

_____

_____

_____

_____

_____

_____

_____

_____

2. State in your own words how the recipients for an organ transplant are chosen.

_____

_____

_____

_____

_____

_____

3. Describe the information found on a uniform donor card.

_____

_____

_____

_____

_____

_____

4. The Uniform Anatomical Gift Act was updated in 1987 and includes many rules. Why was the Act updated? State the rules listed in your textbook that address the following issues:

   a. The exception to a donor's valid statement takes precedence over other individual's wishes.

   _____

   _____

   b. The gift may be refused by the recipient.

   _____

   _____

   c. Survivors, in a specified order of priority, may act on the donor's behalf.

   _____

   _____

5. In 1987, the Social Security Act began to require written protocols from hospitals participating in Medicare or Medicaid to ensure that patients are aware of their options. Explain why you think the Act did this.

_____

_____

_____

_____

_____

_____

_____

_____

6. Compare advance medical directives and durable power of attorney for healthcare. Define each one and explain the differences between the two.

_____

_____

_____

_____

_____

_____

_____

7. Define a living will in relation to life-prolonging declarations.

_____

_____

_____

_____

_____

_____

8. Define hospice. Is it the same thing as a nursing home?

_____

_____

_____

_____

_____

_____

MEDICAL TERMINOLOGY REVIEW

Use a dictionary and highlighted terms in the textbook to define the following terms.

Terms

cadaver _____

_____

hospice _____

_____

ischemia _____

_____

organ _____

_____

palliative _____

_____

tissue _____

_____

Abbreviations

DNR _____

_____

CRITICAL THINKING

1. What do you feel are some of the benefits of hospice?

_____

_____

_____

2. Living donors can donate certain tissues. What are some of the concerns you would have if you were considering being a live donor?

_____

_____

_____

3. Review the Case Study at the beginning of the chapter. Can Ori's mother keep him from being an organ donor on his driver's license? How do you feel about a parent denying an 18-year-old's request to donate?

_____

_____

_____

_____

4. Referring to the same Case Study, how do you feel about the mother's belief that CPR would not be performed on people who were known organ donors because it is less expensive to let the patient die and then harvest the organs?

_____

_____

_____

_____

5. Read the Uniform Anatomical Gift Act and the rules. List any rules that you feel are wrong or unfair, and explain why you think so.

_____

_____

_____

_____

CHAPTER REVIEW TEST

MULTIPLE CHOICE

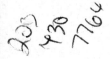

Circle the letter of the correct answer.

1. A medical directive is
   a. not the same thing as a durable power of attorney.
   b. a document in which the physician states his or her plan for medical treatment.
   c. is the same from state to state.
   d. is only for patients who are still able to make their own decisions, i.e., still with the capacity to decide at the time.

2. An organ donor
   a. does not need a removal order if the donor has a signature on his or her driver's license for organ donation.
   b. can only donate bone marrow or stem cells if a live donor.
   c. can be a cadaver or a live person.
   d. can be a patient who is not yet brain dead but is considered to be in a terminal coma.

3. The Uniform Anatomical Gift Act has certain rules. All of the following are included in those rules except:

    a. The donor may revoke the intent to donate.

    b. Financial arrangements can be made for donated organs in a legal way.

    c. The intent to donate must be made in writing.

    d. The donor may designate specific organs or tissue for transplantation.

4. Which statement about hospice is false?

    a. Long-term hospice may be the next step; it is because the patient can no longer be cared for at home.

    b. Family members can care for the patient in hospice when they are able to do so.

    c. The alternative option of hospice care originated in China.

    d. In hospice care, only palliative care is used, which may be pain medication to ease the patient's suffering in his or her last days.

5. Which of the following statements is true with regard to the medical assistant's role in the extended life care of a patient?

    a. The physician is the only one who can answer all questions from the patient.

    b. The MA can direct the patient and family to resources of information.

    c. There will be no documentation for the MA to do.

    d. The MA does not need to know very much about organ and tissue donation as the sensitivity of this subject will be handled by a nurse or the doctor.

6. Which of the following statements are true? (circle all that apply)

    a. One obstacle to donation is family involvement.

    b. Jehovah's Witnesses do not allow blood transfusions but will accept organ and tissue transplants if there is no blood left in the organ or tissue.

    c. Some cultures forbid organ donation.

    d. No religions object to organ donation and transplantation.

7. Which of the following are true of organ and tissue donation? (circle all that apply)

    a. The donor's physician or the physician who pronounces the donor dead is the best physician to be involved in the harvest procedure.

    b. In the United States, the sale and purchase of tissue and organs is prohibited.

    c. The agency that oversees tissue and organ harvest is the United Network for Organ Sharing (UNOS).

    d. The cost of harvesting is passed on to the donor's family.

8. Which of the following resources is not involved in organ donation?

    a. Hospice Foundation of America

    b. The American Association of Organ Donation

    c. The International Association for Organ Donation

    d. The United Network for Organ Sharing

9. Which of the following is not listed as an organ that must be harvested after the patient is pronounced brain dead?

    a. bone

    b. kidney

    c. lung

    d. intestine

10. When decisions about the patient and his or her care are granted to a family member or guardian, the hospital or institution goes in a certain order of relatives. Choose the option that correctly states the first three relatives listed in their priority order.

    a. spouse, parent, grandparent
    b. spouse, adult child, adult sibling
    c. spouse, guardian, adult child
    d. spouse, adult child, either parent

TRUE/FALSE

Indicate whether the statement is true (T) or false (F).

_____ 1. As long as a teenager has a driver's license, he or she can be an organ donor.

F 2. A DNR order stands for Do Not Refuse (treatment).

_____ 3. Some states do not honor living wills as legal documents that recognize a person's right to die naturally under the advanced directive document.

F 4. Corneas are one of the tissues that can be donated by live donors.

_____ 5. A live donor organ or tissue can go to a designated recipient.

_____ 6. It is required that a copy of documentation of a donor's intent must be filed in the medical record only during admission to a hospital.

_____ 7. Cryopreservation is a method of processing donated tissue.

_____ 8. The cost of the harvesting of an organ or tissue is passed on to the donor's family.

_____ 9. The National Conference of Commissioners on Uniform State Laws approved the Uniform Anatomical Gift Act in 1968 to address the inconsistency between various states.

_____ 10. The medical cost of a transplant can include covering the cost of child care.

FILL IN THE BLANK

Using words from the list below, fill in the blanks to complete the following statements.

competent · in a short time · physician

death · inconsistencies · procurement fees

decedent · interest · refusal

decisions · in writing · removal

designated recipient · live · the patient and family members

donation · living will

driver's license · local/regional · tissue

durable power · national · Uniform Anatomical Gift Act

family · naturally

honor that decision · need · waiting

hospital stay · organ donor card

1. The removal of organs or tissues is based on three factors: the source of the _____, the _____ period, and the _____ order.

2. A _____ for health care tells the _____ and the _____ that if the patient is no longer mentally _____, the appointed person with that power of attorney can make _____ for the patient's best _____.

3. When an organ or _____ is donated from a _____ donor, it may be given to a _____.

4. If a _____ prior to death has indicated a _____ to make an organ donation, the institution or health-care provider must _____.

5. Medical costs for transplants can include _____, lost wages for _____, and the _____ and surgical procedures.

6. The National Conference on Uniform State Laws, approved by the _____ in 1968, addresses the _____ among states.

7. When a patient agrees to donate, a request is made to see and document the _____, the_____, and any other documentation of the intent to donate.

8. Organ and tissue distribution was expanded from a _____ system to a _____ system based on _____.

9. A _____ advises the physician of a person's wish to die _____.

10. A living will must have _____ by the attending physician that, for one thing, the patient's _____ will occur _____.

CHAPTER 5

Clinical Environment and Safety in the Medical Office

CHAPTER OUTLINE

Review the Chapter Outline. If any content area is unclear, review that area before beginning workbook exercises.

    A. The Medical Assistant's Role in Office Safety

    B. Personal Safety Measures

    C. General Office Safety

    D. Emergency Plans

    E. OSHA Bloodborne Pathogen Standards

    F. Exposure Control Plan

CHAPTER REVIEW

The following is a summary of the chapter. If any of this material is unclear, review it in the textbook.

Working in the healthcare field has certain elements that can be hazardous to all staff in an office/clinic or any medical facility. Agencies such as OSHA (Occupational Safety and Health Administration) have set regulations to reduce the risks to healthcare workers. Every medical office should have general office safety procedures that all employees are aware of and should follow; there should be an employer-specific Exposure Control Plan that address all regulations set forth by OSHA and other agencies as well. The Bloodborne Pathogen Standard is to be followed as it was designed to reduce employee risk of contracting infectious diseases from blood and all body fluids. All employees must follow the employer's plan for it to be effective. This includes wearing PPE (personal protective equipment) such as gloves, face shields, or moisture-resistant gowns, for example. There must be labels on all chemicals to warn employees of a risk and there must be MSDS (Material Safety Data Sheets) with specifics on each chemical. The safety of personnel and the patients is of utmost importance in the medical field.

LEARNING ACTIVITIES AND STUDY AIDS

Review the following study aids and/or complete the activities to ensure that you have achieved the learning objectives for this chapter.

1. A medical assistant has a role in maintaining office safety. In fact, all healthcare workers and staff should follow procedures that provide a safe environment. List the two major items stated in your textbook that are essential tasks. Then explain in your own words the benefit or reason for strictly complying with your employer's safety requirements.

    _____

    _____

2. List the guidelines of body mechanics as stated in your textbook. Make your statements as brief as possible while retaining the vital information.

_____

_____

_____

_____

_____

_____

_____

_____

3. Review all of the material in the textbook on safety and a safe environment, paying attention to the general office safety measures listed in your textbook for safety in the general office. Recall and list at least four of the measures from your memory of reading the chapter. Write these in one color; then look in the textbook and add in another color the additional measures to complete the list.

_____

_____

_____

_____

_____

_____

_____

_____

4. Go back and reread OSHA's Standards, which require that all employers provide what is needed to keep employees as well as patients as safe as possible. Answer the following specific questions from your review of OSHA's Standards:

   a. On the Internet, research tuberculosis for the cause, how it is spread, and what some of the symptoms are. Use information found there to answer two questions: (1) Why does the Centers for Disease Control suggest TB testing of all health-care workers? (2) Is this to protect the employee or the patient?

   _____

   _____

   _____

   _____

   b. A medical assistant comes to work on a Monday after a weekend of hiking. She received several bug bites while hiking. After scratching them because of severe itching, they now have visible blood and tissue fluids seeping out of them. What should be done in this situation to protect the patients?

5. Study the list of examination room safety items in your textbook. Close the book and write as many of the items as you can recall; even portions of an item should be written. When you have listed all that you can, look in the book again and check your list against those in the book. Write out (in a different color) the ones that you missed from memory and review those again.

_____

_____

_____

_____

_____

_____

_____

6. List two or three guidelines for the three emergencies listed below that you can recall from your textbook. For those you can't recall, determine which actions in general you feel would be appropriate. Once you have finished, go back and review the textbook material to ensure you have these correct. Knowing what to do in an emergency is absolutely vital for health-care workers.

disaster:

_____

_____

fire:

_____

_____

workplace violence:

_____

_____

7. State the major elements addressed by OSHA's Bloodborne Pathogen Standard and include a very brief statement of what is covered in each area. This also provides a good overview of these very important guidelines.

_____

_____

_____

_____

_____

_____

8. Standard Precautions evolved from Universal Precautions, which are guidelines for infection control. List the major areas under Standard Precautions that are covered in your textbook.

_____
_____
_____
_____
_____
_____
_____
_____

9. The disposal of various types and items of biohazardous waste is regulated and there are specific guidelines for disposal.

a. Describe the appropriate container for disposing of potentially infectious blood or tissue.

_____
_____
_____
_____

b. Sharp items such as contaminated needles must be placed in a specific container for disposal as well. What feature must this one have?

_____
_____
_____
_____

MEDICAL TERMINOLOGY REVIEW

Use a dictionary and highlighted terms in the textbook to define the following terms.

Terms

decontamination _____

_____

pathogen _____

_____

Abbreviations

ADA American with Disabilities Act

AIDS acquired immunodeficiency syndrome

HBV Hepatitis B virus

HIV Human immunodefiency virus

MSDS _material safety data sheet_

OPIM _____

OSHA _Occupational Safety and Health Administration_

CRITICAL THINKING

1. What is the main premise of Standard and Universal Precautions and Body Substance Isolation? What impact on patient discrimination do you think this has had?

   _____
   _____
   _____
   _____

2. If you were confronted in the office with an angry patient who is threatening you, you should try to alert another staff member to call the police. What would you do if you were not able to alert someone or if you were alone?

   _____
   _____
   _____
   _____

3. Imagine you are working in the lab doing weekly cleaning tasks at the end of the day. When you reach under the sink to get bleach to mix a 10:1 cleaning solution, the lid to the bottle is loose and some of the bleach splashes in your face and eyes. What would you do *first* according to OSHA's guidelines?

   _____
   _____
   _____
   _____

4. You have a reaction to the powdered gloves at your new job, and your hands are quite itchy from the powder. You ask the office manager to purchase a few boxes of powder-free gloves because of your sensitivity, and the manager says, "No, the doctors want powder and we always buy all of the same kind. If you need a special kind, you will need to purchase them yourself and bring them in to work."

   a. Is it right for your employer to refuse the PPE that you need?

   _____
   _____
   _____

   b. What would you do or say to support your right by OSHA to have PPE provided at no cost to you?

   _____
   _____
   _____
   _____

5. In your clinic, one of the laundry receptacles has a biohazardous label and another is for regular laundry without visible blood or body fluids. Your manager tells you that the laundry services will be a day late due to snow and asks you to take home the regular laundry to do and bring back tomorrow. Would you do this? Explain why or why not.

_____

_____

_____

_____

CHAPTER REVIEW TEST

MULTIPLE CHOICE

Circle the letter of the correct answer.

1. The only time a fire extinguisher should be used is when
   a. there is a real fire.
   b. it is a wood fire as opposed to a chemical fire.
   c. the fire is between you and the door.
   d. there are no electrical cords close to the fire.

2. The regulation of potentially infectious materials includes
   a. vaginal secretions.
   b. cerebrospinal fluid.
   c. amniotic fluid.
   d. all of the above.
   e. none of the above.

3. Radioactive waste from nuclear medicine or radiation
   a. can be poured down a sink or toilet if then flushed thoroughly with water.
   b. does not need to be biohazard labeled as it is always stored in the same place and everyone knows where it is.
   c. can never be incinerated.
   d. can be put in leakproof containers and placed in the biohazard box.

4. Which item below is NOT listed on an MSDS sheet according to your textbook?
   a. storage and disposal requirements
   b. components of the chemical
   c. names of medications that would counteract the chemical
   d. first aid and emergency measures for exposure

5. The use of mercury thermometers has been banned in most offices and communities. Which of the following statements regarding the use of mercury thermometers is *not* true?
   a. The real danger to the patient is that he or she may swallow broken glass if the glass thermometer breaks in the mouth.
   b. Swallowing mercury from a broken glass thermometer is a true emergency and requires either a visit to the ER or a call to the poison control center.
   c. Mercury is a heavy element and is not well absorbed through the skin or cuts.
   d. They are not sanitary enough to use anymore when there are electronic and other types.

6. Which two of the following should be part of an exposure control plan?

    a. postexposure evaluation and follow-up   c. laundry decontamination

    b. surgical procedures   d. HIV testing

7. Which two of the following are listed under General Office Safety in your textbook?

    a. exercise caution when passing through doorways   d. ensure the physician has all needed supplies

    b. always be helpful and nice

    c. keeping food stored and separated from medication in a designated refrigerator and/or cabinet

8. Which of the following statements are true regarding evaluation plans in case of an emergency? Circle all that apply.

    a. Every employee should know where the evacuation routes are posted.   c. Assist all patients from the office or building.

    b. Keep hallways and exit doors free from obstructions.   d. Take all patients 50 feet from the building.

9. Which of the following two statements are true with regard to severe weather events during work hours?

    a. The National Oceanic and Atmospheric Administration (NOAA) issues information about developing dangerous weather events.   c. A *warning* means that there may be an event that could happen.

    b. Patients and staff should go to a basement or inner room without glass windows.   d. A *watch* means that an event is coming and everyone should be watching for it to know when to take cover.

10. Workplace security is an important issue. Which of the following is not true with regard to ensuring safety in your office or facility?

    a. Some employees are given security keys or codes.   c. Account for all prescription pads at the end of the day.

    b. If a key to the facility is lost, a new one must be made immediately.   d. Doors and windows must be kept locked overnight.

TRUE/FALSE

Indicate whether the statement is true (T) or false (F).

__T__ 1. The Americans with Disabilities Act protects the civil rights of the disabled.

__F__ 2. An Accident Report Form is for documenting unusual occurrences and incidents.

__T__ 3. In an earthquake, it is best to evacuate a building and get away from falling debris.

_____ 4. An MSDS sheet can tell you which PPE to wear when working with a certain substance.

_____ 5. OSHA requires TB testing for all healthcare workers.

__F__ 6. Workplace violence only involves patients who are angry.

_____ 7. One of OSHA's standards is called Hazards Communication, which states that all employees will attend seminars to learn the latest changes by OSHA.

_____ 8. Body mechanics pertains only to lifting; carrying and moving are not as dangerous so they are covered under Personal Safety.

_____ 9. Emergency plans should be permanently kept in a policy or procedure manual that should be reviewed regularly by the employees.

_____ 10. An incident report can be good for analyzing an event in order to prevent it from happening again.

FILL IN THE BLANK

Using words from the list below, fill in the blanks to complete the following statements.

accidents	fire departments	physician
all patients	handwashing	prescription pad
banned	HIV or HBV	reduce
chance of exposure	incident	relay services
classifications	law enforcement	review committee
DEA	meeting place	safety
employees	mercury thermometers	spread
evacuation	no charge	telephone
evaluation and treatment	Ongoing Occupational	unusual occurrences
filed	Exposure Risk	

1. Frequent _____ is one of the best ways to _____ the _____ of infection.

2. Post-exposure medical _____ is/are provided by the employer. There is _____ to the employee.

3. Incident reports are used to document _____ or _____ in the medical office.

4. Telecommunications _____ service to the general public must also provide_____, such as TTY.

5. Many facilities are removing _____ from use and some communities have _____ them completely.

6. An employee with _____ should not perform patient care until given advice from a _____ and a medical_____.

7. If an _____ is required of the office and/or building, assist _____ to your assigned_____.

8. Local _____ generally train _____ regarding fire_____ in the office.

9. If a _____ is missing, a/an _____ report should be _____, and _____ and/or the _____ should be notified.

10. In the exposure control plan, there are _____ for employees relating to their _____ to blood or OPIM. A medical assistant or other clinical/lab person is at the classification of _____.

Chapter 6
The Clinical Visit: Office Preparation and the Patient Encounter

CHAPTER OUTLINE

Review the Chapter Outline. If any content area is unclear, review that area before beginning workbook exercises.

    A. The Medical Assistant's Role in the Clinical Visit

    B. The Standard Medical Office

    C. Prepare and Maintain Examination and Treatment Areas

    D. Triage

    E. Consent

    F. Medical Records and Documentation

    G. Charting the Medical History and Clinical Visit

CHAPTER REVIEW

The following is a summary of the chapter. If any of this material is unclear, review it in the textbook.

Medical assisting is truly a multitasking position in both clinical and administrative areas. For the typical office visit, the medical assistant must ensure that rooms are clean, safe, and well-stocked for the day. Good communication techniques must be utilized to attain correct information from each patient, for charting in the medical record, for performing triage by phone or in person, and in questioning patients on the medical history. Another important task that is important for any procedures or surgeries is the informed consent and witness form. It is important that the medical assistant understands this form. Preparing and compiling new patient charts is another task the medical assistant does for the patient, and the although the doctor ultimately determines the diagnosis, prognosis, and a treatment plan, the medical assistant is the support person needed to keep the office running efficiently and to ensure that patients receive the best care.

LEARNING ACTIVITIES AND STUDY AIDS

Review the following study aids and/or complete the activities to ensure that you have achieved the learning objectives for this chapter.

1. Review the section in your textbook regarding the MA's role in the clinical visit. Close the book and write the duties stated there that you can recall. Make another list of duties that medical assistants perform even though not stated in the text.

_____

_____

_____

_____

_____

_____

_____

_____

2. Triage is an important duty and must be accurate to ensure the most severe patients are treated first. What is your explanation of triage? Write a scenario in which two patients both need help at about the same time, and then explain which patient should be treated first and why.

_____

_____

_____

_____

_____

_____

_____

3. Describe the difference between implied consent and informed consent.

_____

_____

_____

_____

_____

_____

_____

4. What does the medical assistant do when obtaining consent?

_____

_____

_____

_____

_____

_____

5. Medical records contain an incredible amount of personal information on a patient and are _legal_ documents. This very important chart is handled by many people who make their own entries. Certain information and requirements are stated in your textbook under the main heading Medical Records and Documentation. Review the items in the book and write them all on one index card.

Review this card often while learning medical records and the documentation within them. Carry this card in your pocket for reference when you are on externship, and perhaps when you are on your new position after graduation.

_____

_____

_____

_____

_____

_____

_____

6. In narrative form instead of a list, write a paragraph describing the guidelines for charting a patient's clinic visit. You should have read the chapter before this activity. Since there are a number of guidelines, go over the list again for review. Make an index card with brief statements of each item so that they will all fit on one card. Then answer the following four questions.

   1. How can you make sure that you spell medical terms correctly?

   _____

   _____

   2. How is an error corrected?

   _____

   _____

   3. Why do you think that missed appointments should be charted?

   _____

   _____

   4. Why is black or blue ink required, and which color is acceptable for allergies?

   _____

   _____

7. When a new patient is seen, the MA will compile a new chart with forms needed. The Patient History Form can be mailed to the patient ahead of time, or he or she can complete it in the office. You have read the chapter in the textbook and are likely to know the components of this history. On one page, design a simple patient history questionnaire with the major categories (for example, family medical history). Write two questions under each section that you feel would be appropriate for that section.

_____

_____

_____

_____

_____

_____

_____

_____

MEDICAL TERMINOLOGY REVIEW

Use a dictionary and highlighted terms in the textbook to define the following terms.

Terms

charting _____

_____

diagnosis _____

_____

implied consent _____

_____

informed consent _____

_____

ophthalmoscope _____

_____

otoscope _____

_____

prognosis _____

_____

sign _____

_____

sphygmomanometer _____

_____

stethoscope _____

_____

symptom _____

_____

thermometer _____

_____

triage _____

_____

Abbreviations

POMR _____

_____

SOAP _____

_____

CRITICAL THINKING

1. If a patient does not speak English very well, how will you ensure that the medical information you collect for the Patient History Form is accurate?

   _____

   _____

   _____

   _____

2. A patient walks into the clinic and is having life-threatening symptoms; however, the doctor is not present in the clinic. The office manager and the RN clinical manager are out to lunch for another 20 minutes, and you are alone covering the phones during this time period. What should you do? List three or four tasks that would be vital.

   _____

   _____

   _____

   _____

3. A patient is in the exam room and you are taking vital signs prior to the physician's examination. As you are taking the blood pressure, you look up at the patient and notice that she is trying to say something but appears to be unable to speak normally and that one side of her face seems to be drooping where it wasn't prior to the start of the vital signs. What is your first thought on what the problem could be? What actions would you take?

   _____

   _____

   _____

   _____

4. Consider that the occupational history of the patient is one of the parts of a patient history. Although not stated in detail in the book, why do you think a patient's past occupation(s) would be important in a medical history? List two examples of occupations that do have an effect on a person's medical state.

   _____

   _____

   _____

   _____

5. You are a new graduate on your first job as a medical assistant. You are in with the physician, a patient, and his wife. The patient was seen for upper abdominal pain, and the physician has diagnosed gallstones. The doctor proposes the removal of the gallbladder. The doctor explains the procedure, why it is needed, and then explains the risks of the surgery. The patient and his wife look at each other and say nothing, but then whisper to each other a little. The patient shakes his head yes and signs the informed consent form. The doctor signs and asks you to sign as a witness. You feel that the patient was not given all the required information for informed consent but are not confident about how to handle this: Should you tell the physician in front of the patient? Sign the form and then tell the doctor later that you did not feel comfortable signing it and why? Ask

another staff member for advice on how to handle it? Refuse to sign it? There are many options. Consider all options you can think of and choose what you feel is best; write an explanation of how you would handle this.

_____

_____

_____

_____

CHAPTER REVIEW TEST

MULTIPLE CHOICE

Circle the letter of the correct answer.

1. Triage is sorting and prioritizing the treatment of patients. Which of the following is not one of the things the MA should do in triaging?
   a. Listen to the complaint and gather the information the patient imparts.
   b. Follow office policy and protocols for additional triage information for severe problems.
   c. Do not bother the RN or the physician as you should be able to triage.
   d. Triaging may be on the phone or in person.

2. Medical records contain a section for filing therapeutic reports. Which two of the following would be under that category?
   a. physical therapy reports
   b. pathology reports
   c. correspondence from a referring physician
   d. emergency room reports

3. Standard equipment in an exam room includes all of the following except:
   a. sphygmomanometer.
   b. portable light.
   c. Snellen eye chart.
   d. audiometer.

4. A sign is
   a. something the patient says his or her problem or pain is (CC).
   b. something the patient feels but is not visible.
   c. something that can be seen.
   d. something that is a condition that will progress to another.

5. A symptom is
   a. what the patient says his or her problem or pain is (CC).
   b. something the patient feels but is not visible.
   c. something that can be seen.
   d. both a and c.
   e. both a and b.

6. The acronym SOAP describes a type of charting. What do the letters stand for?

   a. subjective, objective, assessment, plan
   b. subjective, objective, assessment, prognosis
   c. subjective, objective, allergies, plan
   d. subjective, objective, allergies, prognosis

7. Which of the following would be implied consent? (Circle all that apply)

   a. rolling up the sleeve in preparation for a blood draw
   b. keeping the appointment and allowing the physician to do an exam by putting on the gown
   c. having a cyst removed in the office as a minor surgical procedure
   d. removing shoe and sock for an exam of a swollen ankle

8. What is the difference between a CC and the present illness (PI)? (Choose the two correct statements.)

   a. Nothing. They are the same thing.
   b. The CC will tell the main problem the patient has chronically (i.e., diabetes) and the PI tells the reason that he or she has come in today.
   c. The CC is the brief statement of the reason for today's visit and the PI is an expanded CC. It is more detailed in description of the present symptoms.
   d. The CC states the main problem very briefly (i.e., pain in right knee) and the PI tells the symptoms and other things related to the CC (severe swelling, sharp pain suddenly when the patient fell, cannot put weight on right leg).

9. Which of the following statements about a health genogram is true?

   a. If the patient will complete one, the physician could make a diagnosis with just that.
   b. Shows patterns of illnesses or conditions in the patient's ancestors.
   c. Indicates most diseases a patient may develop as well as those that are hereditary.
   d. Is a computer-generated chart that maps out the patient's entire state of health or disease.

10. Which of the following statements is false about charting procedures?

   a. An MA should not make diagnostic statements.
   b. When charting a patient's words, use quotation marks.
   c. Charting *before* a procedure or treatment is illegal.
   d. Charting information such as collecting a specimen and performing lab tests is not required of the MA as this is not direct patient care or interaction.

TRUE/FALSE

Indicate whether the statement is true (T) or false (F).

_____ 1. POMR stands for Patient Oriented Medical Record.

_____ 2. More and more offices are switching to electronic medical records.

_____ 3. The collection of medical information on the patient's health history involves an oral interview.

_____ 4. The CC and the present illness are the same thing; you can use the terms interchangeably.

_____ 5. *What*, *when*, and *why* are good key words to use to elicit descriptions of symptoms.

_____ 6. Triage is setting the priority of the treatment of patients either by phone or in person at the reception desk.

_____ 7. Used or soiled equipment should be taken to the "dirty" area to be cleaned, disinfected, and or sterilized.

_____ 8. Consent documents for treatment and for releasing medical information are not kept in the patient's medical record but filed in the administrative records.

_____ 9. A patient's medical record, or chart, is a legal document in which accurate entries are critical.

_____ 10. An ophthalmoscope is used to exam both eyes and ears.

FILL IN THE BLANK

Using words from the list below, fill in the blanks to complete the following statements. Note: Some words may be used in more than one statement.

all personnel	incomplete	possible complications
assume	incontinence	predict
before	informed	prognosis
best decisions	jaundice	pull-out
care or treatment	label	respiratory
common sense	laryngitis	risks
condition or disease	legal	severe
cyanosis	liability	sphygmomanometer
diagnosis	medical record	staff member
diagnostic	otoscope	stethoscope
electrocardiogram	outcomes	stirrups
epistaxis	patient teaching	syncope
eructation	phone calls	that is to be done
imaging	policies	thermometer

1. The conclusion about a patient's condition is a _____, which the physician determines after an exam, diagnostics, reports and the patient's history. The physician can anticipate or _____ the outcome of a _____ and the patient's recovery, which is called the _____.

2. Occasionally, equipment may malfunction in the office. It is vital that the MA or any _____ should not forget, ignore, or _____ someone else will take care of the problem. In a court of law, the _____ would be more _____ if it is found that staff knew about it and did not take steps to _____ or get it repaired.

3. A _____ is used to measure the patient's temperature. A _____ is used to listen to internal body sounds. An exam table with _____ and a _____ footrest is best.

 A/An _____ is an instrument to examine ears. To measure blood pressure, a _____ is used.

4. Diagnostic reports that would be filed in the medical record include an _____ and other cardiology reports, _____ therapy reports, _____ reports and other radiology reports, and any additional _____ procedure reports.

5. If a procedure is not charted in the _____, it would be considered _____ by the _____ system.

6. In your textbook, Table 6-3: Common Signs and Symptoms Related by and Observed in Patients, provides medical terms to use for brief statements of the signs and symptoms. Provide the medical term for the definitions that follow:

 belching _____

 yellow color to skin and white parts of the eyes _____

 bluish tint to the skin _____

 inability to hold urine _____

 fainting _____

 nosebleed _____

 loss of voice, hoarseness with little volume _____

7. In the _____ all employees should chart information when providing _____, _____ or _____, among other interactions with the patient.

8. In triage, a good guideline in general is _____. Of course, the policy of the individual workplace is to be followed and _____ _____ must be familiar with these _____ whether they have direct patient care or not.

9. _____ consent must contain four items of information that must be conveyed to the patient so he or she can make the _____ based on all aspects of the treatment, surgery, or procedure _____ giving their consent to it. Those four items are the procedure _____, the expected _____, the _____ and _____ involved.

Procedure 6-1

Prepare and Maintain the Medical Record

Objective: The student will be able to prepare and maintain the medical record.

Supplies: File folder for chart, black or blue ink pen, fasteners, chart dividers, double or triple-hole punch, name and alphabetic, color-coded file labels, preprinted forms such as patient registration record, consent documents, and patient history forms.

Notes to the Student:

_____

_____

_____

_____

_____

_____

Skills Assessment Requirements

Read and familiarize yourself with the procedure; complete the minimum practice requirements (MPRs). Document each MPR using proper charting technique. Complete each procedure within a reasonable amount of time, with a minimum of 85% accuracy.

Name: _____

Date: _____

POINT VALUE ✦ = 3–6 points ⋆ = 7–9 points		PRACTICE TRIAL	GRADED TRIAL # 1	GRADED TRIAL # 2	NOTES:
1. ⋆	Greet and identify the new patient.				
2. ✦	Instruct the patient to complete a registration form if he or she has not mailed one in.				
3. ✦	Upon completion of the registration form, clarify any blanks or illegible handwriting.				
4. ✦	Enter the registration data into the computer.				
5. ✦	Organize forms and dividers according to office requirements and place in the record. Some charts require that forms be double- or triple-hole punched.				
6. ⋆	Label the record and each form with the patient's number, name, and record identification.				
7. ✦	Place the registration form in the record location as directed by office policy.				
8. ⋆	Add an allergy label to the record folder and to appropriate chart forms.				
9. ✦	For each patient return visit, check and place additional forms in the record as necessary.				

Document: Enter the appropriate information in the chart below.

Grading

Points Earned	_____		
Points Possible	_____	63	63
Percent Grade (Points Earned/ Points Possible)	_____		
PASS:	_____	❑ YES ❑ NO ❑ N/A	❑ YES ❑ NO ❑ N/A

Instructor Sign-Off

Instructor: _____ **Date:** _____

Procedure 6-2

Complete a History Form

Objective: The student will be able to complete a Patient History Form.

Supplies: Chart, file folder for chart, patient history form, black or blue ink pen.

Notes to the Student:

_____

_____

_____

_____

_____

_____

Skills Assessment Requirements

Read and familiarize yourself with the procedure; complete the minimum practice requirements. Document each MPR using proper charting technique. Complete each procedure within a reasonable amount of time, with a minimum of 85% accuracy.

POINT VALUE ✦ = 3–6 points ⋆ = 7–9 points		PRACTICE TRIAL	GRADED TRIAL # 1	GRADED TRIAL # 2	NOTES:
1. ⋆	Greet the patient in a formal, age-appropriate manner.				
2. ✦	Explain the health history form. Explain to the patient or parent that additional information beyond the original questions is always important and can be added.				
3. ✦	Observe patient's body language and respond appropriately or tactfully to encourage open sharing of medical information.				
4. ✦	The order of interview for the patient history form follows the order of the form unless office policy dictates otherwise.				
5. ✦	Instruct the patient to fill in the patient identification section. Review it to make sure the information is complete.				
6. ⋆	Use open-ended questions to obtain details of the patient's CC, or present illness, such as: • How long have the symptoms been occurring? • Where do the symptoms occur? • What activity brings on the symptoms or makes the symptoms worse?				

	PRACTICE TRIAL	GRADED TRIAL # 1	GRADED TRIAL # 2	NOTES:
• Do the symptoms occur suddenly or gradually? • What activity helps the symptom(s) disappear or lessen? • When symptoms occur, how long do they last?				
7. ✦ Proceed through the questions about past medical history, family medical history, and social/occupational history as presented on the patient history form.				

Document: Enter the appropriate information in the chart below.

Grading

Points Earned	_____		
Points Possible	_____	48	48
Percent Grade (Points Earned/ Points Possible)	_____		
PASS:	_____	❏ YES ❏ NO ❏ N/A	❏ YES ❏ NO ❏ N/A

Instructor Sign-Off

Instructor: _____ **Date:** _____

Procedure 6-3

Document a Clinical Visit and Procedure

Objective: The student will able to accurately document a clinical visit or procedure.

Supplies: Patient chart, narrative or progress note forms to be added to the chart, black or blue ink pen.

Notes to the Student:

_____

_____

_____

_____

_____

_____

Skills Assessment Requirements

Read and familiarize yourself with the procedure; complete the minimum practice requirements. Document each MPR using proper charting technique. Complete each procedure within a reasonable amount of time, with a minimum of 85% accuracy.

Name: _____

Date: _____

POINT VALUE ✦ = 3–6 points ⋆ = 7–9 points		PRACTICE TRIAL	GRADED TRIAL # 1	GRADED TRIAL # 2	NOTES:
1. ⋆	Verify that the chart is the correct chart for the patient being seen.				
2. ✦	If notes are insufficient for documentation, add the appropriate form.				
3. ✦	With narrative charting or SOAP charting, avoid leaving blank areas.				
4. ✦	Write the date and time in the left hand column of the notes.				
5. ✦	Continue writing in the charting format used by the medical office.				
6. ⋆	Document immediately after performance of procedures.				
7. ✦	Use only standard, accepted abbreviations and describe clinical observations during performance of the procedure.				
8. ✦	Document only facts. DO NOT make diagnoses or judgmental statements.				
9. ⋆	Sign your name and add your title at the end of the documentation.				

Document: Enter the appropriate information in the chart below.

Grading

Points Earned	_____		
Points Possible	_____	63	63
Percent Grade (Points Earned/ Points Possible)	_____		
PASS:	_____	❑ YES ❑ NO ❑ N/A	❑ YES ❑ NO ❑ N/A

Instructor Sign-Off

Instructor: _____ **Date:** _____

CHAPTER 7
Medical Asepsis

CHAPTER OUTLINE

Review the Chapter Outline. If any content area is unclear, review that area before beginning workbook exercises.

  A. The Medical Assistant's Role in Infection Control

  B. The Cycle of Infection

  C. Natural Defenses Against Infection

  D. Asepsis and Infection Control

  E. Infection Control Precautions

  F. Hepatitis

  G. Acquired Immunodeficiency Syndrome (AIDS)

  H. Latex Allergy

CHAPTER REVIEW

The following is a summary of the chapter. If any of this material is unclear, review it in the textbook.

The information covered under the topic of asepsis is vital for all medical assistants to know and to practice consistently. First, handwashing and disinfection were required when it was discovered that infectious diseases were caused by microorganisms. Handwashing is the number one way to prevent the spread of infection. A cycle of infection transmission outlines how the pathogenic microorganisms get into and leave patients and how they are transmitted. This cycle is meant to be broken. People have their own natural defenses, such as the immune system and the skin, but the rise in bloodborne diseases caused OSHA and the CDC to develop Universal and Standard Precautions that, if followed exactly and consistently by every healthcare worker, will significantly lower the spread of infection. The premise of these guidelines is to assume that *all* blood and blood products, tissue, etc., from *all* patients are infectious. The increased use of gloves as the major PPE has also led to an increase in latex allergies and sensitivities. Since a reaction can be severe enough to be life threatening, it is important to know the symptoms of latex allergy. Patient education is important to the health recovery process and the prevention of disease transmission. Those at risk of being exposed to infectious diseases, including healthcare workers, are encouraged to get the vaccine for Hepatitis B. Healthcare workers, including medical assistants, must be committed to following Universal and Standard Precautions and to following all infection control guidelines in place to protect patients and workers.

LEARNING ACTIVITIES AND STUDY AIDS

Review the following study aids and/or complete the activities to ensure that you have achieved the learning objectives for this chapter.

1. Describe five ways that a medical assistant can promote infection control.

   _____

   _____

   _____

   _____

   _____

   _____

   _____

   _____

2. Describe the three main layers of skin, along with five sublayers within one of the main layers. State the functions of the skin. Does the body have any other natural defenses besides the skin?

   _____

   _____

   _____

   _____

   _____

   _____

   _____

   _____

3. Search the Internet for reputable sites that address the anatomy and physiology of the immune system. Use the information found there and in your textbook to explain in your own words the function of the immune system.

   _____

   _____

   _____

   _____

   _____

   _____

4. Explain how a person's general state of health may also be a defense against infection.

   _____

   _____

   _____

   _____

_____

_____

_____

5. In addition to the skin, name the body's other natural defenses against infection.

_____

_____

_____

_____

_____

_____

_____

6. Describe in your own words what asepsis is. What are the differences between medical asepsis and surgical asepsis?

_____

_____

_____

_____

_____

_____

_____

7. Visit the websites of both OSHA and the CDC and look for their statements on their function or role in making and updating infection control guidelines. There may not be one exactly stating that, so try to locate the closest thing to it on their site (Example: There may be a mission statement that includes many other missions than just infection control.)

_____

_____

_____

_____

_____

_____

8. In your own words, explain the importance of Universal and Standard Precautions. Why were they developed? Give five examples of precautions.

_____

_____

_____

_____

_____
_____
_____
_____

9. From memory of your reading of this chapter, list all the items of PPE that you can recall. Then check in your textbook to make sure you listed them all and study those that you missed.

_____
_____
_____
_____
_____
_____
_____
_____

10. Review the section in your textbook about hepatitis. Close the book and do the following from memory: List the routes of transmission and explain the appropriate patient education, since the MA typically does the teaching.

_____
_____
_____
_____
_____
_____
_____
_____
_____

11. As healthcare workers, it is important that medical assistants be thoroughly versed in HIV/AIDS. State the symptoms by stage, how the diagnoses of HIV and AIDS are made, and treatments.

_____
_____
_____
_____
_____
_____
_____

12. Treatment of the HIV/AIDS patient can be very complicated, and infection control measures must be taken. When caring for an HIV/AIDS patient, there are guidelines for the caregiver discussed in the textbook. Reread this section in the chapter then close the book and recall as many as you can. Always go back and check your answers, paying special attention to those that you did not recall.

_____
_____
_____

_____

_____

_____

_____

13. You will learn and practice handwashing in this chapter, and you should have read the theory of handwashing in your textbook by now. Explain the following:

   a. If gloves serve as barriers to the spread of infection, why can't you use gloves *without* washing your hands before and after physical contact with every patient?

   _____

   _____

   _____

   _____

   b. Why must the hands and fingers be kept below the elbows when hand washing?

   _____

   _____

   _____

   _____

14. Nonsterile gloves are used for two major purposes as stated in the theory of this procedure in your text. State the two purposes. The text also provides examples for the use of nonsterile and sterile gloves. Think of an example of your own for wearing nonsterile gloves and then for sterile gloves.

   _____

   _____

   _____

   _____

   _____

   _____

   _____

   _____

15. As a medical assistant, you will undoubtedly find many patients and healthcare workers who are sensitive or allergic to latex. What are the symptoms of a latex allergy? What information can you teach the patient about methods to deal with it?

   _____

   _____

   _____

   _____

   _____

   _____

   _____

   _____

MEDICAL TERMINOLOGY REVIEW

Use a dictionary and highlighted terms in the textbook to define the following terms.

Terms

aerobe _____

_____

anaerobe _____

_____

aseptic technique _____

_____

bactericidal _____

_____

bloodborne pathogens _____

_____

Body Substance Isolation (BSI) _____

_____

carrier _____

_____

Centers for Disease Control (CDC) _____

_____

cilia _____

_____

contamination _____

_____

dermis _____

_____

disinfection _____

_____

epidermis _____

_____

epithelial _____

_____

follicle _____

_____

fomites _____

_____

homeostasis _____

_____

immunity _____

_____

incubation _____

_____

infection _____

_____

integumentary _____

_____

keratinocyte _____

_____

medical asepsis _____

_____

microorganism _____

_____

nonpathogen _____

_____

nosocomial infection _____

_____

personal protective equipment (PPE) _____

_____

phagocytosis _____

_____

Standard Precautions _____

_____

sterile _____

_____

subcutaneous tissue _____

_____

Transmission-Based Precautions _____

_____

Universal Precautions _____

_____

Abbreviations

ELISA _____

_____

CRITICAL THINKING

1. Although not specifically stated in this chapter, explain why hands cannot be sterilized even though we wash them with soap and water. If sterilization is not something you have learned yet, consider what you already know or think about surgery (from TV or personal experience) and offer your best idea.

_____

_____

_____

_____

2. In the Case Study at the beginning of this chapter, list each thing in the last paragraph that Gloria did wrong (that could spread infection).

_____

_____

_____

3. Since OSHA monitors and regulates workplaces for safety and health of the workers, many businesses see OSHA as an unfair regulatory agency. Some labor groups feel that OSHA doesn't do enough. What is your opinion on this? Is the role of OSHA good, bad, could be improved, not necessary, too regulating? Recall the things that you have already learned that OSHA requires. Consider the amount of work and money that many of the requirements would involve for an employer, both big and small. Explain your opinion.

_____

_____

_____

_____

4. A new couple has unprotected sex and then wonders if one of them could have contracted HIV from the other. They go together to a clinic to be tested and both get negative results. However, they still cannot be sure that the initial test proves that they are HIV free. Explain why one HIV test cannot definitely tell the presence of HIV.

_____

_____

_____

_____

5. After reading the section Caring for the HIV/AIDS Patient in this chapter, carefully reread the longest paragraph, which deals with instructing the significant other or family on the more personal aspects of care. There are many more nonmedical things the patient must deal with that a caregiver can help with, such as lack of money because he or she can't work, bills that may be unpaid, driving to appointments and the store, etc. Choose three aspects of the personal effects on the patient and offer at least two things each that a caregiver could help with.

_____

_____

_____

_____

CHAPTER REVIEW TEST

MULTIPLE CHOICE

Circle the letter of the correct answer.

1. Since _____, the United States has been screening all blood transfusions for HIV antibodies.
   - a. 1980
   - b. 1990
   - c. 1978
   - d. 1985

2. The primary stage of HIV infection may last a few weeks and cause _____ symptoms.
   - a. opportunistic
   - b. flulike
   - c. Kaposi's sarcoma
   - d. no symptoms in primary stage

3. The greatest number of microorganisms on the hands are found: (circle all that apply)
   - a. under the nails.
   - b. around the nails.
   - c. in the creases of the palms.
   - d. in rings.

4. The deepest layer of the skin is the
   - a. epidermis.
   - b. subcutaneous.
   - c. stratum corneum.
   - d. statum granulosum.

5. The purpose of medical asepsis is to: (circle all that apply)
   - a. protect the healthcare worker from infections.
   - b. maintain a clean environment.
   - c. teach only handwashing.
   - d. prevent the transmission of disease.

6. The CDC: (circle all that apply)
   - a. works to protect the public health and safety.
   - b. is a state agency of the United States Department of Health and Human Services.
   - c. provides immunization services and health information.
   - d. had the original name of Communicable Disease Center.

7. A 10:1 solution is one part of 10% sodium hypochlorite mixed with nine parts of water. The sodium hypochlorite is actually
   - a. alcohol.
   - b. salt with chloride.
   - c. household bleach.
   - d. none of the above.

8. The personal protective equipment you will wear for various tasks is determined by
   - a. actual or anticipated exposure to microorganisms.
   - b. actual or anticipated exposure to blood and body fluids and OPIM.
   - c. actual or anticipated exposure to nosocomial infections.
   - d. actual or anticipated exposure to hepatitis B or HIV/AIDS.

9. Some states are now requiring _____ to have the series of three HBV immunizations before _____.

   a. men and women, getting married
   b. women, getting pregnant
   c. all healthcare workers, doing direct
      patient care
   d. children, kindergarden

10. HIV can be passed from the infected patient only by contact with their blood or body fluids. It is only when their infected blood or body fluids _____ of someone else that the recipient is infected.

    a. get into the mucous membranes of the
       genitals
    b. get into the bloodstream
    c. get under the skin where they can be
       absorbed and get into the blood
    d. get absorbed into tissue and eventually
       the whole system

TRUE/FALSE

Indicate whether the statement is true (T) or false (F).

_____ 1. Skin is the first line of defense.

_____ 2. The first hepatitis immunization is given, then one month later the second is given, and one month after the second one, the third one is given.

_____ 3. *Bactericidal* means capable of killing bacteria.

_____ 4. An anaerobe survives in an environment with oxygen.

_____ 5. *E. coli* from the colon can cause a urinary infection.

_____ 6. The middle layer of the skin is called the epidermis.

_____ 7. Sneezing and coughing are two of the body's natural defenses against infection.

_____ 8. The two specific types of immunity defenses—cell-mediated and humoral immunity.

_____ 9. The normal pH of gastric juice is alkaline.

_____ 10. Masks and face shields are items of PPE.

FILL IN THE BLANK

Using words from the list below, fill in the blanks to complete the following statements. Note: Some terms may be used in more than one statement.

allergic   inhibit the growth   opportunistic

barrier   integumentary   pathogenic

blood   bloodborne pathogens   irritant

pathogens   IV needles   phagocytosis

body fluids   leukocytes   portal of exit

disease transmission   microorganisms   potentially infectious

gloving   modes   reservoir

healthcare worker   multiple   rubeola

hepatitis   *Mycobacterium tuberculosis*   susceptible

HIV/AIDS   nonpathogenic   unprotected sex

HIV infection   normally harmless   varicella

impaired

1. Microorganisms can be _____ or _____. _____ are those pathogenic and carried in the bloodstream.

2. Universal precautions were established to reduce risk of _____ and _____. All _____, blood products, human tissue and _____ are considered to be _____ materials.

3. Airborne transmission is when the microorganisms move through the air on dust particles. Examples of airborne particles that could cause disease are the _____ and _____ viruses and the _____.

4. The circulatory and lymphatic systems also fight infection by sending out _____ to surround and destroy _____ in a process called _____.

5. The first line of defense against infections is the _____ system. Intact skin serves as a _____ against invasion by the _____ that are normally on our skin.

6. The organisms that cause _____ infections are present in or on humans, and a normal immune system can _____ of these organisms. The _____ immune system of _____ patients is overwhelmed by the _____ organisms.

7. For those patients at risk or those with_____, patient education should include avoiding _____ sex partners and _____, not sharing _____, and avoiding irresponsible behavior that could pass infection to others.

8. Nonsterile _____ is used to prevent _____, and it is primarily for the personal protection of the _____.

9. The most common latex reactions are _____ contact dermatitis and _____ contact dermatitis.

10. The infection cycle begins with a _____ or carrier host, then a _____. There must be vehicles or _____ of transmission, and a _____ host is needed to receive the pathogens.

Procedure 7-1

Hand Washing

Objective: The student, using the supplies and equipment listed below, will demonstrate how to wash hands following medically aseptic technique.

Supplies: Soap (bar or pump), paper towels, waste container, nail brush or cuticle stick.

Notes to the Student:

_____

_____

_____

_____

_____

_____

Skills Assessment Requirements

Read and familiarize yourself with the procedure; complete the minimum practice requirements. Document each MPR using proper charting technique. Complete each procedure within a reasonable amount of time, with a minimum of 85% accuracy.

POINT VALUE ✦ = 3–6 points ✶ = 7–9 points		PRACTICE TRIAL	GRADED TRIAL # 1	GRADED TRIAL # 2	NOTES:
1. ✶	Remove and secure most jewelry. Wedding bands and professional watches are allowed. Push the watch higher than your wrist. Avoid touching the contaminated sink front with your uniform.				
2. ✦	With a paper towel, turn on the water and adjust to a warm temperature. The water should run continuously until you have finished the procedure. Discard the paper towel.				
3. ✦	With your hands and fingers lower than your elbows, wet your wrists and hands.				
4. ✶	Apply soap and scrub lather over the hands and fingers, between the fingers, under and around the nails, and rinse. Apply soap and lather to the wrists and forearms. The purpose of this washing order is to wash the dirtiest areas first. A circular motion and friction rubbing will loosen dirt and microorganisms. If you are using bar soap, rinse it before returning it to the soap dish.				
5. ✦	Use the cuticle stick or nail brush to clean your nails. If you are wearing a wedding band, scrub around it with the nail brush.				

	PRACTICE TRIAL	GRADED TRIAL # 1	GRADED TRIAL # 2	NOTES:
6. ✦ Rinse off the lather, keeping your hands in a downward position. Avoid splashing and touching the sink or faucets.				
7. ✦ Dry your hands with a paper towel and discard it.				
8. ✦ Turn off the faucet with another paper towel and discard it; using a new paper towel prevents the contamination of clean hands.				

Document: Enter the appropriate information in the chart below.

Grading

Points Earned	_____		
Points Possible	_____	54	54
Percent Grade (Points Earned/ Points Possible)	_____		
PASS:	_____	❏ YES ❏ NO ❏ N/A	❏ YES ❏ NO ❏ N/A

Instructor Sign-Off

Instructor: _____ Date: _____

Procedure 7-2

Nonsterile Gloving

Objective: The student, using the supplies and equipment listed below, will demonstrate the application, removal, and disposal of nonsterile gloves following medically aseptic technique.

Supplies: nonsterile gloves, waste receptacle

Notes to the Student:

_____

_____

_____

_____

_____

_____

Skills Assessment Requirements

Read and familiarize yourself with the procedure; complete the minimum practice requirements. Document each MPR using proper charting technique. Complete each procedure within a reasonable amount of time, with a minimum of 85% accuracy.

Name: _____

Date: _____

POINT VALUE ✦ = 3–6 points ⋆ = 7–9 points		PRACTICE TRIAL	GRADED TRIAL # 1	GRADED TRIAL # 2	NOTES:
1. ✦	Wash and dry your hands.				
2. ⋆	Choose gloves of the right size. They should not be so loose that they fall off during a procedure. If they are too tight, they may tear and new gloves will have be applied.				
3. ✦	Take one glove from the box and pull it on over your hand to the wrist.				
4. ✦	Take a second glove and pull it on to the wrist.				
5. ✦	Adjust the gloves so that the wrists are covered.				
6. ✦	To remove the first glove, grasp the outside of the glove at the wrist with the other gloved hand and pull down. This motion will keep the contaminated surface inside and is called the "glove touch glove." Discard the first glove immediately.				
7. ✦	With your ungloved hand, reach inside the second glove. Grasp the inside of the glove and pull it down and off. This second glove removal also keeps the contaminated surface on the inside and is called "ungloved hand touch hand inside before removing." Discard the second glove immediately.				
8. ✦	Wash and dry your hands.				

Name: _____

Date: _____

Document: Enter the appropriate information in the chart below.

Grading

Points Earned	_____		
Points Possible	_____	51	51
Percent Grade (Points Earned/ Points Possible)	_____		
PASS:	_____	❏ YES ❏ NO ❏ N/A	❏ YES ❏ NO ❏ N/A

Instructor Sign-Off

Instructor: _____ **Date:** _____

CHAPTER 8
Surgical Asepsis

CHAPTER OUTLINE

Review the Chapter Outline. If any content area is unclear, review that area before beginning workbook exercises.

    A.   The Medical Assistant's Role in Surgical Asepsis

    B.   Surgical Asepsis

    C.   Sanitization, Disinfection, and Sterilization

    D.   Wrapping Instruments and Preparing Sterile Trays

    E.   Preparing the Surgical Field

    F.   Alcohol-Based Hand Rubs

CHAPTER REVIEW

The following is a summary of the chapter. If any of this material is unclear, review it in the textbook.

The care and safety of the patient is always foremost in healthcare, and correctly using medical or surgical asepsis is a vital part of the medical assistant's job. Sanitization and disinfection are methods of achieving medical asepsis, and sterilization achieves surgical asepsis. Sterilization is most commonly done with an autoclave or chemicals. The MA must also be familiar with a variety of instruments and supplies, know what is sterile and what isn't to prevent contamination, and how to prepare a sterile field for procedures. To prevent infection is the goal of surgical asepsis.

LEARNING ACTIVITIES AND STUDY AIDS

Review the following study aids and/or complete the activities to ensure that you have achieved the learning objectives for this chapter.

1. Search the Internet for more information on the following topics:

    a. pH—What is the normal pH for urine? Blood? Vaginal secretions? The body in general? What level is neutral? Is lower more acidic or more alkaline?

    _____

    _____

    _____

    _____

    b. For the equipment in an office or clinic—endoscope, autoclave, Mayo stands—try to find pictures of each item from a medical supply company, and for your information, notice there are usually several styles and models. It would be beneficial for you to see various kinds as the office you work in may have different models than your classroom.

_____

_____

_____

_____

2. Medical asepsis was covered in Chapter 7. Surgical asepsis is different in some ways from medical asepsis. Review in the textbook the sections on The Medical Assistant's Role in Surgical Asepsis, Surgical Asepsis, and Table 8-1. Close your book and from memory, briefly state in your own words the main principles of surgical asepsis.

_____

_____

_____

_____

_____

_____

3. Differentiate between sanitization, disinfection, and sterilization. How do you know which method to use to properly prepare an instrument? In your textbook, there is a section under Sterilization called Tips for Success: Which Decontamination Steps Should You Perform? Read through this section and make an index card for future reference that will help you determine what decontamination method you should use.

_____

_____

_____

_____

_____

_____

4. Define disinfection and list the various types or ways to disinfect in the medical office.

_____

_____

_____

_____

_____

5. Explain how the autoclave method of sterilization works and include any details that would help someone understand who was unfamiliar with sterilization techniques. Imagine you are telling a friend or family member or anyone who has no medical background.

_____

_____

_____

_____
_____
_____
_____

6. Since you will be practicing and then doing a performance skills check-off for wrapping instruments and preparing sterile trays using sterile technique, use index cards to state the basic steps of wrapping and the preparation of a sterile tray. DO NOT simply list the steps word for word from the book. Be concise, try to fit each procedure on one card, and only state the basic words of the steps. These cards are for your benefit during your externship and your new job after graduation.

_____
_____
_____
_____
_____
_____

7. Use an 81/2 X 11" sheet of plain paper to draw a picture of a sterile field. Based on the information in this chapter about preparing a sterile field, try to draw each instrument or supply item that should be there and label the items. Draw the one-inch border. You can use the instruments listed for one of the three procedures stated in Table 8-4. Look up the instrument(s) if you are unsure of what they look like and do your best to portray each. You are not expected to be an artist or to color it—just a simple drawing that looks like a prepared sterile field. On the back, write in your own words the overall concept of the sterile field—consider such aspects as what the sterile field is for, why everything on it must be sterile, why things are done a certain way.

_____
_____
_____
_____
_____
_____
_____
_____

MEDICAL TERMINOLOGY REVIEW

Use a dictionary and highlighted terms in the textbook to define the following terms.

Terms

antiseptic _____

_____

asepsis, surgical _____

aseptic _____

autoclave _____

autoclave load _____

cold sterilization _____

debris _____

emesis _____

endoscope _____

germicide _____

Mayo stand _____

noncritical _____

pH _____

sanitization _____

spore _____

sterilant _____

sterile _____

sterile field _____

sterilization _____

sterilization indicator _____

ultrasonic cleaning _____

CRITICAL THINKING

1. Picture yourself being sterile and assisting with a minor surgical procedure. In the middle of the procedure, you let your hands go below your waist. What should you do?

_____

_____

_____

_____

2. In the same scenario as above, you have opened a sterile package of instruments and placed them on the tray prior to the procedure, added a small cup of a solution, and draped the tray until the doctor comes in. When you remove the drape so the doctor may begin, you spill the solution on the sterile field. Since the field is sterile and the instruments are sterile, is it all right to proceed? Explain the reasoning behind your answer.

_____

_____

_____

_____

3. In the same scenario as above, following the procedure, you are cleaning up the sterile field. Two of the instruments on the tray were not used and did not touch any blood or body fluids. Do you have to resanitize and disinfect prior to sterilizing them again or can you simply wrap them again? Explain your answer.

_____

_____

_____

_____

4. Read Tips for Success: Which Decontamination Steps Should You Perform? It lists certain items that vary in the way they are decontaminated. Consider the same process for these items: the exam table, a scalpel (nondisposable) to be used for the next incision and drainage procedure, a tourniquet used when drawing blood. Explain how to decontaminate each item below.

   Exam table:

   _____

   Scalpel for surgery:

   _____

   Tourniquet:

   _____

5. You are working on preparing the sterile field and go to the autoclave for the paper-wrapped packs of instruments you ran earlier that day. The tape on the outside of the packs has the darkened stripes so you know that the outside of the pack has been sterilized. The physician is behind schedule and irritated about that. There are no extra instruments for this particular procedure, which is why you planned ahead and autoclaved them before hand. You open all the packs and transfer the contents to the sterile tray and put the sterile cover over it. As you clean up the empty paper and packages, you notice that the sterilization indicator from the inside of the packs had not

changed color. What would you do—say nothing and assume that the tape on outside indicated that the entire package had been sterilized? Tell the doctor that it will take another 40 minutes to reautoclave the items and get them ready for the procedure? Say nothing because you fear the physician's anger or even losing your job?

_____

_____

_____

_____

CHAPTER REVIEW TEST

MULTIPLE CHOICE

Circle the letter of the correct answer.

1. Brand names of glutaraldehyde for disinfection include all of the following except:
   a. Metricide.
   b. Wavicide.
   c. Procide.
   d. Betacide.

2. The order of applying PPE for sterile gowning and other PPE as well as scrubbing is:
   a. mask, hair cover, gown, gloves.
   b. hair cover, scrub, gown, mask, gloves.
   c. mask, hair cover, gown, scrub, gloves.
   d. there is no particular order, as long as scrubbed hands don't get contaminated before putting on the sterile gloves.

3. The phrase "skin to skin, sterile to sterile" is to help you with learning:
   a. aseptic technique.
   b. sterile gowning.
   c. sterile gloving.
   d. surgical asepsis.

4. Are the disinfectants chlorine and compounds phenolics and hydrogen peroxide considered high, moderate, or low level of disinfection?
   a. low
   b. intermediate
   c. high
   d. none of the above

5. The area around the edge of the sterile field is considered contaminated. What size is that area?
   a. one inch
   b. the edge of the Mayo stand beneath the drape
   c. two inches
   d. one-half inch

6. If you must turn your back to the sterile field,
   a. minimize movement to avoid airborne contaminates from getting on the field.
   b. have an extra sterile drape ready to cover the field while you turn from it.
   c. you would have to step out and rewash, regown, reglove, etc.
   d. just keep your hands above your waist, and it would be fine.

7. Which of the following is *not* considered a noncritical item in relation to being disinfected?
   a. blood pressure cuff (sphygmomanometer)
   b. gooseneck lamp
   c. stethoscope
   d. flexible sigmoidoscope

8. Which of the following is true about sterilized packs after being autoclaved? (circle all that apply)
   a. must be removed immediately and allowed to air dry before storing or using
   b. should be allowed to dry in the autoclave before removing them
   c. should be checked for tears or holes
   d. should have tape that has changed color

9. Glassware, such as the jars that hold the cotton balls
   a. cannot be autoclaved.
   b. can be autoclaved if the lid is off.
   c. can be autoclaved if lying on its side.
   d. must be wrapped in the same way instruments are.

10. Sterilization can be accomplished by three methods. Which of the following is *not* a sterilization method?
   a. sanitization plus disinfection with sodium hypochlorite
   b. dry heat
   c. chemicals
   d. steam

TRUE/FALSE

Indicate whether the statement is true (T) or false (F).

_____ 1. When pouring solutions to the sterile field, palming the label avoids staining it and making it illegible.

_____ 2. Some surgical items or equipment cannot be sterilized in the autoclave as they are too delicate or have certain parts that cannot be autoclaved. Those items are always disposable because they cannot be sterilized.

_____ 3. When performing a sterile scrub, remember to open the package with the sterile towel to dry your hands on before scrubbing your hands.

_____ 4. Surgical asepsis removes spores.

_____ 5. Unwrapped instruments can be autoclaved.

_____ 6. Isopropyl alcohol is the best disinfectant used in the medical office.

_____ 7. Sterilization time is the same for all items—it is the temperature that varies.

_____ 8. The air above a sterile field is considered contaminated.

_____ 9. Distilled water must be used in an autoclave to prevent mineral buildup and corrosion.

_____ 10. If the physician needs to draw up medication during a procedure and cannot touch the vial that is not sterile, an MA who is not in sterile gloves holds the vial upside down for the doctor to put the needle in and draw up the medication.

FILL IN THE BLANK

Using words from the list below fill in the blanks to complete the following statements. Note: some terms may be used in more than one statement.

alcohol prep	local anesthetic	sterilant
aseptic	one-inch	sterile
bracelets	penetrate	sterilization
chamber	required	surgical
contaminated	required time	tips
disinfection	rings	touching
distilled water	sanitization	upside down
fingernails	skin	watches
forceps	spores	
invasive	steam	

1. When loading packs into an autoclave correctly, steam must _____ all surfaces for the _____ and at the _____ temperature to kill all microorganisms and their_____.

2. Three ways to clean items of microorganisms are _____, _____, and _____.

3. The autoclave reservoir is filled with _____ to produce _____ for sterilization.

4. There is a _____ perimeter of the sterile field that is considered _____.

5. Prior to assisting with a minor surgical procedure, _____, _____, and _____ should be removed before the _____ hand scrub, and debris should be removed from underneath the _____.

6. To help reduce errors when donning or removing sterile gloves, remembering this simple saying will help: _____ to _____, _____ to _____.

7. Sterile or _____ technique is used at all times during _____ procedures and when _____ integrity is or will be broken.

8. When loading an autoclave, ask yourself some questions, one of which is: Are any of the packs _____ the inside of the autoclave _____?

9. During a surgical procedure, the doctor needs to withdraw _____ from a vial, so the MA uses an _____ to clean the vial top, then holds the vial _____ outside of the sterile field and with the label facing the doctor.

10. Transfer _____, when not in use to prepare a _____ tray, must have the _____ not the handles kept in a chemical _____.

Procedure 8-1

Sanitization

Objective: The student, using the supplies and equipment listed below, will demonstrate performance of manually cleaning and sanitizing of instruments.

Supplies: Contaminated instruments, basin for soaking instruments, examination gloves, utility gloves, neutral low-suds detergent, scrubbing brush, paper towel, cotton towel

Notes to the Student:

_____

_____

_____

_____

_____

_____

Skills Assessment Requirements

Read and familiarize yourself with the procedure; complete the minimum practice requirements. Document each MPR using proper charting technique. Complete each procedure within a reasonable amount of time, with a minimum of 85% accuracy.

POINT VALUE ✦ = 3–6 points ⋆ = 7–9 points		PRACTICE TRIAL	GRADED TRIAL # 1	GRADED TRIAL # 2	NOTES:
1. ⋆	With examination and utility gloves on your hands, place the contaminated instruments in an empty basin, cover it with a cotton towel, and transport it to the cleaning area. Remove the towel and add disinfectant or water with detergent to the basin. After the patient is discharged, clean, disinfect, and supply the room for the next patient.				
2. ✦	In the instrument cleaning area, drain off the disinfectant or detergent and remove the instruments. Carefully wipe away blood and/or any tissue debris. Hold the instruments by their finger openings when possible.				
3. ✦	Place the instruments in a basin with the recommended amount of cleaning agent and water.				
4. ✦	Cleaning one instrument at a time, use a soft brush on all serrated and smooth edges, grooves, and opened hinges.				
5. ✦	Rinse all the instruments with hot water.				
6. ✦	Dry each instrument with a paper towel and allow to air-dry completely on a cotton towel. Lubricate the hinges with a water-based lubricant.				

		PRACTICE TRIAL	GRADED TRIAL # 1	GRADED TRIAL # 2	NOTES:
7. ★	Follow the manufacturer's directions for disposing of cleaning solution. *Do not* reuse.				
8. ✦	Remove the gloves and wash your hands.				
9. ✦	Inspect each instrument for defects and proper function. Package the instruments as needed to ready for sterilization.				
	Ultrasonic Cleansing				
10. ★	With examination and utility gloves on your hands, prepare the cleaning solution for the ultrasonic cleaner as directed by the manufacturer. Observe all MSDS safety and accidental spill precautions.				
11. ✦	Place instruments made of different metals in separate ultrasonic cleaning loads.				
12. ✦	Place the instruments in the ultrasonic cleaner with their hinges open and sharp edges not touching other instruments. Make sure that all the instruments are covered with the ultrasonic cleaning solution. Turn on the ultrasonic cleaner.				
13. ★	When the recommended cleaning time has passed, remove the instruments and rinse each one with hot tap water.				

		PRACTICE TRIAL	GRADED TRIAL # 1	GRADED TRIAL # 2	NOTES:
14. ✦	Dry each instrument with a paper towel and allow to air-dry completely on a cotton towel. Lubricate the hinges with a water-based lubricant.				
15. ✦	Follow the manufacturer's directions for changing the cleaning solution.				
16. ✦	Remove the gloves and wash your hands.				
17. ✦	Inspect each instrument for defects and proper function. Package the instruments as needed to ready for sterilization.				

Document: Enter the appropriate information in the chart below.

Grading

Points Earned	_____		
Points Possible	_____	114	114
Percent Grade (Points Earned/ Points Possible)	_____		
PASS:	_____	❑ YES ❑ NO ❑ N/A	❑ YES ❑ NO ❑ N/A

Instructor Sign-Off

Instructor: _____ **Date:** _____

Procedure 8-2

Disinfection

Objective: The student, using the supplies and equipment listed below, will demonstrate how to perform the steps of disinfection correctly and safely.

Supplies: Contaminated articles, MSDS, disposable gloves, utility gloves, chemical disinfectant, soaking container, paper towels, cotton towel

Notes to the Student:

_____

_____

_____

_____

_____

_____

Skills Assessment Requirements

Read and familiarize yourself with the procedure; complete the minimum practice requirements. Document each MPR using proper charting technique. Complete each procedure within a reasonable amount of time, with a minimum of 85% accuracy.

POINT VALUE ✦ = 3–6 points ⋆ = 7–9 points		PRACTICE TRIAL	GRADED TRIAL # 1	GRADED TRIAL # 2	NOTES:
1. ⋆	Review the MSDS, noting potential hazards, how to clean accidental spills, and whether PPE should be worn.				
2. ✦	Apply disposable gloves to place the contaminated items into the basin. Then apply an additional layer of utility gloves.				
3. ✦	Complete the sanitizing steps in Procedure 8-1. Remember to cover the basin of contaminated instruments with a cloth towel when you move them to the cleaning area.				
4. ⋆	Check the expiration date of the disinfectant and follow the manufacturer's directions for mixing and use.				
5. ✦	With gloves on, completely immerse the contaminated articles in the container of disinfectant. Cover the container and soak the instruments for the length of time recommended by the manufacturer.				
6. ✦	Remove and rinse each instrument thoroughly. Dry the instruments with paper towels.				
7. ✦	Place the disinfected instruments on muslin or into sterilizing packets for the autoclave.				

Document: Enter the appropriate information in the chart below.

Grading

Points Earned	_____		
Points Possible	_____	48	48
Percent Grade (Points Earned/ Points Possible)	_____		
PASS:	_____	❏ YES ❏ NO ❏ N/A	❏ YES ❏ NO ❏ N/A

Instructor Sign-Off

Instructor: _____   **Date:** _____

Procedure 8-3

Wrapping Surgical Instruments for Autoclave Sterilization

Objective: The student, using the supplies and equipment listed below, will demonstrate how to package and wrap instruments and supplies to be placed in the autoclave correctly.

Supplies: Dry wrapping paper, muslin cloth, or sealable bags, sanitize and disinfected items to be sterilized, sterilization indicators for interior and exterior of packages, marker pen.

Notes to the Student:

_____

_____

_____

_____

_____

_____

Skills Assessment Requirements

Read and familiarize yourself with the procedure; complete the minimum practice requirements. Document each MPR using proper charting technique. Complete each procedure within a reasonable amount of time, with a minimum of 85% accuracy.

POINT VALUE ✦ = 3–6 points ⋆ = 7–9 points		PRACTICE TRIAL	GRADED TRIAL # 1	GRADED TRIAL # 2	NOTES:
1. ✦	Place the sanitized items to be sterilized in the center of the dry wrapping paper, muslin, or sealable bag. Place an indicator tape inside the package. The sealable bag may need to be sealed if it is not manufacturer-prepared.				
2. ⋆	For cloth or paper packaging, fold up one corner to cover the items. Double-back a small fold to use as a pull-corner for unwrapping. Do the same fold and double-back fold for the right side and left side. Fold the last side once toward the center and tuck the corner under before applying sterilization indicator tape.				
3. ✦	Use the marker to label the tape with the date, contents, and preparer's initials.				

Name: _____

Date: _____

Document: Enter the appropriate information in the chart below.

Grading

Points Earned	_____		
Points Possible	_____	21	21
Percent Grade (Points Earned/ Points Possible)	_____		
PASS:	_____	❑ YES ❑ NO ❑ N/A	❑ YES ❑ NO ❑ N/A

Instructor Sign-Off

Instructor: _____ **Date:** _____

Procedure 8-4

Loading and Operating an Autoclave

Objective: The student, using the supplies and equipment listed below, will demonstrate loading and operating an autoclave correctly and safely to ensure complete sterilization.

Supplies: Wrapped or unwrapped sanitized and disinfected instruments, distilled water, heat-resistant gloves, manual or automatic autoclave, manufacturer's instruction manual, sterile transfer forceps, storage containers or shelf areas

Notes to the Student:

_____

_____

_____

_____

_____

_____

Skills Assessment Requirements

Read and familiarize yourself with the procedure; complete the minimum practice requirements. Document each MPR using proper charting technique. Complete each procedure within a reasonable amount of time, with a minimum of 85% accuracy.

POINT VALUE ✦ = 3–6 points ⋆ = 7–9 points	PRACTICE TRIAL	GRADED TRIAL # 1	GRADED TRIAL # 2	NOTES:
1. ✦ Wash your hands and assemble materials.				
2. ✦ Check the level of distilled water in the autoclave reservoir and fill as necessary.				
3. ⋆ Load the autoclave, asking yourself the following questions: • Are the autoclave trays 1 inch apart? • Are small packs 1 to 3 inches apart? • Are large packs 2 to 4 inches apart? • Are any of the packs touching the inside of the autoclave chamber? • Are glassware and jars on their sides? • Are dressings and sterilization pouches in a vertical position, on their sides? • Are any materials leaning against plastic items? • For a mixed load of porous and nonporous materials, are materials such as dressings on the top shelf and instruments on the lower shelf?				
4. ✦ Close and latch the door. Turn on the autoclave.				
5. ✦ Sterilization time starts when the correct pressure and temperature has been reached.				

		PRACTICE TRIAL	GRADED TRIAL #1	GRADED TRIAL #2	NOTES:
6. ✦	After steam pressure has been manually or automatically released, open the autoclave door slightly to allow the load to dry. Larger packs with dressings may take 45 to 60 minutes to dry.				
7. ✦	Wearing heat-resistant gloves, remove the dry packages. Inspect for holes, tears, and indicator tape color change. Use the sterile transfer forceps to remove single instruments or items to a clean container. Place sterile items toward the back of the stock so that the oldest dated materials are used first. Avoid storing in cool areas that may cause condensation, make the materials damp, and require additional wrapping and sterilizing.				
8. ✦	Remove the gloves and wash your hands.				
9. ⋆	Record, the date, autoclave load contents, and use of sterilization indicators and quality controls in the sterilization control log.				

Document: Enter the appropriate information in the chart below.

Grading

Points Earned	_____		
Points Possible	_____	60	60
Percent Grade (Points Earned/ Points Possible)	_____		
PASS:	_____	❏ YES ❏ NO ❏ N/A	❏ YES ❏ NO ❏ N/A

Instructor Sign-Off

Instructor: _____ **Date:** _____

Procedure 8-5

Opening a Sterile Surgical Pack to Create a Sterile Field

Objective: The student, using the supplies and equipment listed below, will demonstrate how to use sterile technique to open a sterile surgical pack for a sterile field.

Supplies: Mayo stand, sterile packet(s), sterile transfer forceps, sterile gloves, sterile towels or drapes, waste container

Notes to the Student:

_____

_____

_____

_____

_____

_____

Skills Assessment Requirements

Read and familiarize yourself with the procedure; complete the minimum practice requirements. Document each MPR using proper charting technique. Complete each procedure within a reasonable amount of time, with a minimum of 85% accuracy.

Name: _____

Date: _____

POINT VALUE ✦ = 3–6 points ⋆ = 7–9 points		PRACTICE TRIAL	GRADED TRIAL #1	GRADED TRIAL #2	NOTES:
1. ✦	Wash your hands and assemble the equipment.				
2. ✦	Adjust the height of the Mayo stand to a comfortable working position.				
3. ✦	Position the sterile surgical pack on the Mayo stand so that the top flap will open away from you.				
4. ✦	Remove the sterilization indicator tape from the pack, note whether or not the appropriate color change occurred to indicate sterility, and discard.				
5. ✦	Pull the top flap away from you and down to hang over the edge of the Mayo stand. Pull each of the side flaps away from the packet and over the edge.				
6. ⋆	Without reaching over the sterile field, bring the last flap toward you and down to hang over the edge. Do not touch your body to any part of the sterile field while opening the pack or anytime during a sterile procedure.				

		PRACTICE TRIAL	GRADED TRIAL #1	GRADED TRIAL #2	NOTES:
7. ★	The inside of the pack is now the sterile field. • To move items on the sterile field, use sterile transfer forceps. • To add items to a sterile field, open other packages without touching the inner side of the package or contents, then dump the contents, then dump the contents on the sterile field without crossing or touching it. • To open the inner package of another sterile pack during the procedure, a person with clean hands may open the outer package so that a person with sterile gloves may take the inner packet of instruments and supplies.				
8. ✦	Cover the tray with sterile towels or drape until ready to use. This is done by opening a pack of sterile gloves and a pack of sterile drapes or towels, then put on the sterile gloves to unfold the drape or towel over the sterile field. Some sterile packets come with material for draping the sterile field.				

Document: Enter the appropriate information in the chart below.

Grading

Points Earned	_____		
Points Possible	_____	54	54
Percent Grade (Points Earned/ Points Possible)	_____		
PASS:	_____	❏ YES ❏ NO ❏ N/A	❏ YES ❏ NO ❏ N/A

Instructor Sign-Off

Instructor: _____ **Date:** _____

Procedure 8-6

Using Sterile Transfer Forceps

Objective: The student, using the supplies and equipment listed below, will demonstrate how to move sterile instruments and supplies within a sterile field, onto a sterile field, or into a sterile gloved hand without contaminating.

Supplies: Transfer forceps, sterile tray set upon a Mayo stand, forceps, container 2/3 full of Cidex or other sterilant, sterile 4 x 4 gauze package, instrument or supply pack for use with sterile transfer forceps

Notes to the Student:

_____

_____

_____

_____

_____

_____

Skills Assessment Requirements

Read and familiarize yourself with the procedure; complete the minimum practice requirements. Document each MPR using proper charting technique. Complete each procedure within a reasonable amount of time, with a minimum of 85% accuracy.

Name: _____

Date: _____

Point Value ✦ = 3–6 points ⋆ = 7–9 points		PRACTICE TRIAL	GRADED TRIAL # 1	GRADED TRIAL # 2	NOTES:
1. ✦	Open the 4 x 4 gauze package using sterile technique and lay it on the countertop or Mayo stand.				
2. ✦	Grasp the forceps handles, keeping the tips together. Remove the forceps vertically from the container without touching the sides.				
3. ⋆	Touch the forceps tips to the gauze 4 x 4 to dry them. Do not allow the forceps to touch the sterile field. Holding them vertically, pick up and move an item from the open pack to the sterile field. To move a sterile item on the sterile field, keep the forceps vertical, pick up the item, and lift it to the desired location without touching the sterile field.				
4. ✦	Place the transfer forceps back into the standing container without touching the sides.				

Name: _____

Date: _____

Document: Enter the appropriate information in the chart below.

Grading

Points Earned	_____		
Points Possible	_____	27	27
Percent Grade (Points Earned/ Points Possible)	_____		
PASS:	_____	❏ YES ❏ NO ❏ N/A	❏ YES ❏ NO ❏ N/A

Instructor Sign-Off

Instructor: _____ Date: _____

Procedure 8-7

Performing a Surgical Scrub (Surgical Hand Washing)

Objective: The student, using the supplies and equipment listed below, will demonstrate how to correctly perform surgical hand washing using sterile technique correctly.

Supplies: Germicidal liquid soap in dispenser, large wall clock, sink with hand, knee, or foot on/off controls, sterile towel packet, sterile scrub sponge, orangewood stick or nail file.

Notes to the Student:

_____

_____

_____

_____

_____

_____

Skills Assessment Requirements

Read and familiarize yourself with the procedure; complete the minimum practice requirements. Document each MPR using proper charting technique. Complete each procedure within a reasonable amount of time, with a minimum of 85% accuracy.

POINT VALUE ✦ = 3–6 points ⋆ = 7–9 points		PRACTICE TRIAL	GRADED TRIAL # 1	GRADED TRIAL # 2	NOTES:
1. ✦	Without touching the inside, open the sterile towel packet some distance from potential water spray.				
2. ✦	Remove all jewelry from your hands and wrists. Use an orangewood stick or nail file to remove dirt from under your fingernails.				
3. ✦	Turn on the water with hand, knee, or foot controls and adjust the temperature. Wet your arm from the fingertips to the elbows.				
4. ⋆	Apply liquid soap to your hands and lower arms. For 5 minutes, use a circular motion to create lather, starting from the fingertips and working toward the elbows. Be sure to wash between the fingers and under the fingernails.				
5. ⋆	Rinse the lather from your arm, beginning at the fingertips and proceeding to the elbows. Keep hands above your elbows.				
6. ✦	Repeat the process, applying liquid soap to your hands and lower arms. Scrub from the fingertips to the elbows with the sponge for 3 minutes.				

		PRACTICE TRIAL	GRADED TRIAL # 1	GRADED TRIAL # 2	NOTES:
7. ✦	Rinse thoroughly and leave the water running. Use a sterile towel dry to your hands.				
8. ★	Use the towel to turn off a hand-controlled faucet or, if necessary, use your elbow. Otherwise release the foot pedal or move the knee control to turn off the water.				

Document: Enter the appropriate information in the chart below.

Grading

Points Earned	_____		
Points Possible	_____	57	57
Percent Grade (Points Earned/ Points Possible)	_____		
PASS:	_____	❏ YES ❏ NO ❏ N/A	❏ YES ❏ NO ❏ N/A

Instructor Sign-Off

Instructor: _____   Date: _____

Procedure 8-8

Sterile Gloving and Glove Removal

Objective: The student, using the supplies and equipment listed below, will demonstrate how to apply gloves using sterile technique correctly.

Supplies: Sterile glove pack in correct size

Notes to the Student:

_____

_____

_____

_____

_____

_____

Skills Assessment Requirements

Read and familiarize yourself with the procedure; complete the minimum practice requirements. Document each MPR using proper charting technique. Complete each procedure within a reasonable amount of time, with a minimum of 85% accuracy.

Name: _____

Date: _____

POINT VALUE ✦ = 3–6 points ⋆ = 7–9 points		PRACTICE TRIAL	GRADED TRIAL # 1	GRADED TRIAL # 2	NOTES:
1. ✦	Open the pack of sterile gloves, touching only the outside of the pack. Touching only the outside of the inner packet, turn the cuff end toward you.				
2. ⋆	Open the inner packet by pulling each edge to the side. The gloves will be lying on the sterile field created by opening the inner pack. *Do not* touch the inside of the inner pack.				
3. ✦	Perform a sterile scrub.				
4. ⋆	The following directions are for a right-handed person. Perform the opposite actions if you are left-handed. With the thumb and fingers of the left hand, grasp only the folded-back cuff area (skin to skin: your skin touches what is to be the inside of the glove). While dangling the glove with the left hand, carefully slide the right hand in. *Do not* touch the outside of the glove with your ungloved hand. Keep your hands above your waist and in front of you.				

		PRACTICE TRIAL	GRADED TRIAL # 1	GRADED TRIAL # 2	NOTES:
5. ★	To don the second sterile glove, slide the fingers of your gloved hand under the cuff (sterile to sterile: the outside of the gloved hand is sterile against the sterile outside of the second glove). With the second glove "hooked" by the fingers of you gloved hand; slide your second hand into the glove. Continue to keep your hands above your waist and in front of you.				
6. ✦	Adjust the finger and thumb fit of the gloves (sterile to sterile).				
7. ✦	To remove the gloves, use the fingers of one gloved hand to grasp the other glove at the wrist. Pull the glove over itself and hold it in the palm of the gloved hand. Slide the fingers of the of the ungloved hand under the cuff of the remaining glove, grasp the inside, and pull it down over the glove and off the hand.				
8. ✦	Discard the gloves in a biohazard waste receptacle.				

Document: Enter the appropriate information in the chart below.

Grading

Points Earned	_____		
Points Possible	_____	57	57
Percent Grade (Points Earned/ Points Possible)	_____		
PASS:	_____	❏ YES ❏ NO ❏ N/A	❏ YES ❏ NO ❏ N/A

Instructor Sign-Off

Instructor: _____ **Date:** _____

CHAPTER 9
Pharmacology and Medication Administration

CHAPTER OUTLINE

Review the Chapter Outline. If any content area is unclear, review that area before beginning workbook exercises.

- A. The Medical Assistant's Role in Administering and Dispensing Drugs
- B. Basic Pharmacology
- C. Medication Measurement and Conversion
- D. Safety Guidelines for Administering Medications
- E. The Prescription
- F. Forms and Routes of Medication Administration

CHAPTER REVIEW

The following is a summary of the chapter. If any of this material is unclear, review it in the textbook.

Pharmacology is one of the most important areas of the medical assistant's work, primarily because of the chance of ill effects if errors are made. The MA must study and understand the pharmacology of medications, including aspects such as, but not limited to, the medication actions and absorption, what resources to use for additional information, how to read and write prescriptions and to order refills, the various methods of administration and all routes, and equipment and supplies needed. The controlled substances that may be prescribed or administered in the office are highly regulated and the storage, disposal, and documentation must be done accurately to meet the federal laws that control these substances. The MA should also be familiar with the patients he or she will administer medication to, such as medication allergies, their history, and their state of health. If giving an injection, the size of the patient, the depth to the appropriate tissue, and the size of the syringe and the needle's gauge and length must be determined accurately. The math of medication administration is also a very important aspect as the conversion if necessary and calculations must be accurate in order to administer the ordered amount of medication. Every medical assistant must keep up to date on medications, to know and understand the pharmacology and all aspects of medication administration to ensure patient safety.

LEARNING ACTIVITIES AND STUDY AIDS

Review the following study aids and/or complete the activities to ensure that you have achieved the learning objectives for this chapter.

1. In your textbook, see Table 9-9 of commonly used abbreviations related to pharmacology. Since the MA will use these often, make index cards of these abbreviations and review these cards often. These will be an important reference on an externship or the job and an important study tool.

_____

_____

_____

_____

_____

_____

2. Review the role of the medical assistant in administering and dispensing drugs. Write in your own words, briefly, what that role entails.

_____

_____

_____

_____

_____

_____

_____

3. List and define the various effects of drugs on the body.

_____

_____

_____

_____

_____

_____

_____

4. All medications have their own basic functions. Name those listed in your textbook.

_____

_____

_____

_____

_____

_____

_____

5. In your own words, briefly state the difference between prescription and over-the-counter (OTC) medications.

_____

_____

_____

_____

_____

6. While one name of a medication may be familiar to most people, there are actually three names to every medication. What are the three names? Provide a brief description of each.

_____

_____

_____

_____

_____

_____

7. When an MA needs additional information on a medication, there are various resources available to consult. List those sources.

_____

_____

_____

_____

_____

_____

8. State the simple definition of a drug classification. Then refer to Table 9-4, which is quite extensive. Using index cards, write a classification on each card and include the basic functions as well as examples of each.

_____

_____

_____

_____

_____

_____

9. Why are certain medications controlled by the DEA? The federal Controlled Substances Act (CSA) has established guidelines for the storage, recordkeeping, and safekeeping of these controlled substances. Review this section in your textbook for the various tasks that must be followed since these legal guidelines require strict compliance. Then list the five different schedules that categorize these controlled substances and give a brief description of each as well as one or two examples of medications for each schedule.

_____

_____

_____

10. Drugs must be measured and conversions between systems of measurement are calculated. For example, if a drug is ordered in milligrams (mg) but is supplied in drams, a conversion must be made using one system or the other. State these different systems. What is the reference that makes this easier?

_____

_____

_____

_____

_____

_____

_____

11. Regardless of whether a conversion between measurement systems is needed, briefly describe how drug calculations are made, as stated in your textbook.

_____

_____

_____

_____

_____

_____

_____

12. There are six basic and universal safety guidelines that must be followed when drugs are being administered by any route. Review these six rights in your textbook and study them until they are ingrained because you must use them every time you give a medication. List the six rights here.

_____

_____

_____

_____

_____

_____

13. Every prescription contains seven items of information that must be included. Review the information in your textbook and try to memorize the seven items. Then close your book and list each term here and a very brief explanation of each. Always go back and restudy those that you need to.

_____

_____

_____
_____
_____
_____
_____
_____

14. Prescription pads should be safeguarded due to the potential for theft. List the guidelines an MA can follow to help ensure the pads are not stolen and abused.

_____
_____
_____
_____
_____
_____
_____
_____

15. There are numerous forms of medications, routes or ways the medication is to be given, and ways to administer them. This is also vital for the MA to know since the MA usually is the person who administers medications in the office. Refer to Table 9-10 and again use index cards that are divided into three sections as the tables. Write the form of the medication, its related route of administration, and the procedure of administration. These cards are for your future reference.

_____
_____
_____
_____
_____
_____
_____

16. There are many ways medications can be administered. What is meant by parenteral administration of medications? List a few examples.

_____
_____
_____
_____
_____
_____
_____

MEDICAL TERMINOLOGY REVIEW

Use a dictionary and highlighted terms in the textbook to define the following terms

Terms

chemical name _____

_____

contraindication _____

_____

controlled substance _____

_____

drug _____

_____

generic (nonproprietary) name _____

_____

over-the-counter medication _____

_____

pharmacology _____

_____

side effect _____

_____

sympathemimetic _____

_____

therapeutic effect _____

_____

toxic effect _____

_____

trade (brand, proprietary) _____

_____

Abbreviations

CSA _____

_____

DEA _____

_____

OTC _____

_____

PDR _____

_____

USP-NF _____

_____

CRITICAL THINKING

1. You have received a physician's order to administer 1 mg of a medication to a patient. It is a medication that is injected into the muscle. As soon as you have given the medication, you realize you measured 1 ml instead of calculating 1 mg. What would you do?

   _____

   _____

   _____

   _____

2. A patient has finished seeing the doctor and on her way out, she asks the MA for a sample of Motrin, which is an OTC medication. The MA gives her two packages but does not document this and does not ask the doctor, because the MA felt that since Motrin is an OTC medication, getting it without an order would be appropriate. What is wrong with this scenario? What did the MA do wrong?

   _____

   _____

   _____

   _____

3. A regular patient has come in wanting a new prescription for a medication she has taken for many years, because she is out of refills. The physician is not in the office today, but after checking the medical record and noting that it is the patient's usual medication, the MA calls in a new prescription to the pharmacy and makes a note to have the doctor write the order in the chart when she returns. Is this an appropriate action for the MA, since she used critical thinking to check the chart and felt sure the physician would approve it? Explain your answer.

   _____

   _____

   _____

   _____

4. Explain why IV infusion of medication is the most dangerous method to administer medication and MUST be the right med, strength, and amount. Errors with this route can cause serious problems. All routes of medication administration MUST be done accurately, but there are specific reasons why this route is more risky than the others.

   _____

   _____

   _____

   _____

5. Although a very small of amount of bubbles or air injected into the muscle or the subcutaneous tissue would not be harmful, *the MA must never do it*. Explain why it is not acceptable to have even tiny bubbles within the medication inside the syringe.

   _____

   _____

   _____

   _____

CHAPTER REVIEW TEST

MULTIPLE CHOICE

Circle the letter of the correct answer.

1. Which of the following is not included in Schedule II drugs?

   a. marijuana

   b. morphine

   c. cocaine

   d. Dilaudid

2. An injection into the fatty tissue under the skin is a/an _____ injection.

   a. intramuscular

   b. Z-track

   c. subcutaneous

   d. intradermal

3. The medication abbreviation for twice a day is

   a. b.i.d.

   b. t.i.d.

   c. prn

   d. q2h

4. The oral route of taking/giving medication is the safest route because

   a. it can be absorbed at a slow rate so that the patient can be prepared for any ill effects.

   b. most patients aren't afraid to swallow pills or liquids.

   c. it can be retrieved through emesis immediately if for some reason it is

   determined the patient shouldn't have taken it.

   d. it will dissolve or coat the stomach quickly and avoids nausea.

5. If bubbles are present in the syringe when you are drawing up,

   a. it is all right and you can proceed if they are very small.

   b. tap the ampule neck.

   c. tap the syringe with your finger or a pen to dislodge them and push only that air back into the vial.

   d. push all the med back into the vial and start again as many times as necessary until you can draw with no bubbles.

6. When an injectable medication is in powder form,

   a. mix it with enough tap water to make it thin enough to be injectable.

   b. mix it with sterile water to make it thin enough to be injectable.

   c. mix it with the correct amount of sterile diluent as stated on the label.

   d. mix it with the amount and type of diluent that the doctor specifies.

7. If the doctor orders 4 mg of a certain medication, and the vial states that there are 2 mg in 1 cc, how many cc would you give to deliver 4 mg?

   a. 2 cc

   b. 4 cc

   c. 6 cc

   d. ½ cc

8. If the doctor orders 1 dram of medication to be given and the vial states there are 1 mg in each cc, you must

    a. give 1 cc.

    b. ask the doctor how to determine the number of cc

    c. call the pharmacy first and ask.

    d. convert from apothecary to metric and then calculate the dosage.

9. If a medication has been given in the office but it may have possible side effects a short time following administration, you should

    a. warn the patient to watch for those effects.

    b. ask the patient to wait in the waiting room for a certain period of time.

    c. make sure the patient has a driver to get him or her home.

    d. Tell the patient what those effects could be and to call in immediately if the effects appear.

10. Documenting the administration of medication must include all of the following except:

    a. the name of the medication.

    b. the strength of the medication.

    c. the side effects that could occur.

    d. the route the medication was given.

TRUE/FALSE

Indicate whether the statement is true (T) or false (F).

_____ 1. Therapeutic drugs maintain a healthy state by preventing disease.

_____ 2. Schedule V controlled substances are those with the least potential for abuse.

_____ 3. SC is an abbreviation for subcutaneous, which is one type of tissue to use for injections.

_____ 4. A dermal patch administers a medication sublingually.

_____ 5. A vial of medication for injection has a top that is broken off.

_____ 6. When injecting an intramuscular injection into a young child, the vastus lateralis muscle is used and a maximum amount of 1 ml can be injected there.

_____ 7. An NSAID is an anti-inflammatory drug.

_____ 8. Aspirin is a generic name, and Excedrin is a brand name.

_____ 9. PDR stands for Physician's Desk Reference.

_____ 10. "Sig" for signature on a prescription is for the physician's signature.

FILL IN THE BLANK

Using words from the list below, fill in the blanks to complete the following statements. Note: Some terms may be used in more than one statement.

abbreviations	drug	plants
administration	federal Controlled	potential for abuse
animals	Substance Act	process
any method	function	route
apothecary	general effect	specific organs
area	GI tract	or tissues
basis for dosages	intramuscular	subcutaneous
cells	manufactured	time
DEA	metric	time
decrease or eliminate	minerals	weight
documentation	pain	Z-track
dose	patient	

1. Absorption refers to the _____ and _____ through which a drug reaches the _____.

2. Drugs are classified according to _____ and the _____ of the body they affect. Some affect _____, while others have a more_____.

3. Drugs with a _____ have been identified in the _____, which is enforced by the_____.

4. The six "rights" of medication administration are the right_____, _____, _____, _____, _____, and _____.

5. Some physicians still use _____ in the _____ system, but most are in the _____ system.

6. Drugs are derived from _____, _____, _____, or are _____.

7. The types of injections listed in this chapter are_____, _____, and _____.

8. Parenteral _____ of medication is by _____ other than in the_____.

9. Anesthetic medications _____ sensation of _____.

10. The _____ of a patient can be the _____ of medications.

Procedure 9-1

Demonstrate the Preparation of a Prescription for the Physician's Signature

Objective: The student will be able to prepare a prescription for the physician's signature.

Supplies: physician's order for medication, patient chart, ink pen, computer if Rx is typed, blank prescription

Notes to the Student:

_____

_____

_____

_____

_____

_____

Skills Assessment Requirements

Read and familiarize yourself with the procedure; complete the minimum practice requirements. Document each MPR using proper charting technique. Complete each procedure within a reasonable amount of time, with a minimum of 85% accuracy.

Name: _____

Date: _____

POINT VALUE ✦ = 3-6 points ⋆ = 7-9 points		PRACTICE TRIAL	GRADED TRIAL #1	GRADED TRIAL #2	NOTES:
1. ✦	Gather the equipment.				
2. ✦	Obtain the prescription information (name, dose, amount, frequency, refills) from the physician.				
3. ✦	Correctly write out the prescription according to the information received from the physician.				
4. ⋆	Document the procedure. Include the date, time, medication, strength, dose, frequency, and refills allowed. Some offices will want a photocopy of the written prescription.				

Name: _____

Date: _____

Document: Enter the appropriate information in the chart below.

Grading

Points Earned	_____		
Points Possible	_____	27	27
Percent Grade (Points Earned/ Points Possible)	_____		
PASS:	_____	❏ YES ❏ NO ❏ N/A	❏ YES ❏ NO ❏ N/A

Instructor Sign-Off

Instructor: _____ **Date:** _____

Procedure 9-2

Demonstrate Withdrawing Medication from an Ampule

Objective: The student, using the supplies and equipment listed below, will demonstrate how to withdraw medication from an ampule correctly.

Supplies: Sterile filter needle/syringe set, ampule of medication, sterile gauze 2x4s or 4x4s, alcohol wipes, gloves, sharps container, patient chart

Notes to the Student:

_____

_____

_____

_____

_____

_____

Skills Assessment Requirements

Read and familiarize yourself with the procedure; complete the minimum practice requirements. Document each MPR using proper charting technique. Complete each procedure within a reasonable amount of time, with a minimum of 85% accuracy.

POINT VALUE ✦ = 3-6 points ⋆ = 7-9 points		PRACTICE TRIAL	GRADED TRIAL # 1	GRADED TRIAL # 2	NOTES:
1. ✦	Wash your hands and gather equipment.				
2. ✦	Check to make sure the medication matches the physician's order. Calculate the dosage, if necessary. Look up information relating to the medication's function, usual doses, and side effects. Check for patient allergies.				
3. ✦	Check the medication label a second time against the physician's order.				
4. ⋆	Identify the patient and escort him or her to the treatment area.				
5. ✦	Put on your gloves.				
6. ✦	Dislodge any medication that may be trapped in the ampule neck by holding the ampule by the neck and quickly flicking your wrist in a downward motion.				
7. ✦	Disinfect the ampule with an alcohol swab and check the label again for correct medication and dosage.				
8. ✦	Completely wrap the neck of the ampule with the sterile cotton gauze and snap off the top by pulling it toward you. Discard the top in a sharps container.				

		PRACTICE TRIAL	GRADED TRIAL # 1	GRADED TRIAL # 2	NOTES:
9. ✦	With a filtered needle, withdraw the necessary medication amount. You can withdraw the medication with the ampule either inverted or not.				
10. ⋆	Change needles and discard the filtered needle into a sharps container.				
11. ⋆	Identify the patient.				
12. ✦	Administer the medication according to the physician's orders.				
13. ✦	Discard the used needle into the sharps container.				
14. ✦	Remove the gloves and wash your hands.				
15. ⋆	Document the procedure. Include date, time, site, medication, route, and amount administered. Follow office policy for recording the expiration date and lot number.				

Document: Enter the appropriate information in the chart below.

Grading

Points Earned	_____		
Points Possible	_____	102	102
Percent Grade (Points Earned/ Points Possible)	_____		
PASS:	_____	❏ YES ❏ NO ❏ N/A	❏ YES ❏ NO ❏ N/A

Instructor Sign-Off

Instructor: _____ **Date:** _____

Procedure 9-3

Demonstrate Withdrawing Medication from a Vial

Objective: The student, using the supplies and equipment listed below, will demonstrate accurately withdrawing a medication for injection from a vial.

Supplies: vial of medication, bandage strip(s), sharps container, patient chart.

Notes to the Student:

_____

_____

_____

_____

_____

_____

Skills Assessment Requirements

Read and familiarize yourself with the procedure; complete the minimum practice requirements. Document each MPR using proper charting technique. Complete each procedure within a reasonable amount of time, with a minimum of 85% accuracy.

POINT VALUE ✦ = 3-6 points ⋆ = 7-9 points		PRACTICE TRIAL	GRADED TRIAL #1	GRADED TRIAL #2	NOTES:
1. ✦	Wash your hands and gather equipment.				
2. ⋆	Select the correct-size needle to withdraw the medication. Viscous medications require a greater needle gauge.				
3. ⋆	Check the vial label against the physician's medication order.				
4. ✦	Remove the plastic cap from the vial if necessary. If the vial has already been used, wipe the rubber stopper with an alcohol wipe.				
5. ✦	Inject air into the vial in an amount equal to the medication being removed.				
6. ✦	Place the vial on a firm surface and insert the needle through the rubber stopper.				
7. ✦	Inject air into the vial.				
8. ✦	Invert the vial with the needle tip under the surface of the medication to avoid getting air into the syringe.				
9. ✦	Pull back the plunger to withdraw the necessary amount of medication.				
10. ✦	If air bubbles are present, tap firmly on the syringe to release the bubbles and re-inject them into the vial.				

		PRACTICE TRIAL	GRADED TRIAL #1	GRADED TRIAL #2	NOTES:
11. ✦	Check the level of medication in the vial and withdraw more if needed.				
12. ✦	Withdraw the needle from the vial and replace the cap.				
13. ✦	Remove the needle and discard it in a sharps container.				
14. ✦	Replace the needle with a sharp, sterile needle of appropriate size.				
15. ✦	Inject the medication at the appropriate site.				
16. ✱	Document the procedure. Include the date, time, medication, site, route, and amount administered. Follow office policy for recording the medication expiration date and lot number.				

Document: Enter the appropriate information in the chart below.

Grading

Points Earned	_____		
Points Possible	_____	105	105
Percent Grade (Points Earned/ Points Possible)	_____		
PASS:	_____	❑ YES ❑ NO ❑ N/A	❑ YES ❑ NO ❑ N/A

Instructor Sign-Off

Instructor: _____ Date: _____

Procedure 9-4

Demonstrate the Reconstitution of a Powdered Drug for Injection Administration

Objective: The student, using the supplies and equipment listed below, will demonstrate accurate reconstitution of a powdered medication for injection.

Supplies: Gloves, alcohol wipes, 2 appropriate-size syringes with needles, vial of medication, sterile water, sharps container, fine-tip permanent marker, and patient's chart.

Notes to the Student:

_____

_____

_____

_____

_____

_____

Skills Assessment Requirements

Read and familiarize yourself with the procedure; complete the minimum practice requirements. Document each MPR using proper charting technique. Complete each procedure within a reasonable amount of time, with a minimum of 85% accuracy.

POINT VALUE ✦ = 3-6 points ⋆ = 7-9 points		PRACTICE TRIAL	GRADED TRIAL # 1	GRADED TRIAL # 2	NOTES:
1. ✦	Wash your hands and gather the equipment.				
2. ⋆	Check to make sure the medication matches the physician's order. Calculate the dosage if necessary. Look up information relating to the function of the medication, usual dosage, and side effects.				
3. ✦	Check the medication label again against the physician's order to make sure it is the right medication.				
4. ✦	Remove the protective tops from the diluent (sterile water) and medication and wipe both with alcohol.				
5. ✦	Insert one needle into the diluent, making certain to inject an amount of air equal to the amount of solution you are removing. Withdraw the necessary amount of diluent.				
6. ✦	Inject the diluent into the powdered medication vial.				
7. ✦	Discard the used needle in the sharps container.				
8. ✦	Roll the vial containing the diluent and powder between your palms. It may take several minutes to mix the solution thoroughly. Avoid shaking the vial.				

		PRACTICE TRIAL	GRADED TRIAL #1	GRADED TRIAL #2	NOTES:
9. ★	If the medication will not be used immediately, label the vial with the date and time prepared, your initials, and the expiration date/time.				
10. ✦	With the second needle, draw up the correct amount of prepared medication to give to the patient.				
11. ★	Document the procedure. Include the date, time, medication, site, route, and amount administered. Follow office policy for recording the medication expiration date and lot number.				

Document: Enter the appropriate information in the chart below.

Grading

Points Earned	_____		
Points Possible	_____	75	75
Percent Grade (Points Earned/ Points Possible)	_____		
PASS:	_____	❏ YES ❏ NO ❏ N/A	❏ YES ❏ NO ❏ N/A

Instructor Sign-Off

Instructor: _____ **Date:** _____

Procedure 9-5

Demonstrate the Administration of Medication during Infusion Therapy

Objective: The student, using the supplies and equipment listed below, will demonstrate administering medication through an intermittent infusion device.

Supplies: 3 syringes with needles, medication to be administered, normal saline (0.9%) 4 mL, alcohol wipes, gloves, sharps container, patient chart.

Notes to the Student:

_____

_____

_____

_____

_____

_____

Skills Assessment Requirements

Read and familiarize yourself with the procedure; complete the minimum practice requirements. Document each MPR using proper charting technique. Complete each procedure within a reasonable amount of time, with a minimum of 85% accuracy.

POINT VALUE ✦ = 3-6 points * = 7-9 points		PRACTICE TRIAL	GRADED TRIAL # 1	GRADED TRIAL # 2	NOTES:
1. ✦	Wash your hands and gather the equipment.				
2. *	Check to make sure the medication matches the Physician's order. Calculate the dosage, if necessary. Look up information relating to the medication's function, usual doses, and side effects. Check for patient allergies.				
3. *	Check medication compatibility with the infusion product being used.				
4. ✦	Put on gloves.				
5. ✦	Disinfect the cannula port with the alcohol wipe.				
6. *	Verify that the cannula and vein are freely open, with no blockages.				
7. ✦	With the first of the three syringes, slowly inject 2 mL of the normal saline into the cannula port.				
8. ✦	With the second syringe, administer the medication as prescribed by the physician into the cannula port.				
9. ✦	With the final syringe, inject 2 mL of normal saline into the cannula port.				
10. ✦	Remove the gloves and wash your hands.				
11. *	Document the procedure. Include date, time, site, medication, route, and amount administered.				
12. ✦	Follow office policy for recording the expiration date and lot number.				

Name: _____

Date: _____

Document: Enter the appropriate information in the chart below.

Grading

Points Earned	_____		
Points Possible	_____	84	84
Percent Grade (Points Earned/ Points Possible)	_____		
PASS:	_____	❏ YES ❏ NO ❏ N/A	❏ YES ❏ NO ❏ N/A

Instructor Sign-Off

Instructor: _____ **Date:** _____

Procedure 9-6

Demonstrate the Preparation and Administration of Oral Medication

Objective: The student, using the supplies and equipment listed below, will demonstrate preparation and administration of oral medication.

Supplies: Vial of medication, gloves, patient chart

Notes to the Student:

_____

_____

_____

_____

_____

_____

Skills Assessment Requirements

Read and familiarize yourself with the procedure; complete the minimum practice requirements. Document each MPR using proper charting technique. Complete each procedure within a reasonable amount of time, with a minimum of 85% accuracy.

POINT VALUE ✦ = 3-6 points ✱ = 7-9 points		PRACTICE TRIAL	GRADED TRIAL # 1	GRADED TRIAL # 2	NOTES:
1. ✦	Wash your hands and gather equipment.				
2. ✦	Put on gloves.				
3. ✱	Check to make sure the medication matches the physician's order. Calculate the dosage, if necessary. Look up information relating to the medication's function, usual doses, and side effects.				
4. ✦	Check for patient allergies.				
5. ✦	Check the medication label a second time against the physician's order.				
6. ✱	Identify the patient and escort him or her to the treatment area.				
7. ✦	Pour the correct amount of medication.				
8. ✱	*For pills, capsules, and tablets:* Pour the correct amount from the container directly into a medicine cup. *For liquids and suspensions:* If the ingredients are not evenly mixed, shake the bottle gently but thoroughly. Allow time for any bubbles to disappear. When pouring, hold the medication bottle with your palm over the label and hold the medicine cup at eye level.				
9. ✦	Check a third time to match the medication against the physician's order.				

		PRACTICE TRIAL	GRADED TRIAL # 1	GRADED TRIAL # 2	NOTES:
10. ✦	If at any time you have doubts about the function of the medication, the dosage or route of administration, or the possibility of an allergic reaction, immediately consult the physician.				
11. ✦	Give the medicine cup to the patient. Have drinking water available for pills, capsules, and tablets, as well as for liquids or suspensions, if necessary.				
12. ✦	Observe as the patient takes the medication to ensure that it is swallowed completely, without difficulty.				
13. ✦	Dispose of the used medication cup and preparation supplies. Wash your hands and return the multiple-use medication bottle to the storage shelf.				
14. ∗	Document the procedure. Include date, time, site, medication, route, and amount administered. Follow office policy for recording the expiration date and lot number.				

Document: Enter the appropriate information in the chart below.

Grading

Points Earned	_____		
Points Possible	_____	96	96
Percent Grade (Points Earned/ Points Possible)	_____		
PASS:	_____	❏ YES ❏ NO ❏ N/A	❏ YES ❏ NO ❏ N/A

Instructor Sign-Off

Instructor: _____   **Date:** _____

Name: _____

Date: _____

Procedure 9-7

Demonstrate the Administration of a Subcutaneous Injection

Objective: The student, using the supplies and equipment listed below, will demonstrate correctly administering a subcutaneous injection.

Supplies: gloves, alcohol wipes, syringe with needle, vial or ampule of medication, bandage strip(s), sharps container, patient chart.

Notes to the Student:

_____

_____

_____

_____

_____

_____

Skills Assessment Requirements

Read and familiarize yourself with the procedure; complete the minimum practice requirements. Document each MPR using proper charting technique. Complete each procedure within a reasonable amount of time, with a minimum of 85% accuracy.

POINT VALUE ✦ = 3-6 points * = 7-9 points		PRACTICE TRIAL	GRADED TRIAL # 1	GRADED TRIAL # 2	NOTES:
1. ✦	Wash your hands and gather the equipment.				
2. *	Check to make sure the medication matches the physician's order. Calculate dosage if necessary. Look up information relating to the function of the medication, usual dosage, and side effects.				
3. ✦	Check the medication label again against the physician's order to make sure it is the right medication.				
4. *	Identify the patient and escort to treatment area.				
5. ✦	Select the subcutaneous site Put on gloves. Loosen the cap of the needle so that you can drop it on the counter just before you withdraw medication from the ampule or vial. Cleanse the skin site with an alcohol wipe and allow it to thoroughly air-dry.				
6. ✦	Withdraw the correct amount of medication. If necessary, cover the needle by the slide cap method. Otherwise, if the patient is nearby, do not recap the needle.				
7. ✦	Check a third time to match the medication against the physician's order.				
8. ✦	If you have any doubts, consult the physician immediately before administering the medication.				

		PRACTICE TRIAL	GRADED TRIAL # 1	GRADED TRIAL # 2	NOTES:
9. ✦	Lightly stretch the skin immediately surrounding the injection site with your nondominant hand.				
10. ⋆	Quickly insert the needle at a 45-degree angle. Hold the barrel of the syringe with your nondominant hand and pull (aspirate) the plunger with your dominant hand. If no blood appears in the syringe barrel, move your nondominant hand to the skin position and hold the syringe with your dominant hand. Push the plunger down with your index finger.				
11. ✦	Withdraw the needle and blot the area gently with an alcohol wipe. Discard the syringe into the sharps container. Apply a bandage strip to protect the patient's clothing.				
12. ✦	Remove the gloves and wash your hands.				
13. ⋆	Document the procedure. Include the date, time, medication, site, route, and amount administered. Follow office policy for recording the medication expiration date and lot number.				

Name: _____

Date: _____

Document: Enter the appropriate information in the chart below.

Grading

Points Earned	_____		
Points Possible	_____	90	90
Percent Grade (Points Earned/ Points Possible)	_____		
PASS:	_____	❏ YES ❏ NO ❏ N/A	❏ YES ❏ NO ❏ N/A

Instructor Sign-Off

Instructor: _____ **Date:** _____

Procedure 9-8

Demonstrate the Administration of a Intramuscular Injection to Adults and Children

Objective: The student, using the supplies and equipment listed below, will demonstrate correctly administering an intramuscular injection to an adult or child.

Supplies: gloves, alcohol wipes, syringe with needle, vial or ampule of medication, bandage strips, sharps container, patient chart.

Notes to the Student:

_____

_____

_____

_____

_____

_____

Skills Assessment Requirements

Read and familiarize yourself with the procedure; complete the minimum practice requirements. Document each MPR using proper charting technique. Complete each procedure within a reasonable amount of time, with a minimum of 85% accuracy.

POINT VALUE ✦ = 3-6 points ⋆ = 7-9 points		PRACTICE TRIAL	GRADED TRIAL #1	GRADED TRIAL #2	NOTES:
1. ✦	Wash your hands and gather the equipment.				
2. ⋆	Check to make sure the medication matches the physician's order. Calculate dosage if necessary. Look up information relating to the function of the medication, usual dosage, and side effects.				
3. ✦	Check the medication label again against the physician's order to make sure it is the right medication.				
4. ⋆	Identify the patient and escort to treatment area. Ask parents to identify the child patient.				
5. ✦	Select the intramuscular site. Put on gloves. Loosen the cap of the needle so that you can drop it on the counter just before you withdraw medication from the ampule or vial. Cleanse the skin site with an alcohol wipe and allow it to thoroughly air-dry.				
6. ✦	Follow the procedure for withdrawing medication from a vial or ampule. Withdraw the correct amount. If necessary, cover the needle by the slide cap method. Otherwise, do not recap the needle.				

		PRACTICE TRIAL	GRADED TRIAL #1	GRADED TRIAL #2	NOTES:
7. ✦	Check a third time to match the medication against the physician's order.				
8. ✦	If you have any doubts, consult the physician immediately before administering the medication.				
9. ✦	Grasp the skin immediately surrounding the injection site with your nondominant hand. For a small child, ask another clinical staff person to hold the child, then grasp the upper outer quadrant area of the vastus lateralis muscle.				
10. ★	Quickly but lightly thrust the needle at a 90-degree (perpendicular) angle. Hold the barrel of the syringe with your nondominant hand and with your dominant hand pull (aspirate) the plunger. If no blood appears in the syringe barrel, move your nondominant hand to the skin position and hold the syringe with your dominant hand. Push the plunger down with your index finger.				

	PRACTICE TRIAL	GRADED TRIAL # 1	GRADED TRIAL # 2	NOTES:
11. ✦ Withdraw the needle and apply pressure with an alcohol wipe. Massage the muscle unless contraindicated. Discard the syringe into the sharps container. Apply a bandage strip to protect the patient's clothing.				
12. ✦ Remove the gloves and wash your hands.				
13. ✶ Document the procedure. Include the date, time, medication, site, route, and amount administered. Follow office policy for recording the medication expiration date and lot number.				

Name: _____

Date: _____

Document: Enter the appropriate information in the chart below.

Grading

Points Earned	_____		
Points Possible	_____	90	90
Percent Grade (Points Earned/ Points Possible)	_____		
PASS:	_____	❏ YES ❏ NO ❏ N/A	❏ YES ❏ NO ❏ N/A

Instructor Sign-Off

Instructor: _____ Date: _____

Procedure 9-9

Demonstrate the Administration of a Z-Track Injection

Objective: The student, using the supplies and equipment listed below, will demonstrate correctly how to administer a Z-track injection.

Supplies: gloves, alcohol wipes, tuberculin syringe with needle, vial of medication, bandage strips, sharps container, patient chart.

Notes to the Student:

_____

_____

_____

_____

_____

_____

Skills Assessment Requirements

Read and familiarize yourself with the procedure; complete the minimum practice requirements. Document each MPR using proper charting technique. Complete each procedure within a reasonable amount of time, with a minimum of 85% accuracy.

POINT VALUE ✦ = 3-6 points ⋆ = 7-9 points		PRACTICE TRIAL	GRADED TRIAL # 1	GRADED TRIAL # 2	NOTES:
1. ✦	Wash your hands and gather the equipment.				
2. ⋆	Identify the patient and escort to the treatment area.				
3. ✦	Select the appropriate intramuscular site. Put on the gloves.				
4. ✦	Cleanse the skin with an alcohol wipe and allow to thoroughly air-dry.				
5. ✦	Cleanse the top of the medication vial with an alcohol wipe and allow to air-dry. Withdraw the correct dosage from the vial and hold the syringe in your dominant hand.				
6. ✦	With your nondominant hand, pull the skin laterally toward the side opposite the site.				
7. ⋆	Quickly but lightly thrust the needle into the site at a 90-degree (perpendicular) angle. While still holding the skin away from the needle site, inject the medication and wait for 10 seconds.				

		PRACTICE TRIAL	GRADED TRIAL # 1	GRADED TRIAL # 2	NOTES:
8. ★	After 10 seconds, quickly withdraw the needle and allow the skin to track back over the original injection site.				
9. ✦	Blot the area gently with an alcohol wipe. Discard the syringe into the sharps container. Apply a bandage strip to protect the patient's clothing.				
10. ★	Do not massage the injection site. Document the procedure. Include the date, time, medication, site, route, and amount administered. Follow office policy for recording the medication expiration date and lot number.				

Document: Enter the appropriate information in the chart below.

Grading

Points Earned	_____		
Points Possible	_____	72	72
Percent Grade (Points Earned/ Points Possible)	_____		
PASS:	_____	❏ YES ❏ NO ❏ N/A	❏ YES ❏ NO ❏ N/A

Instructor Sign-Off

Instructor: _____ Date: _____

CHAPTER 10
Vital Signs

CHAPTER OUTLINE

Review the Chapter Outline. If any content area is unclear, review that area before beginning workbook exercises.

    A. The Medical Assistant's Role in the Initial Clinical Visit

    B. Vital Signs

    C. Preparing the Patient for a Physical Examination

    D. Assessment Methods Used in an Examination

CHAPTER REVIEW

The following is a summary of the chapter. If any of this material is unclear, review it in the textbook.

Numerous times a day the medical assistant measures height, weight, and vital signs as well as maintains the exam room, prepares patients for exams, and assists the physician during those examinations. The results of the four vital signs along with height and weight can give the provider a large amount of information to help with diagnosis and treatment. Each measurement can indicate a variety of conditions when it is higher or lower than the normal ranges appropriate for the age of the patient. Preparation of the room, equipment, instruments, and supplies in advance of a patient's clinical visit should all be anticipated by the MA. The patient must be prepared and assisted as necessary, measurements taken, a history and reason for the visit taken, and all is charted. While assisting the physician during the physical exam, the medical assistant may play an active role, passing instruments and positioning the patient, or the MA may simply be in the exam room as a chaperone. For each clinical visit, the efficient MA anticipates the needs of the patient and the physician.

LEARNING ACTIVITIES AND STUDY AIDS

Review the following study aids and/or complete the activities to ensure that you have achieved the learning objectives for this chapter.

1. Explain the principles of vital signs and state normal values for various age groups.

    _____

    _____

    _____

    _____

    _____

    _____

2. Most patients come in for recurrent clinic visits. State the things the medical assistant would do in these types of visits.

_____

_____

_____

_____

_____

_____

_____

3. Body temperature, as the other vital signs, may change from normal, and this can indicate various things about the patient. Discuss the significance of these changes in temperature. Some variations may be acceptable—such as those due to age—some may not. Cover them all, including elevated and lowered.

_____

_____

_____

_____

_____

_____

_____

4. State what the pulse rate is then list what factors affect pulse rates. This is addressed in the text and in Table 10-4. What does the term *systole* represent?

_____

_____

_____

_____

_____

_____

_____

5. In your own words, state the significance of the respiratory rate in patient assessment. What are the three things that should be assessed when measuring respirations?

_____

_____

_____

_____

_____

6. What is the role of the blood pressure measurement in patient assessment? What is *diastole*? (You have stated systole's meaning in question 4.)

_____

_____

_____

_____

_____

_____

_____

7. What does the weight and height of a patient state about his or her health status? Is there one normal value for patients based on age as in the vital signs?

_____

_____

_____

_____

_____

_____

_____

_____

8. During an examination of the patient, there are various methods of assessment. List them and briefly describe what is performed by the examiner.

_____

_____

_____

_____

_____

_____

9. Review Procedure 10-12 regarding the medical assistant's tasks in assisting the physician during the physical examination. Discuss how the MA helps, including patient preparation, gowning, positioning, and draping. List the various positions.

_____

_____

_____

_____

_____

MEDICAL TERMINOLOGY REVIEW

Use a dictionary and highlighted terms in the textbook to define the following terms.

Terms

accommodation _____

_____

apical _____

_____

aural _____

_____

auscultation _____

_____

axillary _____

_____

blood pressure _____

_____

conduction _____

_____

convection _____

_____

diaphoresis _____

_____

diastolic _____

_____

hypertension _____

_____

hypotension _____

_____

inspection _____

_____

malignant hypertension _____

_____

mensuration _____

_____

oral _____

_____

palpation _____

_____

percussion _____

_____

radial _____

_____

rhythm _____

_____

sublingually _____

_____

systolic _____

_____

temperature _____

_____

turgor _____

_____

Abbreviations

BPM _____

_____

CV _____

_____

TPR _____

_____

CRITICAL THINKING

1. During a patient clinical visit, whether for a physical or other reason, the MA does some inspection assessment of the patient. Think of what may be visible about the patient that the MA may note.

_____

_____

_____

2. If a patient walks in without an appointment and presents as extremely short of breath (SOB) and appears weak, do you think that you should spend the time doing weight, height, and all the vitals before alerting the doctor of the patient's immediate condition?

_____

_____

_____

3. If a patient is not able to be in the knee-chest position due to a physical reason such as a back problem or is too elderly, etc., what alternative position would work for a rectal examination?

_____

_____

_____

_____

4. A 9-year-old child comes into the office with a temperature of 99.0°F orally, a pulse of 116, respiration of 24, and blood pressure of 112/58. Circle the vitals that are out of normal range. In those that do not have a range stated in the textbook, look on the Internet or in another textbook and list all vital normal ranges on an index card. State briefly in your own words why two people can have different vital sign measurements and still both will be considered normal.

_____

_____

_____

_____

5. You are assisting a physician with a physical exam, you have prepared all the supplies and have any equipment ready. The patient is a female and will be having a pelvic exam with the physical exam. Although the physician does not need you to assist him, you are expected to be present with the doctor anyway. State why the MA would be present in this situation. Would the same be true if the patient were a male? Would the same be true if the doctor was a female and the patient were a male?

_____

_____

_____

_____

CHAPTER REVIEW TEST

MULTIPLE CHOICE

Circle the letter of the correct answer.

1. Draping a patient during an examination provides all of the following except:
   a. warmth.
   b. comfort.
   c. position.
   d. modesty.

2. The average pulse rate for elderly adults is
   a. 80–120 bpm.
   b. 80–90 bpm.
   c. 110–130 bpm.
   d. 50–70 bpm

3. Before taking a temperature, you should ask the patient two things. Circle the two correct answers.
   a. Has he or she smoked before coming into the office?
   b. Has he or she had any hot or cold liquids immediately before coming into the office?
   c. What is his or her usual temperature?
   d. Which thermometer would he or she prefer to be used?

4. Which of the following factors can influence a patient's body temperature? (circle all that apply)
   a. pregnancy
   b. emotions
   c. increased food intake
   d. physical activity

5. An instrument used to more thoroughly assess hearing than a tuning fork is:
   a. audiostomer.
   b. audiomanometer.
   c. audiometer.
   d. otoscope.

6. One of the vital signs can be controlled by the patient, and the MA should make sure the patient doesn't know when it is being measured. This is:
   a. pulse.
   b. respiration.
   c. temperature.
   d. blood pressure.

7. A sphygmomanometer is used for
   a. assessing the sounds of underlying organs.
   b. taking blood pressure.
   c. testing a patient's electrical system of the heart.
   d. taking an apical pulse.

8. The term for exhaling carbon dioxide during respiration is
   a. breathing.
   b. expiration.
   c. exhalation.
   d. inspiration.

9. Choose the two correct names for the parts of the stethoscope that are used against the patient's skin to auscultate.
   a. bell
   b. chestpiece
   c. palpitator
   d. diaphragm

10. Which of the following factors can affect the heart rate and rhythm? (circle all that apply)
    a. physical condition
    b. medications
    c. gender
    d. age

TRUE/FALSE

Indicate whether the statement is true (T) or false (F).

_____ 1. The normal axillary temperature range is 96.6 – 98.6 F.

_____ 2. Mensuration means measurement.

_____ 3. In measuring pulse, you should note the rate, the rhythm, and the volume.

_____ 4. Accommodation means listening to internal body sounds.

_____ 5. Rectal temperature is considered the most accurate measurement of temperature.

_____ 6. Pulse rates in newborns and infants are much slower than adults.

_____ 7. Respiration should be counted without the patient's being aware of it.

_____ 8. A reason for making an error in blood pressure is failing to center the cuff over the brachial artery.

_____ 9. Dehydration can cause a weaker heartbeat.

_____ 10. An apical pulse must taken by using a stethoscope over the apex of the heart.

FILL IN THE BLANK

Using words from the list below, fill in the blanks to complete the following statements. Note: Some terms are used in more than one statements.

assess	medical condition	respirations
auscultates	nares	rhythm
bladder	otoscope	sitting erect
bowel sounds	pelvic exams	speculum
depth	percussion	tuning fork
Fowler's	physical examination	underlying organs
hearing	pulse	volume
lightly but sharply	rate	vision
lithotomy	rectal	visual acuity

1. A _____ temperature is taken only when the patient's _____ dictates it.

2. The three aspects to note when taking _____ are _____, _____, and _____.

3. The three aspects to note when taking a _____ are _____, _____, _____.

4. _____refers to the physician's tapping the fingertips _____ against various areas of the body to _____the size and location of _____.

5. The _____ position is used for _____and Pap smears.

6. Emptying the _____ makes the patient feel more comfortable during the _____.

7. The ears are examined with an _____, usually with a disposable _____; a larger _____ can be attached to the otoscope to examine the _____.

8. When the physician _____ the abdomen, he or she is listening to _____.

9. The _____ position is when the patient is _____ on the table.

10. The _____ is used to assess _____, and _____ is the assessment of the clarity of a patient's _____.

Procedure 10-1

Perform an Oral Temperature with a Digital Electric Thermometer

Objective: The student, using the supplies and equipment listed below, will demonstrate correctly measuring oral temperature with a digital, electronic thermometer.

Supplies: Electronic digital thermometer, thermometer probe covers, watch with second hand (for pulse and respiration count), examination gloves.

Notes to the Student:

_____

_____

_____

_____

_____

_____

Skills Assessment Requirements

Read and familiarize yourself with the procedure; complete the minimum practice requirements. Document each MPR using proper charting technique. Complete each procedure within a reasonable amount of time, with a minimum of 85% accuracy.

Name: _____

Date: _____

POINT VALUE ✦ = 3-6 points ⋆ = 7-9 points		PRACTICE TRIAL	GRADED TRIAL # 1	GRADED TRIAL # 2	NOTES:
1. ⋆	Identify the patient, escort to the examination room, and offer a place to sit on a chair or the examination table.				
2. ✦	Wash your hands and apply gloves.				
3. ⋆	Ask the patient if he or she has had hot or cold drinks or food or smoked a cigarette within the last 10 minutes. If so, wait 10 minutes. If not, proceed with taking the oral temperature.				
4. ✦	Remove the electronic thermometer from its charge base and place a cover on the probe.				
5. ✦	Place the probe under the tongue near the frenulum linguae. Instruct the patient to close the mouth around the thermometer.				
6. ✦	Explain to the patient that the thermometer will need to stay in place until the beep sounds. You may count pulse and respirations now (see Procedures 7-6 through 7-8) or after the temperature is taken.				

		PRACTICE TRIAL	GRADED TRIAL # 1	GRADED TRIAL # 2	NOTES:
7. ✦	When the beep sounds, remove the thermometer from the patient's mouth, note the temperature, and discard the probe cover in a waste receptacle.				
8. ✦	Remove the gloves and wash your hands. Return the thermometer to its charge base.				
9. ★	Record the temperature in the appropriate place on the chart. Return the thermometer to its designated storage location. This task should be completed within the time limit set by the instructor.				

Document: Enter the appropriate information in the chart below.

Grading

Points Earned	_____		
Points Possible	_____	63	63
Percent Grade (Points Earned/ Points Possible)	_____		
PASS:	_____	❑ YES ❑ NO ❑ N/A	❑ YES ❑ NO ❑ N/A

Instructor Sign-Off

Instructor: _____   **Date:** _____

Procedure 10-2

Perform an Axillary Temperature with a Digital Electric Thermometer

Objective: The student, using the supplies and equipment listed below, will demonstrate accurately measuring an axillary temperature with a digital electronic thermometer.

Supplies: Digital electronic thermometer, thermometer probe cover, watch with second hand (for pulse and respiration count), examination gloves.

Notes to the Student:

_____

_____

_____

_____

_____

_____

Skills Assessment Requirements

Read and familiarize yourself with the procedure; complete the minimum practice requirements. Document each MPR using proper charting technique. Complete each procedure within a reasonable amount of time, with a minimum of 85% accuracy.

POINT VALUE ✦ = 3-6 points ⋆ = 7-9 points		PRACTICE TRIAL	GRADED TRIAL # 1	GRADED TRIAL # 2	NOTES:
1. ⋆	Identify the patient, escort to the examination room, and offer a place to sit on a chair or the examination table. Have the patient either unbutton or take off his or her shirt to allow access to the axilla.				
2. ✦	Wash your hands and apply gloves.				
3. ⋆	Observe the axillary area for dryness or diaphoresis. Pat the area dry with a washcloth or towel if it is diaphoretic.				
4. ✦	Remove the electronic thermometer from its charge base and place a cover on the probe.				
5. ✦	Ask the patient to raise an arm. Place the thermometer in direct contact with the skin of the axilla and have the patient lower the arm against the side of the chest.				
6. ✦	Explain that the thermometer will need to stay in place until the beep sounds. You may count pulse and respirations now or after the temperature is taken.				

	PRACTICE TRIAL	GRADED TRIAL # 1	GRADED TRIAL # 2	NOTES:
7. ✦ When the beep sounds, remove the thermometer and discard the probe cover in a waste receptacle.				
8. ✦ Remove the gloves and wash your hands. Return the thermometer to its charge base.				
9. ＊ Record the temperature (Figure 10-7), pulse, and respirations in the appropriate place on the chart. Write "A" after the temperature to indicate that the axillary route was used.				
10. ✦ Return the thermometer to its designated storage location.				

Document: Enter the appropriate information in the chart below.

Grading

Points Earned	_____		
Points Possible	_____	69	69
Percent Grade (Points Earned/ Points Possible)	_____		
PASS:	_____	❏ YES ❏ NO ❏ N/A	❏ YES ❏ NO ❏ N/A

Instructor Sign-Off

Instructor: _____ **Date:** _____

Procedure 10-3

Perform a Rectal Temperature with a Digital Electric Thermometer

Objective: The student, using the supplies and equipment listed below, will demonstrate accurately measure a rectal temperature with a digital thermometer.

Supplies: Digital electronic thermometer (rectal) and probe covers, lubricant, tissue, examination gloves

Notes to the Student:

_____

_____

_____

_____

_____

_____

Skills Assessment Requirements

Read and familiarize yourself with the procedure; complete the minimum practice requirements. Document each MPR using proper charting technique. Complete each procedure within a reasonable amount of time, with a minimum of 85% accuracy.

POINT VALUE ✦ = 3-6 points ⋆ = 7-9 points		PRACTICE TRIAL	GRADED TRIAL #1	GRADED TRIAL #2	NOTES:
1. ⋆	Identify the patient and escort to the examination room. Assist the patient in removing clothing from the waist down. Keeping the patient draped, assist him or her into a left side-lying position (Sim's position) on the examination table. Drape for exposure of the buttocks only.				
2. ✦	Wash your hands and apply gloves.				
3. ✦	Remove the electronic thermometer from its charge base and place a cover on the probe.				
4. ✦	Place a small amount of lubricant on a tissue next to the patient. Dip the tip of the probe cover in the lubricant.				
5. ⋆	Inform the patient of procedure before you insert the rectal probe. For an adult, insert the lubricated probe cover approximately 1 1/2 inches into the anus. For an infant, insert it 1/4 to 1/2 inch, and for a child, 1/2 to 1 inch.				
6. ✦	Hold the thermometer in place until it beeps. Remove the thermometer and discard the probe cover in a waste receptacle.				

		PRACTICE TRIAL	GRADED TRIAL # 1	GRADED TRIAL # 2	NOTES:
7. ✦	Remove the gloves and wash your hands. Return the thermometer to its charge base.				
8. ⋆	Record the temperature in the appropriate place on the chart. Write an "R" after the measurement to indicate the rectal route.				
9. ✦	Return the thermometer to its designated storage location.				

Document: Enter the appropriate information in the chart below.

Grading

Points Earned	_____		
Points Possible	_____	63	63
Percent Grade (Points Earned/ Points Possible)	_____		
PASS:	_____	❏ YES ❏ NO ❏ N/A	❏ YES ❏ NO ❏ N/A

Instructor Sign-Off

Instructor: _____ **Date:** _____

Procedure 10-4

Perform a Aural Temperature with a Tympanic Electric Thermometer

Objective: The student, using the supplies and equipment listed below, will demonstrate accurately taking an aural temperature according to the patient's age.

Supplies: Tympanic thermometer and probe covers and examination gloves

Notes to the Student:

_____

_____

_____

_____

_____

_____

Skills Assessment Requirements

Read and familiarize yourself with the procedure; complete the minimum practice requirements. Document each MPR using proper charting technique. Complete each procedure within a reasonable amount of time, with a minimum of 85% accuracy.

POINT VALUE ✦ = 3-6 points ⋆ = 7-9 points		PRACTICE TRIAL	GRADED TRIAL # 1	GRADED TRIAL # 2	NOTES:
1. ⋆	Identify the patient, escort to the examination room, and offer a place to sit on a chair or the examination table. If the patient is a child, encourage the parent to sit and hold the child.				
2. ✦	Wash your hands and apply gloves.				
3. ✦	Explain the basic procedure to the patient or parent. Assess whether the patient has had an aural temperature before. Depending on the patient's age and previous experience or knowledge of the procedure, you may need to assure him or her that the procedure is painless or demonstrate on the parent before taking a child's temperature.				
4. ✦	Remove the tympanic thermometer from its charge base and place a cover on the probe.				
5. ⋆	For an adult, pull the outer ear in an upward direction. For a child or infant, pull the outer ear in a downward direction.				
6. ✦	With your hand insert the probe-covered earpiece of the thermometer into the ear canal and press the scan button to obtain the temperature reading.				

	PRACTICE TRIAL	GRADED TRIAL # 1	GRADED TRIAL # 2	NOTES:
7. ✦ When the thermometer beeps, withdraw it from the patient's ear and pop the probe cover into the waste receptacle. Read the temperature reading in the thermometer's display window.				
8. ✦ Remove the gloves and wash your hands. Return the thermometer to its charge base.				
9. ＊ Record the temperature on the patient's chart, followed by a "T" to indicate tympanic temperature.				
10. ✦ Return the tympanic thermometer to its designated storage location.				

Document: Enter the appropriate information in the chart below.

Grading

Points Earned	_____		
Points Possible	_____	69	69
Percent Grade (Points Earned/ Points Possible)	_____		
PASS:	_____	❏ YES ❏ NO ❏ N/A	❏ YES ❏ NO ❏ N/A

Instructor Sign-Off

Instructor: _____ **Date:** _____

Procedure 10-5

Perform a Dermal Temperature with a Disposable Thermometer

Objective: The student, using the supplies and equipment listed below, will demonstrate accurately measuring a dermal temperature with a disposable thermometer.

Supplies: Disposable dermal strips; clean, dry washcloth; examination gloves

Notes to the Student:

_____

_____

_____

_____

_____

_____

Skills Assessment Requirements

Read and familiarize yourself with the procedure; complete the minimum practice requirements. Document each MPR using proper charting technique. Complete each procedure within a reasonable amount of time, with a minimum of 85% accuracy.

Name: _____

Date: _____

POINT VALUE ✦ = 3-6 points ⋆ = 7-9 points		PRACTICE TRIAL	GRADED TRIAL # 1	GRADED TRIAL # 2	NOTES:
1. ⋆	Identify the patient, escort to the examination room, and offer a place to sit on a chair or the examination table.				
2. ✦	Wash your hands and apply gloves.				
3. ✦	Observe the forehead for dryness or diaphoresis. Pat the area dry with a washcloth if it is diaphoretic.				
4. ✦	Carefully unwrap the dermal strip without touching the chemical dots and place it on the forehead.				
5. ⋆	Leave the strip on the forehead for the length of time recommended by the manufacturer, usually about 15 seconds.				
6. ✦	After noting the temperature of the last color-changed dot, remove and dispose of the dermal thermometer in a waste receptacle.				
7. ✦	Remove the gloves and wash your hands.				
8. ⋆	Record the temperature on the patient's chart, followed by the word "dermal." This task must be completed within the time limit set by the instructor.				

Name: _____

Date: _____

Document: Enter the appropriate information in the chart below.

Grading

Points Earned	_____		
Points Possible	_____	57	57
Percent Grade (Points Earned/ Points Possible)	_____		
PASS:	_____	❏ YES ❏ NO ❏ N/A	❏ YES ❏ NO ❏ N/A

Instructor Sign-Off

Instructor: _____ Date: _____

Procedure 10-6

Perform a Radial Pulse Count

Objective: The student, using the supplies and equipment listed below, will demonstrate accurately measuring a radial pulse.

Supplies: Watch with second hand.

Notes to the Student:

_____

_____

_____

_____

_____

_____

Skills Assessment Requirements

Read and familiarize yourself with the procedure; complete the minimum practice requirements. Document each MPR using proper charting technique. Complete each procedure within a reasonable amount of time, with a minimum of 85% accuracy.

Name: _____

Date: _____

POINT VALUE ✦ = 3-6 points * = 7-9 points		PRACTICE TRIAL	GRADED TRIAL # 1	GRADED TRIAL # 2	NOTES:
1. *	The patient has been identified, escorted to the examination room, and offered a place to sit on a chair or the examination table.				
2. ✦	Wash your hands (unless you have already done so prior to taking the temperature).				
3. ✦	Explain the procedure to the patient (unless you have already done so prior to taking the temperature). Do not mention that you will be counting respirations after taking the pulse.				
4. ✦	Position the patient's arm at about heart level, with the palm facing down. Identify the radial artery with the three middle fingertips by feeling pulsation through the arterial wall.				
5. ✦	Palpate for the pulsation of the radial artery on the inside of the wrist below the thumb. Note the strength and rhythm of the pulse. Do not palpate the pulse with your thumb.				

		PRACTICE TRIAL	GRADED TRIAL # 1	GRADED TRIAL # 2	NOTES:
6. ★	Looking at your watch, start counting the pulse beats when the second hand is at 3, 6, 9, or 12. Count for one full minute. While still holding the wrist, observe the patient's respiratory efforts and count as instructed in Procedure 10-8.				
7. ★	Document the rate, strength, and rhythm of the pulse on the chart.				
8. ✦	Wash your hands.				

Name: _____

Date: _____

Document: Enter the appropriate information in the chart below.

Grading

Points Earned	_____		
Points Possible	_____	57	57
Percent Grade (Points Earned/ Points Possible)	_____		
PASS:	_____	❑ YES ❑ NO ❑ N/A	❑ YES ❑ NO ❑ N/A

Instructor Sign-Off

Instructor: _____ Date: _____

Procedure 10-7

Perform an Apical Pulse Count

Objective: The student, using the supplies and equipment listed below, will demonstrate accurately performing an apical pulse count.

Supplies: Stethoscope, alcohol prep, watch with a second hand.

Notes to the Student:

_____

_____

_____

_____

_____

_____

Skills Assessment Requirements

Read and familiarize yourself with the procedure; complete the minimum practice requirements. Document each MPR using proper charting technique. Complete each procedure within a reasonable amount of time, with a minimum of 85% accuracy.

POINT VALUE ✦ = 3-6 points ⋆ = 7-9 points	PRACTICE TRIAL	GRADED TRIAL # 1	GRADED TRIAL # 2	NOTES:
1. ⋆ The patient has already been identified, and you have washed your hands to obtain vital signs.				
2. ✦ Explain the procedure to the patient. Do not mention that you will be counting respirations after you have noted the apical pulse.				
3. ✦ Wipe the stethoscope earpieces with the alcohol prep. With the earpieces pointed toward the nose, place the stethoscope earpieces in your ears. Place the bell or diaphragm on the patient's chest in the area of the apex of the heart.				
4. ✦ Begin counting heartbeats (each "lub-dub" counts as one heartbeat) when the second hand of the watch is at 3, 6, 9, or 12.				
5. ✦ Count for one full minute. Note the quality and regularity of the heartbeat.				
6. ⋆ Chart the rate, rhythm, and any other pertinent information. If the radial pulse is also documented, write "RP" before the radial pulse rate and "AP" before the apical pulse rate. This task must be complete within the time limit specified by the instructor.				

Name: _____

Date: _____

Document: Enter the appropriate information in the chart below.

Grading

Points Earned	_____		
Points Possible	_____	42	42
Percent Grade (Points Earned/ Points Possible)	_____		
PASS:	_____	❏ YES ❏ NO ❏ N/A	❏ YES ❏ NO ❏ N/A

Instructor Sign-Off

Instructor: _____ Date: _____

Procedure 10-8

Perform a Respiration Count

Objective: The student, using the supplies and equipment listed below, will demonstrate accurately performing a respiratory count without the patient being aware that the MA is doing this count.

Supplies: Watch with second hand.

Notes to the Student:

_____

_____

_____

_____

_____

_____

Skills Assessment Requirements

Read and familiarize yourself with the procedure; complete the minimum practice requirements. Document each MPR using proper charting technique. Complete each procedure within a reasonable amount of time, with a minimum of 85% accuracy.

POINT VALUE ✦ = 3-6 points ⋆ = 7-9 points		PRACTICE TRIAL	GRADED TRIAL # 1	GRADED TRIAL # 2	NOTES:
1. ⋆	This procedure is a continuation of the radial or apical pulse count. The patient has been identified and you have washed your hands.				
2. ✦	After counting the radial or apical pulse and mentally noting the rate, continue holding the patient's wrist or holding the stethoscope chestpiece in place.				
3. ✦	Watch the patient's chest rise (inspiration) and fall (expiration) and count the respiratory cycles for 30 seconds. Observe the regularity and depth of the respirations. Make a mental note of the respiratory rate				
4. ⋆	Multiply the 30-second count by two and record that figure as the respiratory rate. Record the pulse as well. Add any appropriate comments about the regularity or depth of the respirations on the chart. This task must be completed within the time limit specified by the instructor.				

Name: _____

Date: _____

Document: Enter the appropriate information in the chart below.

Grading

Points Earned	_____		
Points Possible	_____	30	30
Percent Grade (Points Earned/ Points Possible)	_____		
PASS:	_____	❏ YES ❏ NO ❏ N/A	❏ YES ❏ NO ❏ N/A

Instructor Sign-Off

Instructor: _____ Date: _____

Procedure 10-9

Measure Blood Pressure

Objective: The student, using the supplies and equipment listed below, will demonstrate obtaining an accurate blood pressure reading.

Supplies: Stethoscope, 70% isopropyl alcohol wipes, sphygmomanometer (aneroid or mercury)

Notes to the Student:

_____

_____

_____

_____

_____

_____

Skills Assessment Requirements

Read and familiarize yourself with the procedure; complete the minimum practice requirements. Document each MPR using proper charting technique. Complete each procedure within a reasonable amount of time, with a minimum of 85% accuracy.

POINT VALUE ✦ = 3-6 points ⋆ = 7-9 points		PRACTICE TRIAL	GRADED TRIAL #1	GRADED TRIAL #2	NOTES:
1. ✦	Wash your hands and assemble the equipment. Squeeze the bladder of the sphygmomanometer cuff to make sure it is completely deflated.				
2. ⋆	Identify the patient and escort to a central area or patient examination room. Have the patient sit either on a chair or on the examination table. Explain the procedure to the patient.				
3. ✦	Cleanse the earpieces, diaphragm, and bell of the stethoscope with the alcohol wipes.				
4. ✦	Expose the patient's upper arm and ask the patient to extend the arm with the palm facing upward. You may have to assist the patient in rolling up the sleeve.				
5. ✦	Place the sphygmomanometer cuff around the patient's upper arm and secure it snugly, centering over the brachial artery.				
6. ✦	Palpate the brachial pulse.				
7. ✦	Hold the arm with the attached sphygmomanometer at heart level.				
8. ✦	Place the sphygmomanometer gauge where you can monitor it easily or ask the patient to hold it.				

		PRACTICE TRIAL	GRADED TRIAL # 1	GRADED TRIAL # 2	NOTES:
9. ✦	Place the stethoscope earpieces in your ears. Place the diaphragm of the stethoscope over the location where you felt the brachial pulse. Hold the bell of the stethoscope in place with the thumb of your non-dominant hand while supporting the elbow with your fingers.				
10. ✦	With your dominant hand, close the thumbscrew on the hand bulb by turning it clockwise. Quickly and evenly pump the bulb to inflate the cuff.				
11. ✦	Slowly turn the thumbscrew counterclockwise, releasing air at approximately 2–3 mm per second.				
12. ✶	Listen and mentally note when you hear the first pulsation. Slowly continue to release air until the pulsation sounds cease, and make a mental note of that reading.				
13. ✦	Quickly release the rest of the air, deflating the cuff. Remove the cuff.				
14. ✦	If it is necessary to check the blood pressure reading because of an error in the procedure or an abnormally high or low reading, wait one minute before retaking the blood pressure on the same arm.				

		PRACTICE TRIAL	GRADED TRIAL # 1	GRADED TRIAL # 2	NOTES:
15. ✦	Clean the earpieces and diaphragm with 70% ethyl alcohol. Return the sphygmomanometer and stethoscope to their usual storage place.				
16. ✦	Wash your hands.				
17. ＊	After recording the date and time, document the first pulsation sounds as systolic and the last sounds as diastolic readings. Write the systolic over diastolic readings in fraction format. If the blood pressure was taken with the patient standing or lying down, specify the position in the chart. If the patient asks for the reading and office policy allows it, you may inform the patient of the reading. This task must be completed within the time limit specified by the instructor.				

Name: _____

Date: _____

Document: Enter the appropriate information in the chart below.

Grading

Points Earned	_____		
Points Possible	_____	111	111
Percent Grade (Points Earned/ Points Possible)	_____		
PASS:	_____	❏ YES ❏ NO ❏ N/A	❏ YES ❏ NO ❏ N/A

Instructor Sign-Off

Instructor: _____ Date: _____

Name: _____

Date: _____

Procedure 10-10

Taking Height and Weight Measurements

Objective: The student, using the supplies and equipment listed below, will demonstrate accurately obtaining height and weight measurements.

Supplies: Upright balance scales with height bar, paper towel.

Notes to the Student:

_____

_____

_____

_____

_____

_____

Skills Assessment Requirements

Read and familiarize yourself with the procedure; complete the minimum practice requirements. Document each MPR using proper charting technique. Complete each procedure within a reasonable amount of time, with a minimum of 85% accuracy.

Name: _____

Date: _____

POINT VALUE ✦ = 3-6 points ⋆ = 7-9 points		PRACTICE TRIAL	GRADED TRIAL # 1	GRADED TRIAL # 2	NOTES:
1. ⋆	Identify the patient and escort him or her to the examination room.				
2. ✦	Wash your hands.				
3. ✦	Explain the procedure to the patient. Explain that most personal items may be left in the room, although a female patient may want to take her purse. Escort the patient to the scales.				
4. ⋆	Balance the scales to read zero.				
5. ✦	Instruct the patient to step on the scales. You may need to place a paper towel on the scale for patients who wish to remove their shoes. Assist the patient onto the scales and provide support as needed.				
6. ✦	Instruct the patient to stand still. Move the weights until the scale balances.				
7. ⋆	Note the weight and return the balance weights to zero.				
8. ✦	Ask the patient to step off the scales, assisting as necessary.				
9. ✦	Help the patient to step on the scales backwards so that his or her back is against the scale. Ask the patient to stand erect, eyes looking ahead.				

		PRACTICE TRIAL	GRADED TRIAL # 1	GRADED TRIAL # 2	NOTES:
10. ★	Raise the height bar in a collapsed position above the patient's head. Extend the bar and slowly bring it down until it touches the top of the patient's head. Note the height.				
11. ◆	Raise the entire height bar up over the patient's head, collapse it, and return it to its original position.				
12. ◆	Ask the patient to step off the scales, assisting as necessary.				
13. ★	Record the height and weight on the patient's chart.				

Name: _____

Date: _____

Document: Enter the appropriate information in the chart below.

Grading

Points Earned	_____		
Points Possible	_____	93	93
Percent Grade (Points Earned/ Points Possible)	_____		
PASS:	_____	❏ YES ❏ NO ❏ N/A	❏ YES ❏ NO ❏ N/A

Instructor Sign-Off

Instructor: _____ **Date:** _____

Name: _____

Date: _____

Procedure 10-11

Demonstrate Patient Positions Used in a Medical Examination

Objective: The student, using the supplies and equipment listed below, will demonstrate correctly assisting the patient into the sitting, supine, Sims', prone, dorsal recumbent, and lithotomy positions.

Supplies: Patient gown, pants, and drapes; examination table paper

Notes to the Student:

_____

_____

_____

_____

_____

_____

Skills Assessment Requirements

Read and familiarize yourself with the procedure; complete the minimum practice requirements. Document each MPR using proper charting technique. Complete each procedure within a reasonable amount of time, with a minimum of 85% accuracy.

Name: _____

Date: _____

		PRACTICE TRIAL	GRADED TRIAL #1	GRADED TRIAL #2	NOTES:
POINT VALUE ✦ = 3-6 points ⋆ = 7-9 points					
1. ⋆	Identify the patient and escort him or her to the examination room.				
2. ✦	Wash your hands.				
3. ✦	Explain the procedure to the patient. Ask the patient to completely undress and to put on a patient gown. For a breast examination, instruct the patient to tie the gown in the front.				
4. ✦	Instruct the patient to sit on the examination table, assisting as necessary. Cover the patient with the drape.				
5. ✦	Assist the patient into the supine position.				
6. ✦	Assist the patient into the Sim's position.				
7. ✦	Assist the patient into the prone position.				
8. ✦	Assist the patient back into the supine position, then into the dorsal recumbent position.				
9. ✦	Assist the patient into the lithotomy position.				

		PRACTICE TRIAL	GRADED TRIAL #1	GRADED TRIAL #2	NOTES:
10. ✦	Assist the patient in returning to the sitting position and stepping off the examination table.				
11. ✶	After the examination has been completed and the physician has discussed the procedure with the patient, clean the examination room. Remove the used paper from the examination table and replace it with clean paper for the next patient.				
12. ✶	Wash your hands and complete documentation in the patient's chart.				

Name: _____

Date: _____

Document: Enter the appropriate information in the chart below.

Grading

Points Earned	_____		
Points Possible	_____	93	93
Percent Grade (Points Earned/Points Possible)	_____		
PASS:	_____	❏ YES ❏ NO ❏ N/A	❏ YES ❏ NO ❏ N/A

Instructor Sign-Off

Instructor: _____ Date: _____

Procedure 10-12

Assisting the Physician with the Physical Examination

Objective: The student, using the supplies and equipment listed below, will demonstrate correctly assisting the physician with the physical examination.

Supplies: Examination table with clean covering (sheet) and stirrups if pelvic examination is to be performed, patient gown and appropriate drapes, pillow with disposable cover, scales with height rod, Snellen chart and color vision charts, disposable gloves, lubricant and tissues, emesis basin, alcohol swabs, laryngeal mirror, nasal and ear speculums, ophthalmoscope and otoscope, pen light, reflex hammer, sphygmomanometer and stethoscope, tape measure, thermometer, tongue depressors, tuning fork, urine specimen container, gooseneck lamp.

Notes to the Student:

_____

_____

_____

_____

_____

_____

Skills Assessment Requirements

Read and familiarize yourself with the procedure; complete the minimum practice requirements. Document each MPR using proper charting technique. Complete each procedure within a reasonable amount of time, with a minimum of 85% accuracy.

Name: _____

Date: _____

POINT VALUE ✦ = 3-6 points ⋆ = 7-9 points		PRACTICE TRIAL	GRADED TRIAL #1	GRADED TRIAL #2	NOTES:
1. ⋆	Equip each examination room with the necessary supplies, equipment and instruments. Ensure that instruments are in working order and the room temperature is comfortable.				
2. ⋆	Identify the patient and escort him or her to the examination room.				
3. ✦	Wash your hands.				
4. ✦	Obtain the patient's weight and height, usually in a semiprivate but central location in the clinical area				
5. ✦	Obtain vital signs and pain assessment.				
6. ✦	Instruct the patient to remove necessary clothing and to put on the gown or cover. Offer to assist the patient if necessary and explain where to place removed clothing.				
7. ✦	Instruct the patient to sit on the examination table and provide a drape.				
8. ✦	Obtain the patient history through interview and review of the complete forms.				
9. ✦	Gather the instruments the physician will need.				
10. ✦	Notify the physician that the patient is ready.				

		PRACTICE TRIAL	GRADED TRIAL # 1	GRADED TRIAL # 2	NOTES:
11. ★	When the physician is ready, assist with positioning the patient and the physical examination. Be prepared to gather additional supplies and assist the physician with any instruments or supplies necessary for the examination.				
12. ✦	Upon completion of the examination, assist the patient from the examination table.				
13. ★	Prepare specimens for examination and/or transport by labeling and completing appropriate forms.				
14. ✦	Remove soiled instruments and equipment to the dirty utility room for cleaning				
15. ✦	Clean the room and dispose of any waste. Wash your hands.				
16. ✦	Prepare the room for the next patient.				

Document: Enter the appropriate information in the chart below.

Grading

Points Earned	_____		
Points Possible	_____	108	108
Percent Grade (Points Earned/ Points Possible)	_____		
PASS:	_____	❑ YES ❑ NO ❑ N/A	❑ YES ❑ NO ❑ N/A

Instructor Sign-Off

Instructor: _____ Date: _____

CHAPTER 11
Minor Surgery

CHAPTER OUTLINE

Review the Chapter Outline. If any content area is unclear, review that area before beginning workbook exercises.

A. The Medical Assistant's Role in Office Surgery

B. Surgeries Performed in the Medical Office

C. Implied and Informed Consent

D. Preoperative Care and Patient Preparation

E. Assisting During Minor Surgery

F. Recovery/Postoperative Care

CHAPTER REVIEW

The following is a summary of the chapter. If any of this material is unclear, review it in the textbook.

The medical assistant has many responsibilities in minor surgery, from scheduling the procedure, obtaining insurance precertification, preparing the room and instruments (preoperative care) and assisting with the procedure (intraoperative care) to instructing and dismissing the patient (postoperative care). The role of the MA can be either as the scrub assistant or as the circulating assistant in a wide variety of procedures that can be performed in the medical office setting, such as biopsy, incision and drainage, and suturing a laceration or other type of wound. All surgeries require informed consent to be given by the patient, and the medical assistant usually signs the form as the witness. The medical assistant must follow strict sterile techniques, know the various instruments used along with their functions, and the appropriate dressings to use and the phases of wound healing. Following the postoperative recovery, patient instruction, and dismissal of the patient, the MA must accurately and thoroughly document his or her part of the procedure.

LEARNING ACTIVITIES AND STUDY AIDS

Review the following study aids and/or complete the activities to ensure that you have achieved the learning objectives for this chapter.

1. In minor surgery performed in the office, the MA may perform either scrub or circulating assistant duties during the procedure. Describe what these two roles involve for that medical assistant in the surgery room. Then list five examples of the MA's varied duties during the pre-, intra-, and postoperative periods of patient care.

_____

_____

_____

_____

_____

_____

_____

_____

2. From your reading you have learned about various minor surgery procedures. After reviewing the chapter's section on types of surgeries performed in the medical office, list those surgeries that are discussed in the bulleted list, even though there are many more listed in Table 11-1: Simple Surgical Procedures That May Be Performed in a Medical Office or Surgical Clinic. Then, think of procedures and surgeries you know about either from personal experience, TV shows, the news, or elsewhere. List five of those you know of—briefly state the name and purpose of each one.

_____

_____

_____

_____

_____

_____

_____

3. Give an example of implied consent. State the elements included on an informed consent form.

_____

_____

_____

_____

_____

_____

_____

4. Preoperative patient care could start a week or more before the actual procedure. Review the related section of the chapter and notice the short bulleted list at the beginning. Study this list, then close your book and list the four items from memory. Do not include any "day-of" preparation of the room and instruments, as that is addressed in question 5.

_____

_____

_____

_____

_____

_____

5. You are starting your day in the clinic, and after checking the day's schedule at about 8:30 A.M., you see that an I & D is scheduled at 11:00 A.M. In your own words, describe in one paragraph the

duties or tasks involved when setting up the room. Do not include things that are preoperative *patient care* as discussed in question 4.

_____

_____

_____

_____

_____

_____

_____

6. List the functions of surgical instruments which determine their classification. Include one example of an instrument with each function.

_____

_____

_____

_____

_____

_____

_____

7. Various patient positions for exams were presented in Chapter 10. Surgical patients must be positioned as well depending on the procedure to be performed, most often using those same positions. Draping for an exam and for a surgical procedure are done for different reasons, and the drapes are positioned differently. Explain in your own words the draping principles for minor surgery.

_____

_____

_____

_____

_____

_____

8. List the three methods of local anesthesia used during surgery in the medical office. Create a table similar to that in your chapter of the three types but now separate the information into the following columns: Method, example medication names, strength of example meds (if any), any notations about medications.

9. A minor surgery performed in the office usually requires at least one assistant for the physician doing the procedure. Summarize in a paragraph the tasks required for the MA from the explanation in the textbook.

_____

_____

_____

_____

_____

_____

_____

10. Some average suture sizes are stated in your chapter. Which size is thicker: 6-0 or 2-0? What is one reason for using 10-0 or 11-0? Where are absorbable sutures used?

_____

_____

_____

_____

_____

_____

_____

11. The recovery time following a minor surgical procedure is much shorter than for a major operation as an inpatient but is no less important. The postoperative care for a patient in the office falls into two basic categories depending on whether the patient received local anesthesia or general anesthesia. State the postoperative care during recovery for a minor procedure and that for a general anesthesia patient.

_____

_____

_____

_____

_____

_____

12. What instructions during patient teaching would you give to a minor surgery postoperative patient? Relate what is involved in the discharge of a post-op patient.

_____

_____

_____

_____

_____

13. List the three phases of healing that a wound goes through and describe what happens during each phase.

_____

_____

_____

_____

_____

_____

_____

14. There are many, many types of dressings and bandages used in medical office surgical procedures. On the Internet, search for "dressings and bandages," "medical supplies," or "surgical supplies." Try to find a site from a medical supply source/store that offers a number of various dressings. Make a list of five dressings and state a use or unique feature for each.

_____

_____

_____

_____

_____

_____

_____

_____

MEDICAL TERMINOLOGY REVIEW

Use a dictionary and highlighted terms in the textbook to define the following terms.

Terms

abrasion _____

_____

anesthesia _____

_____

approximation _____

_____

avulsion _____

_____

biopsy _____

_____

cannula _____

closed wound _____

colposcopy _____

contraction _____

cryosurgery _____

cutting _____

dissection _____

distal _____

drainage _____

elective surgery _____

electrocautery _____

emergency surgery _____

granulation _____

hemostat _____

incision _____

inflammatory _____

intraoperative _____

laceration _____

local anesthesia _____

Mayo stand _____

open wound _____

_____

optional surgery _____

_____

postoperative (post-op) _____

_____

preoperative (pre-op) _____

_____

puncture _____

_____

Abbreviations

D & C _____

_____

I & D _____

_____

CRITICAL THINKING

1. You are the circulating nonsterile MA during a procedure. You are holding a vial of anesthetic upside down with the label facing the physician, and the doctor accidentally touches the metal rim around the top and not the rubber section as he or she should have. Would the needle then be contaminated, even though you would have wiped the top with alcohol before holding up for the physician? If it is not contaminated, explain why not. If it is contaminated, what would need to be done at that point?

_____

_____

_____

2. In the same scenario as in question 1, you are holding the vial, and the physician accidentally sticks your finger instead of the rubber section. Are you at risk of being infected with a disease? Why or why not?

_____

_____

_____

3. Almost all patient instruction should be given both orally and in writing, especially postoperative patients who may not understand or remember your instructions due to the anesthesia. Many errors can be made by the patient if instructions are not clear. Come up with a scenario or example of something harmful that could result from a patient's not remembering the oral instructions and not having anything written to refer to.

_____

_____

_____

4. While you are sterile and assisting the physician with a cyst removal procedure, the physician reaches up to scratch her head briefly. She is wearing a surgical cap and there is no visible body fluid on her gloves. There is one major problem here and possibly several other minor ones. Think this through and determine what you think the problems are. Explain in a paragraph what you feel is wrong and why.

_____

_____

_____

_____

5. A patient has had general anesthesia in a minor surgical procedure today and has been monitored appropriately during recovery. The patient seems to be fully awake, vitals are all normal, and the patient does fine when sitting up and then getting off the table with your help. During patient teaching, the patient seems to understand and repeats the instructions back to you correctly. According to office policy, the patient may be discharged. However, the patient does not have a driver to take him home, and you tell him he should call someone or offer to call a taxi for him. The patient states he is fine and can drive and insists he must get home to feed his pets. You ask him to wait but he refuses and leaves, once again insisting he is fine.

Part 1: on a separate page, write out the chart note you think would be appropriate from the time you did the last vital signs check and the patient stood up from the table (the rest was charted on a Postoperative Care and Discharge Sheet). Remember from an earlier chapter that "if it isn't charted, it didn't happen."

Note to Student: The chart note should have the date and time on the left side, followed by your note in narrative format. At the end, sign your first initial, your last name, and your title, "MA."

Part 2: three hours later the office receives a call from a local hospital that the patient was killed in a motor vehicle accident on his way home from your office. The caller want to know his condition when he left. Does your chart note cover all details that would likely relieve your office of legal liability for his death? Underline things in your chart note that would be supportive of your (and the doctor's and the practice's) defense.

_____

_____

_____

_____

CHAPTER REVIEW TEST

MULTIPLE CHOICE

Circle the letter of the correct answer.

1. Wound healing occurs in three major phases. Which of the following is the phase in which a scar begins to lighten and small blood vessels are absorbed?
   a. inflammatory
   b. granulation
   c. contraction
   d. fibroblastic

2. Which two of the following are alternatives to suture wound closures?
   a. wire staples
   b. dressing and bandage
   c. cartridge
   d. adhesive skin closure strips

3. When removing a dressing, the chapter states five main signs to assess the wound. Which one of the following is not one of those signs?
   a. color
   b. edema
   c. pain
   d. approximation

4. A fenestrated drape is one that
   a. can be connected to other drapes to cover a large area.
   b. always has a plastic backing.
   c. is always made of muslin.
   d. none of the above.

5. The textbook discusses surgical instruments in three major categories by their function. Which of the following is not one of those three categories?
   a. clamping and grasping
   b. repair and restructure
   c. dilating, probing, and visualizing
   d. cutting

6. The three basic steps of skin preparation include all of the following except:
   a. apply antiseptic solution to the surgical area.
   b. scrub with an antiseptic soap and rinse.
   c. air dry the skin prior to cleansing.
   d. shave as necessary.

7. Which of the following is not one of the indications of infection as discussed in your text?
   a. warmth
   b. odor of drainage
   c. hardness at surgical site
   d. decreased drainage

8. Sutures on the face are usually removed in
   a. 3–5 days.
   b. 1–3 days.
   c. 5–10 days.
   d. 0 days; absorbable suture is used on the face to minimize scarring.

9. The medical assistant working in the room with the physician for a minor surgical procedure could be: (circle all that apply)
   a. circulating and sterile.
   b. circulating and nonsterile.
   c. preparatory and semisterile.
   d. assisting and sterile.

10. It is typically considered to be the job of the MA during a minor surgery to maintain and keep close by the: (circle all that apply)
    a. drug tray.
    b. emergency cart.
    c. emergency lighting.
    d. fire extinguisher.

TRUE/FALSE

Indicate whether the statement is true (T) or false (F).

_____ 1. During removal, a suture should be cut near the knot where most of the microorganisms are.

_____ 2. A patient reaction to a local anesthetic can be as serious anaphylactic shock.

_____ 3. It is for a legal reason that you should not leave the treatment room once the sterile tray(s) have been set up. It is your responsibility to keep the sterility of the field and you are accountable.

_____ 4. Draping the patient and the area around the surgical site is for the modesty and dignity of the patient.

_____ 5. The scrub assistant is sterile and the circulating assistant is not.

_____ 6. A swaged needle is one that is attached to the suture material.

_____ 7. The main reason to shave the surgical site preoperatively is to make a straight incision difficult.

_____ 8. A local anesthetic is one that is given by the doctor before and during the procedure instead of an anesthetic that is administered by an anesthesiologist.

_____ 9. A sponge is a piece of gauze.

_____ 10. A circulating assistant during a procedure can add sterile supplies to the sterile field.

FILL-IN THE BLANK

Using words from the list below, fill in the blanks to complete the following statements. Note: Some of the terms may be used in more than one statement.

any reason	hang over the edge	pulled down
antiseptic	injection	positioning and draping
burn	local	reaching
consciousness	local anesthetics	reduce pain
contamination	medical condition	significant other
cardiac	medications	skin
cleansed	oximeter	sterile field
family member	patient teaching	suture
general	possibility of infection	tissue
healing	prevent infection	

1. Avoid _____ across the _____ for _____ during the procedure.

2. On a surgical sterile field, the sterile wrapper edges must _____ of the Mayo stand to protect both the _____ and the operator from _____.

3. A wound must be _____ and repaired to _____, arrest any bleeding, promote _____, and _____.

4. When removing a _____, it should be cut as close to the _____ on one side so that no exposed, contaminated suture is _____ through the _____ and out the other side.

5. To prevent the _____, an _____ should be used before and after sutures or staples are removed.

6. If a patient's level of _____ is altered, the patient is placed on a _____ monitor and a pulse _____.

7. The physician determines which local anesthetic to use based on the patient's _____, history, and other _____ the patient takes.

8. Injected _____ tend to _____ for about 10 seconds after the _____.

9. In pre- and postoperative care, it is good practice in the _____ to include a _____ or _____.

10. _____ usually occurs before _____ anesthesia takes place but typically not before _____ anesthesia.

Procedure 11-1

Prepare the Skin for a Surgical Procedure

Objective: The student, using the supplies and equipment listed below, will demonstrate how to prepare the patient's skin for a surgical procedure with a surgical scrub and shave.

Supplies: shave prep kit, including razor, sterile basin pack, antiseptic germicidal soap, sterile 4 × 4s, sterile applicators, sterile sponge forceps, Mayo stand or side tray, sterile water or saline, waste receptacle, hazardous waste container, plastic bags for disposal of contaminated material, sterile gloves, sterile towels, sterile drapes, antiseptic.

Notes to the Student:

_____

_____

_____

_____

_____

Skills Assessment Requirements

Read and familiarize yourself with the procedure; complete the minimum practice requirements. Document each MPR using proper charting technique. Complete each procedure within a reasonable amount of time, with a minimum of 85% accuracy.

Name: _____

Date: _____

		PRACTICE TRIAL	GRADED TRIAL # 1	GRADED TRIAL # 2	NOTES:
1. ✦	Wash your hands thoroughly. Gather equipment and supplies.				
2. ⋆	Identify the patient and guide him or her to the treatment area. Explain the entire procedure to the patient.				
3. ✦	Instruct the patient to void if necessary.				
4. ✦	Have the patient remove appropriate clothing and wear a patient gown until it is time for positioning and draping.				
5. ⋆	Unwrap the outer wraps of all packs. Unwrap the basin pack. Following correct technique for pouring liquids in a sterile field, pour germicidal soap into one basin, sterile water or saline into the second basin, and germicidal solution into the third basin.				
6. ✦	Wash your hands and apply sterile gloves. Position the patient and remove the gown as necessary.				
7. ✦	You may need to shave the area before it is surgically scrubbed. If so, apply soap solution to the area.				
8. ✦	Remove the razor from the shave prep pack that has been placed outside the sterile field.				

		PRACTICE TRIAL	GRADED TRIAL # 1	GRADED TRIAL # 2	NOTES:
9. ✦	Pull the skin gently taut at the surgical site. Shave in the direction of hair growth.				
10. ✦	Rinse the skin with sterile saline or water in an outward circular motion, then pat the area dry.				
11. ✦	Wash your hands and put on sterile gloves.				
12. ✦	Apply soapy solution to the patient's skin in a circular motion with a sterile sponge, starting at the center of the surgical site and moving outward. During the application the circles should not overlap each other or repeat over the same area.				
13. ✦	Cleanse the skin by continuing from the center of the circle making your way to the outer rim. During the application the circles should not overlap each other or repeat over the same area.				
14. ✦	Rinse the area in the same circular manner with new sterile sponges				
15. ✦	Allow area to air dry.				
16. ✦	Apply germicidal solution in concentric circles with a sterile sponge or cotton-tipped applicators.				

		PRACTICE TRIAL	GRADED TRIAL # 1	GRADED TRIAL # 2	NOTES:
17. ✦	After allowing the prep area to completely air-dry, drape 3 to 5 inches above and below the surgical site with sterile towels.				
18. ✦	Drape the prepared surgical site with a sterile towel. If the patient must be left unattended at any time after the surgical scrub, another medical assistant or scrub float will need to cover the prepped area with a sterile towel.				
19. ✶	If the physician did not participate in the patient prep or setting up the surgical tray, alert him or her that the patient has been prepped.				
20. ✶	Document the scrub procedure with patient education notes.				

Name: _____

Date: _____

Document: Enter the appropriate information in the chart below.

Grading

Points Earned	_____		
Points Possible	_____	132	132
Percent Grade (Points Earned/Points Possible)	_____		
PASS:	_____	❏ YES ❏ NO ❏ N/A	❏ YES ❏ NO ❏ N/A

Instructor Sign-Off

Instructor: _____ **Date:** _____

Name: _____

Date: _____

Procedure 11-2

Set Up a Surgical Tray and Assist the Physician with Minor Surgical Procedures

Objective: The student, using the supplies and equipment listed below, will demonstrate how to assist the physician with minor surgery by preparing for the procedure, anticipating physician needs, and providing or reinforcing instruction to the patient or significant other(s).

Supplies: sterile surgical pack, including two pairs of sterile gloves, towel pack, 4 × 4 sponge pack, sterile drapes, needle pack and suture materials, sterile instrument pack, sterile syringe pack, two sterile surgical basins, and sterile specimen containers, Mayo stand and/or a surgical instrument table, transfer forceps and holder, waste container lined with plastic bag, sharps disposal container, biohazard waste container, local anesthetic, alcohol preps

Notes to the Student:

_____

_____

_____

_____

_____

_____

Skills Assessment Requirements

Read and familiarize yourself with the procedure; complete the minimum practice requirements. Document each MPR using proper charting technique. Complete each procedure within a reasonable amount of time, with a minimum of 85% accuracy.

POINT VALUE ✦ = 3-6 points ⋆ = 7-9 points		PRACTICE TRIAL	GRADED TRIAL # 1	GRADED TRIAL # 2	NOTES:
1. ✦	Determine scrub and float assistant staffing needs for the procedure.				
2. ✦	Wash your hands.				
3. ✦	Sanitize and disinfect a Mayo instrument stand by using a 4 × 4 gauze square that has been soaked in 70% isopropyl alcohol. Starting from the middle of the tray, use a circular motion to cleanse the entire tray, including the rim.				
4. ✦	If your place of employment uses sterile disposable drapes, place the package on a counter and carefully peel back the top layer to expose the fan folded drape. Grasping only the corner of the drape with your thumb and forefinger, raise it quickly to a height that allows it to carefully unfold, without touching the counter top, or any portion of your body. If your place of employment uses sterile towels, they will be folded in the same manner and placed inside towel canisters. Sterile towels will be removed the same way.				

		PRACTICE TRIAL	GRADED TRIAL #1	GRADED TRIAL #2	NOTES:
5. ✦	With the drape held firmly with the thumb and forefinger of one hand well above waist level, take your other hand and pinch the opposite corner of the drape between your thumb and forefinger. Both corners along the shortest side of the drape are now firmly held.				
6. ✦	With the drape held above waist level, carefully reach over the Mayo stand and pull the drape towards you as you lay it on the stand. It is critical that the bottom edge of the drape does not touch the stand as you are reaching across. The drape must also not swing and touch any portion of your body at any time.				
7. ✦	At this point in the procedure the tray is now considered sterile. It must not be left unattended, reached over, or touched. If the sterile drape needs to be adjusted, you may reach under and use the draping portions to make minor adjustments.				
8. ✦	Gather the appropriate supplies needed for the procedure. If you gather items that are wrapped twice you must apply them in a sterile manner.				

		PRACTICE TRIAL	GRADED TRIAL #1	GRADED TRIAL #2	NOTES:
9. ✦	Position the package in your non-dominant hand with the flap facing up. The package should look like an envelope, with the envelope opening on top and towards your fingertips. You may adjust the package as needed at this point, as this outer wrapping is not sterile and neither is your hand.				
10. ✦	Pull open the top flap by gently grasping it with your other hand and pulling it up and underneath, ticking it into the fingers of the non-dominant hand.				
11. ✦	Follow the same procedure, pulling the right flap to the right and the left flap to the left, without crossing over your non-dominant hand. This method allows the inner package to remain sterile while it is being exposed for removal. Gathering the loose ends into your fingers prevents them from being dragged across the sterile field or folding back onto the sterile package before it is placed on the tray.				
12. ✦	Carefully apply the package to the sterile field by holding it well above the tray and letting it carefully fall onto the tray.				
13. ✦	Items that have been sterilized in plastic pouches must also be applied in a sterile manner.				

		PRACTICE TRIAL	GRADED TRIAL #1	GRADED TRIAL #2	NOTES:
14. ✦	Carefully peel apart the package and allow the instrument to fall onto the sterile field.				
15. ✦	Do not allow the package to touch the sterile field and do not allow the instruments to slide or bounce as they land on the tray.				
16. ⋆	Once all items have been applied to the sterile field, you may wash your hands using a surgical scrub and apply sterile gloves. With sterile gloves on you may open the previously applied sterile package and verify its contents. You may also arrange the items on the tray according to physician preference. *Note:* If you drop your hands below your waist or touch any item outside of the sterile area you are once again contaminated. You must also pay very close attention to your clothes as scrubs that are worn too loosely will fall forward and contaminate the sterile tray. Once you have verified that all items are present and arranged according to physician preference you must cover the sterile tray. To cover the sterile tray follow the instructions for set up, but instead of crossing over the field and pulling the drape to you, you must hold the drape in front of you at a level so that the top towel and bottom towel are even and carefully lay it over the tray.				

	PRACTICE TRIAL	GRADED TRIAL # 1	GRADED TRIAL # 2	NOTES:
17. *	Identify the patient and guide him or her to the treatment area. Explain the entire procedure to the patient.			
18. ✦	Instruct the patient to void if necessary. Provide draping or a gown for the patient as required for the procedure. Sometimes a patient will disrobe and gown in another room before entering the treatment area.			
19. ✦	Assist the patient onto the examination table.			
20. *	Perform a skin prep as described in Procedure 8-1.			
21. ✦	Assist the physician in scrubbing, gowning, and gloving as needed.			
22. ✦	The physician may want you to open the packet of sterile gloves and place the packet where it can be easily accessed at the start of the procedure. (Depending on the duties of the scrub assistant during the procedure, you may be designated to scrub, and to gown, mask, and glove.)			

		PRACTICE TRIAL	GRADED TRIAL # 1	GRADED TRIAL # 2	NOTES:
23. ✦	When the physician is ready to proceed, he or she may remove the drapes from the tray setups without contaminating the trays or the sterile field. If you are directed to do this, grasp the towel or drape at the distal corners (away from the center). Lift the towel toward you without reaching over the tray and unprotected sterile field.				
24. ✦	In anticipation of soiled dressings, place a bag or container to the side for the physician to discard them into. *Note:* You may fulfill the role of scrub assistant or circulating assistant, depending on the procedure and the needs of the physician.				
25. ∗	Observe closely and anticipate the physician's needs. If a specimen container is needed, hold it to receive a specimen.				
26. ✦	In most cases the physician will prefer to apply the first sterile dressing but occasionally may direct the scrub to do it. You will reinforce or anchor the dressing.				

	PRACTICE TRIAL	GRADED TRIAL # 1	GRADED TRIAL # 2	NOTES:
27. ✦ When the procedure has been completed, collect all soiled instruments in a basin and remove them from the patient's view. Dispose of soiled dressings in biohazard containers.				
28. ✦ Remove your gloves and discard. Wash your hands.				
29. ∗ If specimen containers have been contaminated, use clean gloves to place and tighten lids on them. Label and bag specimens before transporting or sending them to the lab.				
30. ∗ Obtain and chart vital signs following office policy and document your recovery observations, including mental status, changes in drainage and size of drainage on dressings, and ability to ambulate and urinate. (Observation requirements may vary according to the medical office specialty.)				
31. ✦ Review your observations with the physician. When the physician determines discharge readiness, he or she discusses care instructions with the patient and significant other(s).				

		PRACTICE TRIAL	GRADED TRIAL # 1	GRADED TRIAL # 2	NOTES:
32. ★	Give the patient a printed copy of the physician's discharge instructions, and review and reinforce them with the patient. Before the patient leaves the facility, help with any additional paperwork, such as follow-up appointments.				
33. ✦	Assist or transport the patient to significant others or, in some cases, to the car.				
34. ★	Chart the results of patient instruction immediately.				
35. ✦	Don appropriate PPE to clean and sanitize the room for the next patient.				
36. ✦	Wash your hands.				

Name: _____

Date: _____

Document: Enter the appropriate information in the chart below.

Grading

Points Earned	_____		
Points Possible	_____	240	240
Percent Grade (Points Earned/Points Possible)	_____		
PASS:	_____	❏ YES ❏ NO ❏ N/A	❏ YES ❏ NO ❏ N/A

Instructor Sign-Off

Instructor: _____ Date: _____

Procedure 11-3

Assist the Physician with Suturing

Objective: The student, using the supplies and equipment listed below, will demonstrate sterile technique when assisting with suture repair of an incision.

Supplies: sterile packs, including patient drapes, towels, and 4 × 4s, scalpels with blades or blades (size according to physician's preference), suture and needle pack (according to physician's preference), sterile suture pack, including scalpel handle, thumb forceps, needle holder, scissors, hemostats, Mayo stand and side stand or table, anesthetic (usually local), sterile transfer forceps and holder, sterile basins, sterile saline or water, sterile gloves, needle and syringe pack, waste container with plastic bag liner, biohazard waste container sharps container.

Notes to the Student:

_____

_____

_____

_____

_____

_____

Skills Assessment Requirements

Read and familiarize yourself with the procedure; complete the minimum practice requirements. Document each MPR using proper charting technique. Complete each procedure within a reasonable amount of time, with a minimum of 85% accuracy.

Name: _____

Date: _____

		PRACTICE TRIAL	GRADED TRIAL # 1	GRADED TRIAL # 2	NOTES:
POINT VALUE ✦ = 3-6 points ✶ = 7-9 points					
1. ✦	Wash your hands.				
2. ✶	Identify the patient and guide him or her to the treatment area. Explain the entire procedure to the patient.				
3. ✦	Position the patient on the exam table so that the area to be sutured is exposed.				
4. ✦	Drape to cover the patient's clothing. Follow the guidelines for prepping the skin and draping it for minor surgery.				
5. ✶	Perform a 5-minute sterile scrub.				
6. ✦	Put on sterile gloves.				
7. ✦	Take a position standing opposite the physician.				
8. ✦	Place two sterile sponges near the wound site.				
9. ✦	Have additional sponges ready as needed.				
10. ✶	Pass instruments to the physician as requested, with a firm "snap" into the palm of the physician's hand.				
11. ✶	Prepare a scalpel handle with blade according to the physician's preference. Pass the scalpel to the physician when necessary.				
12. ✦	Sponge the area as necessary and as directed by the physician.				
13. ✦	Pass other instruments, such as toothed forceps, as necessary.				

		PRACTICE TRIAL	GRADED TRIAL # 1	GRADED TRIAL # 2	NOTES:
14. ★	Place the needle in the needle holder. Pass the needle holder, needle, and suture to the physician, keeping the suture material within the sterile field.				
15. ◆	Keep a hold on the distal end of the suture until the physician sees it and takes it.				
16. ◆	With suture scissors, cut sutures as directed by the physician 1/8 to 1/4 inch above the knot.				
17. ◆	Sponge the closed wound during suturing and discard the soiled sponges.				
18. ◆	Place used instruments in a disinfectant-filled instrument basin immediately.				
19. ◆	Add unused sterile instruments to the disinfectant at the same time, or use another disinfectant-filled instrument basin.				
20. ◆	Remove the gloves and discard. Wash your hands				
21. ◆	Apply dressings as instructed by the physician.				
22. ◆	Help the patient into a comfortable position. Monitor vital signs according to office procedures.				
23. ★	Provide the patient with both oral and written postoperative instructions, including the date and time of the follow-up appointment.				

		PRACTICE TRIAL	GRADED TRIAL #1	GRADED TRIAL #2	NOTES:
24. ✦	Make sure the patient is stable for discharge.				
25. ✶	Complete requisitions for specimens. Transport them to the laboratory or secure them for courier transport to the laboratory.				
26. ✦	Inspect instruments for residual tissue or body fluids and remove any material you discover. Then, clean, sanitize, and sterilize the instruments.				
27. ✦	Clean and sanitize the room for the next patient.				
28. ✦	Wash your hands.				

Name: _____

Date: _____

Document: Enter the appropriate information in the chart below.

Grading

Points Earned	_____		
Points Possible	_____	189	189
Percent Grade (Points Earned/Points Possible)	_____		
PASS:	_____	❏ YES ❏ NO ❏ N/A	❏ YES ❏ NO ❏ N/A

Instructor Sign-Off

Instructor: _____ **Date:** _____

Name: _____

Date: _____

Procedure 11-4

Assist the Physician with Suture or Staple Removal

Objective: The student will be able to assist the physician with suture or staple removal.

Supplies: suture removal kit, including suture scissors, thumb forceps, and sterile 4 × 4 gauze, or staple removal kit, including staple remover and sterile 4 × 4 gauze; antiseptic swabs; sterile 4 × 4 gauze; gloves; surgical tape; biohazard waste container; sharps container, if necessary

Notes to the Student:

_____

_____

_____

_____

_____

_____

Skills Assessment Requirements

Read and familiarize yourself with the procedure; complete the minimum practice requirements. Document each MPR using proper charting technique. Complete each procedure within a reasonable amount of time, with a minimum of 85% accuracy.

POINT VALUE ✦ = 3-6 points ⋆ = 7-9 points		PRACTICE TRIAL	GRADED TRIAL # 1	GRADED TRIAL # 2	NOTES:
1. ✦	Wash your hands.				
2. ⋆	Identify the patient and guide him or her to the treatment area. Explain the entire procedure to the patient.				
3. ✦	Describe the sensation of pulling or tugging normally felt as the sutures or staples are removed.				
4. ✦	Apply gloves.				
5. ✦	Remove any dressing present. Moisten adhered dressing with sterile saline or hydrogen peroxide before removal, if necessary.				
6. ✦	Grasp the edge of the dressing and lift it halfway to the point of the suture line. Then lift the other edge in the same manner. Once the dressing is free of the suture area, it can be disposed of in a biohazard container.				
7. ✦	Cleanse the suture or staple area and surrounding skin.				
8. ✦	Open the sterile suture or staple removal kit.				
9. ✦	Wash your hands and put on sterile gloves.				

		PRACTICE TRIAL	GRADED TRIAL # 1	GRADED TRIAL # 2	NOTES:
	For Sutures:				
10. ⋆	With the thumb forceps, grasp the suture knot. Gently lift the knot upward.				
11. ⋆	With your other hand, slip the notched edge of the suture scissors under the suture as close to the skin as possible. Close the scissors to cut the suture.				
12. ⋆	Gently pull on the knot and pull the unexposed suture through the skin. Place it on the 4 × 4 gauze.				
13. ✦	Continue until all the sutures are removed. Check the patient chart for total number of sutures applied to verify that all sutures have been removed. If the count is inconsistent you must report this to the physician for further instructions.				
14. ✦	Cleanse the skin with an antiseptic swab.				
15. ✦	Allow the skin to air-dry and apply adhesive skin closures or dressing as the physician directs.				
	For Staples:				
16. ⋆	Slide the bottom jaw of the staple remover under the staple.				
17. ⋆	Squeeze the staple remover handles together. The staple will bend slightly into a "V" shape				

		PRACTICE TRIAL	GRADED TRIAL # 1	GRADED TRIAL # 2	NOTES:
18. ★	Carefully lift the staple from the skin. Place it on the 4 × 4 gauze.				
19. ✦	Continue the process until all the staples are removed.				
20. ✦	Cleanse the skin with antiseptic swab.				
21. ✦	Allow the skin to air-dry and apply adhesive skin closures or dressing as the physician directs.				
	Clean-up for Both Procedures:				
22. ✦	Dispose of contaminated materials in a biohazard or sharps container as appropriate.				
23. ✦	Remove the gloves and discard.				
24. ✦	Wash your hands.				
25. ★	Document the procedure.				

Name: _____

Date: _____

Document: Enter the appropriate information in the chart below.

Grading

Points Earned	_____		
Points Possible	_____	174	174
Percent Grade (Points Earned/Points Possible)	_____		
PASS:		❏ YES	❏ YES
		❏ NO	❏ NO
		❏ N/A	❏ N/A

Instructor Sign-Off

Instructor: _____ Date: _____

Procedure 11-5

Change a Sterile Dressing

Objective: The student, using the supplies and equipment listed below, will demonstrate a sterile dressing change.

Supplies: Prepackaged dressing pack, including sterile gauze or sponges, sterile thumb forceps, sterile dressings, adhesive tape (or tape most appropriate for skin condition and dressing function); Mayo stand and side tray; antiseptic solution; sterile transfer forceps; sterile gloves; scissors; sterile basins; thumb forceps; disposable gloves; waste container with plastic bag liner, biohazard waste container.

Notes to the Student:

_____

_____

_____

_____

_____

_____

Skills Assessment Requirements

Read and familiarize yourself with the procedure; complete the minimum practice requirements. Document each MPR using proper charting technique. Complete each procedure within a reasonable amount of time, with a minimum of 85% accuracy.

Name: _____

Date: _____

POINT VALUE ✦ = 3-6 points ✴ = 7-9 points		PRACTICE TRIAL	GRADED TRIAL #1	GRADED TRIAL #2	NOTES:
1. ✴	Identify the patient and guide him or her to the treatment area. Explain the entire procedure to the patient.				
2. ✦	Wash your hands.				
3. ✦	Assemble the equipment on the Mayo stand or side table, using aseptic technique. Arrange the supplies and equipment.				
4. ✦	Apply non-sterile gloves, then remove the dressing by pulling it in the direction of the wound.				
5. ✦	Place the removed dressing into a biohazard bag, without touching the outside of the bag. Be careful not to pass it over your sterile tray.				
6. ✴	Arrange the supplies and equipment. Inspect the patient's wound and make a mental note to later document in the chart. A description of the wound size, shape, and any indication of infection, such as pus or inflammation should be noted.				
7. ✦	Hold the antiseptic container with your palm covering the label. Pour some of the antiseptic into a sink or waste container. As the solution flows across the edge of the container, the edge will be disinfected. Pour the antiseptic into the sterile basin.				

		PRACTICE TRIAL	GRADED TRIAL #1	GRADED TRIAL #2	NOTES:
8. ✦	Wash your hands with a surgical scrub and apply sterile gloves.				
9. ✦	Using sterile forceps and sterile cotton balls or sterile gauze pads, depending on the size of the wound, cleanse the wound. Disposable materials can be discarded in biohazard, and reusable items will be cleaned at the end of the procedure.				
10. *	Cleanse the wound by moving from the inside to the outside, wiping from the top of the wound to the bottom, one time. The cotton ball must be changed with each stroke.				
11. *	Apply the sterile dressing to the wound and remove your gloves. Verify that your patient does not have an allergy to adhesives. If any allergy is present, secure the dressing with non-adhesive disposable bandage wrap such as Coban.				
12. ✦	Secure the dressing with adhesive tape. Tape should cover the entire dressing or be wrapped completely around the extremity.				

		PRACTICE TRIAL	GRADED TRIAL # 1	GRADED TRIAL # 2	NOTES:
13. ⋆	Provide the patient with written and verbal instructions on wound care, signs of infection, and when the patient should follow up with the physician.				
14. ✦	When the patient has exited the procedure area you may apply non-sterile gloves and clean the room in preparation for the next patient.				

Name: _____

Date: _____

Document: Enter the appropriate information in the chart below.

Grading

Points Earned	_____		
Points Possible	_____	99	99
Percent Grade (Points Earned/Points Possible)	_____		
PASS:	_____	❑ YES	❑ YES
		❑ NO	❑ NO
		❑ N/A	❑ N/A

Instructor Sign-Off

Instructor: _____ **Date:** _____

Chapter 12
Diagnostic Procedures

CHAPTER OUTLINE

Review the Chapter Outline. If any content area is unclear, review that area before beginning workbook exercises.

    A. The Medical Assistant's Role in Diagnostic Testing

    B. Clinical Laboratory Improvement Amendments (CLIA)

    C. Regulations and Laboratory Safety

    D. Hospital Laboratory Setting

    E. The Physician Office Laboratory

    F. Ordering Diagnostic Tests

CHAPTER REVIEW

The following is a summary of the chapter. If any of this material is unclear, review it in the textbook.

Diagnostic testing results play a vital role in diagnosing disease or confirming wellness. Accuracy, safety, adherence to regulations, and ensuring payment by obtaining precertification are major factors in the process of diagnostic testing, which spans from the physician's initial order through the receipt, follow-up, and filing of the results. The medical assistant needs to understand and comply with various regulations from agencies and organizations including the FDA, the EPA, OSHA, and JCAHO. An MA may work in a physician's office laboratory (POL) or in a hospital or reference lab. All are regulated by CLIA, which developed quality standards and various levels of test complexity that a lab can perform. The waived level of performing lab tests is most common for the medical assistant's duties and can require the use of many different items of equipment in the lab. It is commonly the medical assistant who ensures payment prior to diagnostic testing by obtaining a precertification from third party or insurance providers, scheduling tests and instructing patients in test preparation, reviewing results when they come in to compare the patient's results to the normal range, flagging abnormal results for the physician, performing follow-up as directed, and finally filing the lab report in the patient's medical record.

LEARNING ACTIVITIES AND STUDY AIDS

Review the following study aids and/or complete the activities to ensure that you have achieved the learning objectives for this chapter.

1. The medical assistant may work in a hospital or reference laboratory or may work in a Physician's Office Laboratory (POL). To define the role of the medical assistant, state the duties that would be

performed in all facilities, the duties for the MA working in a POL, and the duties for the MA working in a hospital or reference laboratory.

_____

_____

_____

_____

_____

_____

2. Clinical Laboratory Improvement Amendments (CLIA) set the standards for laboratory testing. Explain in your own words how CLIA sets those standards.

_____

_____

_____

_____

_____

_____

_____

3. The test categories of waived, PPMP, moderate-complexity, and high-complexity tests allow for various tests to be performed under each category. Explain the differences between each of the above listed categories.

_____

_____

_____

_____

_____

_____

_____

4. State the purpose of quality control and quality assurance and explain the difference between the two.

_____

_____

_____

_____

_____

_____

_____

5. Three major agencies have roles that relates to laboratory testing—the FDA, the EPA, and OSHA. State the purpose of each agency's involvement in such testing as explained in your textbook.

_____

_____

_____

_____

_____

_____

6. The Joint Commission on Accreditation of Healthcare Organizations has an important role in the hospital setting. Answer the following regarding JCAHO:

   a. Is this a federal agency?

   _____

   _____

   _____

   b. What has JCAHO done regarding the quality of care?

   _____

   _____

   _____

7. What is the purpose of the Safe Medical Devices Act and what are the major requirements of it?

   _____

   _____

   _____

   _____

   _____

   _____

8. Diagnostic testing in hospital laboratories is provided for both inpatients (surgical and anatomical) and outpatients (clinical). Review Table 12-2: Hospital Laboratory Functional Areas. Close your book, then, writing in two columns as the table appears, list as many of the departments as you can recall. Review the table in your textbook again and check for any that you may have missed.

   _____

   _____

   _____

   _____

   _____

9. Since there are many tests that can be performed in a POL, there are many items of equipment as well. List three pieces of equipment that were discussed in the textbook.

_____

_____

_____

_____

_____

_____

10. A physician's order is needed for a lab test to be performed. Answer the following questions:

    a. Is a verbal order acceptable? Explain your answer.

_____

_____

_____

    b. What are three primary tasks for the MA when an order is initiated?

_____

_____

_____

    c. Nine items of information required for the diagnostic test request form are listed in your textbook. From memory or from critical thinking, state any five of those nine items.

_____

_____

_____

11. Why is a precertification obtained?

_____

_____

_____

_____

_____

_____

12. When scheduling diagnostic tests for a patient with an outside agency, what factors should be considered and discussed with the patient before contacting the agency?

_____

_____

_____

_____

_____

_____
_____
_____

13. Screening and following up on test results is the final part of the entire process of lab testing. In your own words and from your memory of reading this chapter, tell what the MA would do in this task.

_____
_____
_____
_____
_____
_____
_____
_____
_____

MEDICAL TERMINOLOGY REVIEW

Use a dictionary and highlighted terms in the textbook to define the following terms.

Terms

centrifuge _____
_____

glucometer _____
_____

hematocrit _____
_____

hemoglobin _____
_____

photometer _____
_____

Abbreviations

BUN _____
_____

CBC _____
_____

CLIA _____
_____

CO_2 _____
_____

CPT _____
_____

C & S _____

_____

diff _____

_____

DOB _____

_____

ESR _____

_____

Hct _____

_____

HFCA _____

_____

Hgb _____

_____

ICD-9-CM _____

_____

POL _____

_____

PPMP _____

_____

PT _____

_____

PTT _____

_____

RBC _____

_____

SSN _____

_____

WBC _____

_____

CRITICAL THINKING

1. As you are ordering supplies for the office, you see a flyer in the mail for a sale on syringes and needles that are not safety devices. Would you try to save money on supplies or order the more expensive safety syringes and needles? Explain the reasons for your decision.

_____

_____

_____

_____

2. Your physician verbally (for now) gave you an order for a lab test that required a 7 ml purple top tube of blood, which you have already drawn. Now you cannot recall which test the physician wanted, and she has already left the office for the day. What are two ways you could find out? How can you prevent this from happening in the future?

_____

_____

_____

_____

3. You have scheduled a test at an outside agency for a patient who is not in the office at this time. You call the patient to tell her that you were able to get it booked for tomorrow at noon and that she should fast after midnight tonight. The patient becomes upset, stating that she is elderly and cannot fast until noon and that she would not have a ride to the test tomorrow as her son is working then. What could you have done differently to avoid this problem?

_____

_____

_____

_____

4. You are working in an office and precepting a medical assisting student extern. A patient who is in her seventh month of pregnancy comes in, and you want the student to room the patient and perform the prenatal duties, but she doesn't do a urine glucose and protein dipstick. When asked, she tells you it is because there was no written order from the doctor. Explain in your own words and as if you were talking to the student what a standing order is.

_____

_____

_____

_____

5. Your physician ordered a bone marrow biopsy to be done on a patient, which you scheduled and assisted with about three months ago. It is brought up today when the patient called the billing department. Someone came to you saying the patient was very angry because he has been billed for the procedure. He states his insurance company told him there was no precertification obtained prior to the procedure so it will not pay. You check the chart and realize you did not call to obtain the precertification before scheduling the biopsy. Consider some things you could do at this point (not what you would say to the patient) that are not specifically listed in the textbook but that seem to be logical steps to resolve this problem.

_____

_____

_____

_____

CHAPTER REVIEW TEST

MULTIPLE CHOICE

Circle the letter of the correct answer.

1. There are five types of CLIA Certificates. Which of the following is not one of those types?
   a. Certificate of Registration
   b. Certificate of Waiver
   c. Certificate of Comparison
   d. Certificate for PPMP

2. Which of the following fall under the Hematology Department of a lab? (circle all that apply)
   a. white blood cell count
   b. glucose level
   c. hemoglobin and hematocrit
   d. a BUN level

3. A glucometer uses a _____ to reflect the light through the patient sample to determine the test result.
   a. urinometer
   b. photometer
   c. lightometer
   d. focusometer

4. Lab test results may be sent to the physician by (circle all that apply)
   a. phone.
   b. fax
   c. regular mail
   d. email

5. What laboratory area would a throat specimen go to based on the information in this chapter of your textbook?
   a. chemistry
   b. microbiology
   c. hematology
   d. immunology

6. When calling a patient about lab results or a request to return to the clinic to discuss them, you may get an answering machine. Which of the following are appropriate to leave on that machine?
   a. your name
   b. your phone number
   c. your office or doctor's name
   d. what tests the results are for (not the results themselves)

7. Which of the following choices are true about a reference laboratory? (circle all that apply)
   a. It is under the same regulations and guidelines as a POL.
   b. It can perform high-level testing.
   c. It is independently owned.
   d. It cannot have contracts with insurance providers and managed care providers.

8. Laboratories performing waived tests only apply for a
   a. Certificate of Accreditation.
   b. Certificate of Compliance.
   c. Certificate for PMPP.
   d. Certificate of Waiver.

9. Those who do the fewest amount of waived tests are: (circle all that apply)
   a. medical assistants.
   b. physicians.
   c. medical lab technologists.
   d. medical lab technicians.

10. An example of quality control would be: (circle all that apply)
   a. drawing blood from the patient.
   b. confirming that the patient has followed the required preparation.
   c. checking the accuracy of a glucometer.
   d. selecting the appropriate container or system to collect the sample in.

TRUE/FALSE

Indicate whether the statement is true (T) or false (F).

_____ 1. Many CLIA-waived tests are visual color comparison.

_____ 2. CLIA is a federal agency as are the FDA and the EPA.

_____ 3. JCAHO is a government agency under the FDA.

_____ 4. The MA should not leave any patient information on an answering machine when calling with test results.

_____ 5. POL indicates that a lab is actually in the office and specimens are tested on the premises.

_____ 6. A lab requisition is an order form for the tests the physician wants performed on a patient's specimen(s).

_____ 7. Mark open vials of quality control solutions with the "open" and "discard" dates.

_____ 8. When performing a quality control test, record it in the patient's chart.

_____ 9. A waived laboratory with a PPMP certificate can perform tests using a microscope.

_____ 10. Both reference and physician office laboratories are governed by the same regulations and guidelines.

FILLIN THE BLANK

Using words from the list below fill in the blanks to complete the following statements Note: Some terms may be used in more than one statement.

asked to return

called

Clinical Laboratory
    Improvement
    Amendments

diabetes

discuss them

Environmental
    Protection Agency

error or risk

facilities

federal

Food and Drug
    Administration

glucometer quality
    control

implementation

insurance carrier

least complex

may be performed

microbiology

obtaining specimens

OSHA

other body fluids

POL

quality control

responsibility

safety standards

scheduling

scope of your training

test results

urine

waived

waived tests

wound drainage

1. The _____ and the _____ are two _____ agencies that enforce _____.

2. The _____ department identifies microorganisms in specimens such as blood, _____, stool, nose and throat tissues or mucus, _____, and _____.

3. Before _____ a diagnostic test, the medical office must contact the _____ to confirm coverage and the _____ where the test _____.

4. Depending on the nature of the _____, the patient may be _____ with the results or _____ to _____ in the office.

5. As an MA working in a _____, you may perform _____, provide patient education about _____, and collect specimens within the _____ and physician supervision.

6. When using equipment, you will be required to follow _____ and _____ guidelines.

7. _____ of CLIA was the _____ of the Health Care Financing Administration (HCFA).

8. The objective of _____ is to ensure reliable and valid _____.

9. Emphasize the importance of _____ in the treatment of _____.

10. _____ tests are the _____ tests to perform, so there is little danger of _____ to the patient.

Procedure 12-1

Check the Accuracy of Glucometer Results Using Quality Control Methods

Objective: The student, using the supplies and equipment listed below, will demonstrate how to perform quality control testing of the glucometer.

Supplies: quality control log book, glucometer, quality controls specific to brand of glucometer.

Notes to the Student:

_____

_____

_____

_____

_____

_____

Skills Assessment Requirements

Read and familiarize yourself with the procedure; complete the minimum practice requirements. Document each MPR using proper charting technique. Complete each procedure within a reasonable amount of time, with a minimum of 85% accuracy.

POINT VALUE ✦ = 3-6 points ✶ = 7-9 points		PRACTICE TRIAL	GRADED TRIAL #1	GRADED TRIAL #2	NOTES:
1. ✦	Wash your hands and assemble materials.				
2. ✶	Perform control testing as recommended by the manufacturer and per office policy.				
	a. Check unsealed quality control vials and test strips for open and discard dates and expiration dates. Label the control vials and test strips if you are opening them for the first time.				
	b. If you are changing code strips, calibrate and change the number per manufacturer's instructions.				
3. ✦	Record the test results in a quality control log. If control results are abnormal, report them to the supervisor. Label the glucometer "Repair" and remove it from the clinical area to prevent other staff from using it. Return the glucometer to the clinical area only after the problem has been corrected.				
4. ✦	Dispose of waste materials in the appropriate container.				
5. ✦	Wash your hands and return the glucometer and quality test control equipment to the designated storage area.				

Name: _____

Date: _____

Document: Enter the appropriate information in the chart below.

Grading

Points Earned	_____		
Points Possible	_____	33	33
Percent Grade (Points Earned/Points Possible)	_____		
PASS:	_____	❏ YES ❏ NO ❏ N/A	❏ YES ❏ NO ❏ N/A

Instructor Sign-Off

Instructor: _____ Date: _____

Procedure 12-2

Obtain a Precertification by Telephone

Objective: The student, using the supplies and equipment listed below, will complete the precertification.

Supplies: precertification log book, telephone and telephone number, tickler file containing contact information, blue or black ink pen

Notes to the Student:

_____

_____

_____

_____

_____

_____

Skills Assessment Requirements

Read and familiarize yourself with the procedure; complete the minimum practice requirements. Document each MPR using proper charting technique. Complete each procedure within a reasonable amount of time, with a minimum of 85% accuracy.

POINT VALUE ✦ = 3-6 points ⋆ = 7-9 points		PRACTICE TRIAL	GRADED TRIAL # 1	GRADED TRIAL # 2	NOTES:
1. ⋆	Gather the patient chart and insurance contact information.				
2. ✦	Telephone the insurance carrier and follow voice prompts if given.				
3. ✦	When the telephone receptionist or voice prompt asks if the claim question is from a physician, medical office, or patient, state the physician's name or the medical office's name.				
4. ⋆	Ask the person at the insurance company for his or her full name. Document the name, time of telephone contact, and date in the precertification log book.				
5. ✦	Give the necessary information: diagnosis, procedure(s) anticipated, treatment location, and whether it is an inpatient or outpatient procedure.				
6. ✦	Document the precertification number in the log book as it is given and repeat the number to your contact person to verify. Thank the insurance contact person.				

		PRACTICE TRIAL	GRADED TRIAL #1	GRADED TRIAL #2	NOTES:
7. ★	In the designated area of the patient chart, following office policy, document the name of the insurance contact person, the time, precertification number(s) given for the procedures anticipated, treatment location, and whether it is an inpatient or outpatient procedure.				
8. ✦	Complete, whether it is an inpatient or outpatient procedure, necessary forms.				
9. ★	Make a copy and give it to the patient. Place the original forms on the chart.				

Name: _____

Date: _____

Document: Enter the appropriate information in the chart below.

Grading

Points Earned	_____		
Points Possible	_____	66	66
Percent Grade (Points Earned/Points Possible)	_____		
PASS:	_____	❑ YES ❑ NO ❑ N/A	❑ YES ❑ NO ❑ N/A

Instructor Sign-Off

Instructor: _____   Date: _____

Procedure 12-3

Demonstrate Screening and Follow-Up of Test Results

Objective: The student, using the supplies and equipment listed below, will demonstrate how to screen and follow up on returned laboratory results.

Supplies: returned laboratory reports, patient chart, blue or black ink pen, telephone

Notes to the Student:

_____

_____

_____

_____

_____

_____

Skills Assessment Requirements

Read and familiarize yourself with the procedure; complete the minimum practice requirements. Document each MPR using proper charting technique. Complete each procedure within a reasonable amount of time, with a minimum of 85% accuracy.

Name: _____

Date: _____

	PRACTICE TRIAL	GRADED TRIAL #1	GRADED TRIAL #2	NOTES:
POINT VALUE ✦ = 3-6 points ⋆ = 7-9 points				
1. ✦ Sort lab reports according to physician.				
2. ✦ Sort the reports according to patient's last name, first name, and initial for each physician.				
3. ✦ Match patient identification numbers in cases where names are similar.				
4. ⋆ Attach the new reports to the patient chart and place them in a designated area for the physician to read and interpret. The physician will initial each laboratory test that he or she reads.				
5. ⋆ Call patients with their laboratory results or set up appointments to discuss the results as designated by the physician. If an answering machine or voicemail is activated, do not include patient information in your message. Leave a phone number for the patient to return the call.				
6. ✦ Place the laboratory reports in the chart according to office procedure.				
7. ✦ On a tickler file, note the next scheduled date for routinely scheduled laboratory procedures.				
8. ✦ Work with the patient to schedule the next appointment if the laboratory procedure is weekly or monthly.				

Document: Enter the appropriate information in the chart below.

Grading

Points Earned	_____		
Points Possible	_____	54	54
Percent Grade (Points Earned/Points Possible)	_____		
PASS:	_____	❏ YES ❏ NO ❏ N/A	❏ YES ❏ NO ❏ N/A

Instructor Sign-Off

Instructor: _____ Date: _____

CHAPTER 13
Microscopes and Microbiology

CHAPTER OUTLINE

Review the Chapter Outline. If any content area is unclear, review that area before beginning workbook exercises.

    A. The Medical Assistant's Role in Specimen Collection

    B. Microscopes

    C. Microbiology

    D. Preparing Specimens for Microscopic Examination

    E. Specimen Collection, Storage, and Transport

CHAPTER REVIEW

The following is a summary of the chapter. If any of this material is unclear, review it in the textbook.

The field of microbiology offers many opportunities for the medical assistant to use a variety of skills. The MA knows how to use a microscope and is aware of the five different types, although most often a compound or bright field type is utilized in a POL. The medical assistant will prepare specimens after collecting and instructing patients on proper collection, such as for a Gram stain, wet mounts, and culture and sensitivity testing. Specimens can be collected for microbiological examinations on the throat, a wound, urine, and stools. It is important that the MA is knowledgeable of normal and pathogenic flora, bacteria and other pathogenic microorganisms, and the significance of gram-negative and gram-positive gram stain results.

LEARNING ACTIVITIES AND STUDY AIDS

Review the following study aids and/or complete the activities to ensure that you have achieved the learning objectives for this chapter.

1. Describe the medical assistant's role in the areas of microbiological testing and specimen collection.

_____

_____

_____

_____

_____

_____

_____

_____

2. Your textbook presents five types of microscopes. Review the information in the text and in Table 13-1: Types of Microscopes. Explain briefly the use of each type listed below:

Compound or bright field

_____

_____

Phase contrast

_____

_____

Dark field

_____

_____

Fluorescence compound

_____

_____

Electron

_____

_____

3. There are seven basic parts of a microscope. Review them in your textbook then close the book and list as many of the seven as you can from memory. Then go back to the book and check any that you may have forgotten, add them to your list, and then briefly state in your own words the function of each of the seven parts.

_____

_____

_____

_____

_____

_____

_____

4. The MA must know how to use a microscope if working in the lab area. Review Procedure 13-1: Demonstrate Using a Microscope a few times. Make a flash card that states each step of the procedure. You don't have to use every word as stated for this procedure, just state the minimum amount you would need to jog your memory sufficiently to allow you to correctly perform this task on the externship or job. Having a short list of steps to refer to when practicing or performing the use of a microscope (or any procedure) can be very helpful.

_____

_____

_____

_____

_____

_____

_____

5. Name the three major classification groups for microorganisms and give a brief definition of each. In the two-name system for prokaryotic and eukaryotic microorganisms, each of the two words of the name represents something. In the example of *Staphylococcus aureus*, which represents the genus and which is the species?

_____

_____

_____

_____

_____

_____

_____

6. Define normal flora. Review Table 13-2: Normal Flora in Body Systems, which lists this flora in the skin, respiratory, and gastrointestinal tracts. Since spelling of many of the terms used in the table is difficult, make a flash card for each of the three body systems with the system on one side and the types of normal flora for that system on the other side. Close the book, put away the card, and try to list as many of the types of flora for each system that you can recall. Follow up by checking the book or your recently made card when you are finished and spend some extra time studying those you may have forgotten.

_____

_____

_____

_____

_____

_____

_____

_____

7. Bacteria, parasites, and viruses cause disease. Read through the information in your textbook to determine how each of the three pathogenic microorganisms cause disease, then write a paragraph explaining the information in your own words.

_____

_____

_____

_____

_____

_____

_____

8. Because the MA will likely prepare a specimen smear, review Procedure 13-2: Preparing a Specimen Smear for Microbiological Examination. Prepare a flash card as in question 4 above. Do not write the things you are sure you will remember—try to be concise so this can be a quick reference on the job. Review this card as you practice your procedures.

_____

_____

_____

_____

_____

_____

_____

9. What is gram staining and what is it used for?

_____

_____

_____

_____

_____

_____

_____

10. What are three ways to prepare wet mount slides? List the three types and give one example of what each one can differentiate.

_____

_____

_____

_____

_____

_____

_____

_____

11. List three reasons a stool specimen would be taken. Name four basic factors in the proper collection of stool so that results will be accurate.

_____

_____

_____

_____

_____

_____

12. Explain culture and sensitivity testing.

_____

_____

_____

_____

_____

_____

_____

13. Describe how urine culture specimens are collected. Differentiate between the two methods of collection.

_____

_____

_____

_____

_____

_____

_____

_____

MEDICAL TERMINOLOGY REVIEW

Use a dictionary and highlighted terms in the textbook to define the following terms.

Terms

binocular _____

_____

eukaryotes _____

_____

microbiology _____

_____

monocular _____

_____

morphology _____

_____

mycology _____

_____

normal flora _____

_____

ocular _____

_____

opportunistic pathogen _____

_____

organelle _____

_____

parasitology _____

_____

pathogenicity _____

_____

prokaryotes _____

_____

serology _____

_____

staph _____

_____

strep _____

_____

ultramicroscopic _____

_____

virology _____

_____

viruses _____

_____

Abbreviations

KOH _____

_____

QNS _____

_____

QS _____

_____

UTI _____

_____

CRITICAL THINKING

1. In the clinic, you are collecting urine from a patient using a catheter. As you are inserting the catheter, it slips from your hands and touches the patient's leg. What would you do and why?

_____

_____

_____

2. A patient has been instructed to collect three stool specimens for occult blood. The patient brings the specimens into the office but tells you he was not able to do them on different days, and they were all collected on the same day. Is this acceptable? Why or why not?

_____

_____

_____

3. You need to prepare a wet mount and set it up on the microscope for the doctor. As you look through the high power lens, it appears to be cloudy and has a lot of artifacts. When you move the slide slightly, you notice that the artifacts do not move with the slide. What do you think the problem could be? What would you do to correct this?

_____

_____

_____

_____

4. If a patient had been treated with antibiotics for 10 days for a bladder infection and yet the infection was still present after the course of medication, what test do you think the physician might order at this point? Why?

_____

_____

_____

_____

5. You are preparing a specimen smear for a microbiological examination by the doctor. You heat fix the slide but you realize you have heated it too much as it becomes hard to hold. What does this do to the specimen if this happens and what would you do?

_____

_____

_____

_____

CHAPTER REVIEW TEST

MULTIPLE CHOICE

Circle the letter of the correct answer.

1. There are five types of microscopes described in your textbook. Which of the following is not one of those five types?
   a. phase contrast
   b. phase field
   c. electron
   d. dark field

2. Which of the following are dyes used in a gram stain? (circle all that apply)
   a. iodine
   b. sassafrass
   c. crystal violet
   d. gentian stain
   e. none of the above

3. KOH is
   a. saline.
   b. indica ink.
   c. potassium hydroxide.
   d. normal saline.

4. Another term for stool guaiac is
   a. hemorrhoidal bleeding.
   b. fecal occult blood test.
   c. stool specimen.
   d. enteric pathogens.

5. A needle can be used to collect the exudate from _____ for a culture.
   a. a wound
   b. the throat
   c. blood
   d. the genitals

6. Urine cultures can be obtained from three methods of urine collection as stated in your textbook. Which of the following is not one of those three?
   a. clean-catch
   b. clean voided
   c. voided
   d. catheterized

7. Stool cultures are performed to
   a. diagnose bacterial infections in the GI tract.
   b. diagnose occult blood.
   c. determine the presence of microorganisms.
   d. diagnose ova, parasites, and other organisms in the GI tract.

8. Which type of urine catheter is only used for a urine culture collection? (circle all that apply)
   a. a straight or curved catheter
   b. temporary catheter
   c. in and out catheter
   d. indwelling catheter

9. Unrefrigerated urine should be received in the lab's testing area within
   a. one hour.
   b. two hours.
   c. 24 hours.
   d. up to four hours.

10. The magnification of an object by a microscope is accomplished by the interaction of
    a. the degree of lens curvature and the size of the lens.
    b. visible light and the lens systems.
    c. light and the magnifier in the oculars.
    d. the condenser and the iris.

TRUE/FALSE

Indicate whether the statement is true (T) or false (F).

_____ 1. A binocular microscope has one ocular lens.

_____ 2. The condenser is located on the substage of a microscope.

_____ 3. Oil immersion is used with the 10x lens to increase the power to 100x.

_____ 4. *E. coli* can cause a bladder infection (or other UTI).

_____ 5. There are three types of microscopes in addition to the five listed in your textbook.

_____ 6. Viruses are ultramicroscopic.

_____ 7. There are two focus knobs—for low power and high power.

_____ 8. The bacteria *Staphylococcus aureus* is always on our skin as normal flora.

_____ 9. When you are finished working with a microscope, you must clean the lenses with any soft cloth or paper.

_____ 10. Viruses carry DNA or RNA.

FILL IN THE BLANK

Using words from the list below, fill in the blanks to complete the following statements.

bacteria	image to be viewed	prokaryotic organisms
contaminated	in reverse	random
culture	microbiological specimens	specimens of three stool specimens
documented in the log	mirrors that reflect light	
documented in the patient chart	occult blood	slide
enteric pathogens	pathogenic bacteria	tissue or secretion
examined	pathogenic microorganisms	types of bacteria
Gram stain	positive or negative	upside down
harmless	prepared media	urinalysis tests

1. The tube of a microscope contains a series of _____ and the _____.

2. When looking through a microscope, remember that you are viewing the image _____ and _____.

3. Operating the microscope is not _____, but the maintenance, cleaning, and repairs to it are _____.

4. _____ are the most important group of _____.

5. Normal flora are generally _____ but potentially _____ that colonize in the human body.

6. A _____ is a simple diagnostic test that identifies _____ by _____ classification.

7. _____ must be properly prepared on a _____ before they can be _____ under the microscope.

8. The physician may ask a patient to collect a stool specimen, or a _____ for a number of a reasons, including microscopic examination for _____, ova and parasite examination, and _____ detection.

9. The term _____ refers to a process in which a direct specimen of _____ is cultivated in _____; once it is grown, it is examined for _____.

10. _____ urine specimens commonly used for routine _____ are not used for cultures as they may be _____.

Name: _____

Date: _____

Procedure 13-1

Demonstrate Using the Microscope

Objective: The student, using the supplies and equipment listed below, will demonstrate how to use the microscope and focus all three objectives.

Supplies: microscope, lens paper, lens cleaner, prepared slide (with or without cover slip), immersion oil, disposable gloves, tissues

Notes to the Student:

_____

_____

_____

_____

_____

_____

Skills Assessment Requirements

Read and familiarize yourself with the procedure; complete the minimum practice requirements. Document each MPR using proper charting technique. Complete each procedure within a reasonable amount of time, with a minimum of 85% accuracy.

Name: _____

Date: _____

POINT VALUE

✦ = 3-6 points

★ = 7-9 points

		PRACTICE TRIAL	GRADED TRIAL # 1	GRADED TRIAL # 2	NOTES:
1. ✦	Wash your hands and put on disposable gloves.				
2. ✦	Remove the cover from the microscope.				
3. ✦	Check that the microscope is clean and in working order. Replace the light bulb if necessary.				
4. ✦	Turn the light off until you are ready to focus the objectives on the specimen slide.				
5. ✦	Clean the lenses and eyepieces (oculars) with lens paper. Use lens cleaner as necessary, but do *not* oversaturate the glue holding the lens in place.				
6. ✦	Secure the slide on the stage with the slide clips.				
7. ✦	Revolve the low-power objective into place until it is seated or you hear a click.				
8. ✦	Adjust the oculars so that you see only one field rather than separate left and right views.				
9. ✦	Using the coarse adjustment control knob, raise the body tube of the microscope and swivel the 10X objective into place.				
10. ✦	Turn the light on.				
11. ✦	Lower the body tube with the coarse adjustment control knob, to bring the slide into general focus.				

		PRACTICE TRIAL	GRADED TRIAL # 1	GRADED TRIAL # 2	NOTES:
12. ✦	With the iris controls, adjust the light to cover the slide. It is not important at this point to achieve clear focus.				
13. ✦	Observing from the side, lower the body tube to bring the objective closer to the slide without touching it.				
14. ✦	Look through the oculars, using the coarse adjustment to bring the specimen into focus. Adjust the iris if you need more light.				
15. ✦	Observing from the side, switch to the high-power objective without touching the slide. The body tube may need to be adjusted during this process.				
16. ✦	When the high-power objective (40X) is in place, adjust the fine focus controls to bring the specimen into clear focus.				
17. ✦	If the slide specimen is dry and does not have a cover slip, apply a drop of oil and turn the oil immersion objective into place. Lower the objective until it is covered with oil.				
18. ✦	After the specimen has been examined, lower the stage.				

		PRACTICE TRIAL	GRADED TRIAL #1	GRADED TRIAL #2	NOTES:
19. ✦	Remove the slide specimen and dispose of it in a biohazard waste receptacle.				
20. ✦	Turn off the light.				
21. ✦	Clean the lenses with lens cleaner and lens paper. Clean the stage.				
22. ✦	Rotate the objectives to return the low-power objective directly above the stage.				
23. ✦	Cover the microscope.				
24. ✦	Clean the work area.				
25. ✦	Dispose of the gloves and wash your hands.				

Name: _____

Date: _____

Document: Enter the appropriate information in the chart below.

Grading

Points Earned	_____		
Points Possible	_____	150	150
Percent Grade (Points Earned/Points Possible)	_____		
PASS:	_____	❏ YES ❏ NO ❏ N/A	❏ YES ❏ NO ❏ N/A

Instructor Sign-Off

Instructor: _____ Date: _____

Procedure 13-2

Prepar a Specimen Smear for Microbiological Examination

Objective: The student, using the supplies and equipment listed below, will demonstrate how to prepare a slide for microscopic examination.

Supplies: glass slide (preferably with frosted edge), disposable gloves, sterile distilled water, inoculating loops or specimen swabs, flamesource, biohazardous waste container, sharps container

Notes to the Student:

_____

_____

_____

_____

_____

_____

Skills Assessment Requirements

Read and familiarize yourself with the procedure; complete the minimum practice requirements. Document each MPR using proper charting technique. Complete each procedure within a reasonable amount of time, with a minimum of 85% accuracy.

POINT VALUE ✦ = 3-6 points ⋆ = 7-9 points		PRACTICE TRIAL	GRADED TRIAL # 1	GRADED TRIAL # 2	NOTES:
1. ✦	Wash your hands.				
2. ✦	Gather equipment and supplies.				
3. ✦	Wash your hands again and put on disposable gloves.				
4. ⋆	Write the patient information on the frosted edge of the slide.				
5. ✦	Prepare a thin film, or smear, on the slide.				
	For a specimen from a swab:				
6. ✦	Roll and turn the swab across the slide.				
	For a specimen from a Petri dish:				
7. ✦	Gather sterile distilled water with a sterile inoculating loop and place it on the slide.				
8. ✦	Use the inoculating loop to gather the microbial specimen, without gathering any culture medium.				
9. ✦	Mix the specimen into the distilled water on the slide.				
10. ✦	Sterilize the loop over the flame.				

		PRACTICE TRIAL	GRADED TRIAL #1	GRADED TRIAL #2	NOTES:
	For a specimen from a liquid:				
11. ✦	Dip the inside of the sterile inoculating loop in the culture until it appears covered with a film.				
12. ✦	Touch the film to the center of the slide.				
13. ✦	Allow the specimen on the slide to air-dry completely.				
14. ✦	Hold and pass the slide through the flame several times. The slide is now ready to stain.				
15. ✶	Clean the work area.				
16. ✦	Dispose of the gloves and wash your hands.				

Name: _____

Date: _____

Document: Enter the appropriate information in the chart below.

Grading

Points Earned	_____		
Points Possible	_____	102	102
Percent Grade (Points Earned/Points Possible)	_____		
PASS:	_____	❑ YES ❑ NO ❑ N/A	❑ YES ❑ NO ❑ N/A

Instructor Sign-Off

Instructor: _____ Date: _____

Name: _____

Date: _____

Procedure 13-3

Preparing a Gram Stain

Objective: The student, using the supplies and equipment listed below, will demonstrate how to prepare a slide for microscopic examination of Gram-negative and Gram-positive bacteria.

Supplies: disposable gloves, slide with fixed smear, crystal violet dye, Gram's iodine, alcohol/acetone mixture, safranin dye, wash bottle filled with distilled water, rack and tray for slide staining, forceps, paper towel, biohazardous waste container, sharps container

Notes to the Student:

_____

_____

_____

_____

_____

_____

Skills Assessment Requirements

Read and familiarize yourself with the procedure; complete the minimum practice requirements. Document each MPR using proper charting technique. Complete each procedure within a reasonable amount of time, with a minimum of 85% accuracy.

POINT VALUE ✦ = 3-6 points ⋆ = 7-9 points		PRACTICE TRIAL	GRADED TRIAL #1	GRADED TRIAL #2	NOTES:
1. ✦	Wash your hands. Gather equipment, supplies, and the prepared slide.				
2. ✦	Wash your hands again and put on disposable				
3. ✦	Lay the slide on the slide rack and tray.				
4. ⋆	Pour crystal violet on the slide and allow it to stain for 1 minute.				
5. ✦	Rinse the slide gently with water from the wash bottle.				
6. ✦	Lay the slide on the slide rack and tray.				
7. ⋆	Pour Gram's iodine, also known as mordant, on the slide. Allow it to stain for 2 minutes.				
8. ✦	Lift the slide diagonally with the forceps and rinse gently with water from the wash bottle.				
9. ✦	Maintaining the vertical hold, gently pour the acetone/alcohol decolor-izing mixture over the slide. Pour until the runoff is clear (approximately 1 minute).				
10. ✦	Lay the slide on the slide rack and tray.				
11. ⋆	Pour safranin dye on the slide and allow it to stain for 30 seconds.				
12. ✦	Lift the slide angled vertically with the forceps and rinse gently.				
13. ✦	Let the slide air-dry vertically, or blot—do not wipe—the stained area with a paper towel				

		PRACTICE TRIAL	GRADED TRIAL #1	GRADED TRIAL #2	NOTES:
14. ✦	Mount the slide on the microscope for examination.				
15. ✦	Return supplies to storage.				
16. *	Clean the work area.				
17. ✦	Dispose of biohazardous waste and sharps in the appropriate containers.				
18. ✦	Dispose of the gloves and wash your hands.				

Name: _____

Date: _____

Document: Enter the appropriate information in the chart below.

Grading

Points Earned	_____		
Points Possible	_____	120	120
Percent Grade (Points Earned/Points Possible)	_____		
PASS:	_____	❏ YES ❏ NO ❏ N/A	❏ YES ❏ NO ❏ N/A

Instructor Sign-Off

Instructor: _____ Date: _____

Procedure 13-4

Instruct a Patient in Collecting a Fecal Specimen for Occult Blood or Culture Testing

Objective: The student, using the supplies and equipment listed below, will demonstrate how to provide verbal and written instruction to the patient.

Supplies: *Fecal Occult Blood:* patient chart, testing kit, clean and dry large-mouth container with spatula, patient label and laboratory requisition form, if needed, disposable gloves, black ink pen. *Fecal Culture Testing:* patient chart, specimen container for transport, spatula, patient label and laboratory requisition form, if needed, disposable gloves, black ink pen.

Notes to the Student:

_____

_____

_____

_____

_____

_____

Skills Assessment Requirements

Read and familiarize yourself with the procedure; complete the minimum practice requirements. Document each MPR using proper charting technique. Complete each procedure within a reasonable amount of time, with a minimum of 85% accuracy.

POINT VALUE ✦ = 3-6 points ⋆ = 7-9 points		PRACTICE TRIAL	GRADED TRIAL # 1	GRADED TRIAL # 2	NOTES:
1. ✦	Wash your hands.				
2. ✦	Gather supplies.				
3. ✦	Check the kit to make sure it has not expired.				
4. ⋆	Greet and identify the patient. Escort him or her to the examination room.				
5. ✦	Ask the patient what he or she understands about the reason(s) for the test. Clarify the information as needed to help the patient understand.				
6. ✦	Inform the physician if further discussion would benefit the patient.				
7. ⋆	Provide verbal instructions for fecal occult blood or culture testing. Reinforce them by giving the patient a written copy of the instructions and the appropriate test kit supplies, lab requisitions, and patient identification labels.				
	For *fecal occult blood specimen collection*, instruct the patient as follows.				
8. ✦	Using the spatula provided for each slide, place a thin smear over the first square (labeled A).				
9. ✦	Take a small specimen from a different area and smear it over the second square (labeled B).				
10. ✦	Close the flap covering the slide.				

		PRACTICE TRIAL	GRADED TRIAL #1	GRADED TRIAL #2	NOTES:
11. ✦	Allows the slide to air-dry.				
12. ✦	Repeat these steps for the remaining two slides, according to the physician's order.				
13. ✦	Return the three slides to the medical office as soon as possible.				
	For *fecal culture specimen collection*, instruct the patient as follows.				
14. ✦	After collecting the specimen in a clean, dry container, tighten the container lid.				
15. ✦	Transport the specimen immediately or transfer it to a preservative container.				
16. ⋆	Document on the chart the instructions you gave and the patient's understanding.				
17. ✦	Wash your hands.				

Document: Enter the appropriate information in the chart below.

Grading

Points Earned	_____		
Points Possible	_____	111	111
Percent Grade (Points Earned/Points Possible)	_____		
PASS:	_____	❏ YES ❏ NO ❏ N/A	❏ YES ❏ NO ❏ N/A

Instructor Sign-Off

Instructor: _____ Date: _____

Procedure 13-5

Perform a Wound or Throat Culture Using Sterile Swabs

Objective: The student, using the supplies and equipment listed below, will perform swab culture collection and prepare it for transport and processing.

Supplies: *Wound*: patient chart, single- or double-swab collection device (one swab for culture inoculation and one for Gram stain), setup for anaerobic culture (for nonsuperficial wound, if physician ordered), specimen label, disposable gloves. *Throat*: patient chart, tongue depressor, sterile swab and transport device, specimen label, disposable gloves

Notes to the Student:

_____

_____

_____

_____

_____

_____

Skills Assessment Requirements

Read and familiarize yourself with the procedure; complete the minimum practice requirements. Document each MPR using proper charting technique. Complete each procedure within a reasonable amount of time, with a minimum of 85% accuracy.

Name: _____

Date: _____

POINT VALUE ✦ = 3-6 points ⋆ = 7-9 points		PRACTICE TRIAL	GRADED TRIAL # 1	GRADED TRIAL # 2	NOTES:
1. ✦	Wash your hands.				
2. ✦	Gather supplies.				
3. ⋆	Identify and greet the patient, then escort him or her to the examination room. Explain the process of specimen collection.				
4. ✦	Wash your hands again and put on disposable gloves.				
	Wound specimen collection:				
5. ✦	Mentally note the type and amount of drainage; any redness, warmth, or swelling in the surrounding area; any other abnormalities.				
6. ✦	Swab the inside of the wound. Do not swab the surrounding skin area.				
7. ✦	Place the swab in the transport container and medium, if used.				
	Throat culture specimen collection:				
8. ✦	Ask the patient to open the mouth wide and extend the tongue forward.				
9. ✦	Examine the throat and observe for redness, swelling of throat tissue, amount and type of drainage, or the presence of white patches or pustules.				
10. ✦	Place the tongue depressor firmly on the tongue and press down.				

	PRACTICE TRIAL	GRADED TRIAL # 1	GRADED TRIAL # 2	NOTES:
11. ✦ Swab the posterior pharynx between the tonsillar pillars. Note: be careful not to touch the sterile swab to the teeth, tongue, or roof of mouth.				
12. ✦ Place the swab in the transport container and medium, if used.				
13. ★ Label the container with the patient's name (first and last), date and time of collection, and source of specimen.				
14. ✦ Dispose of any waste materials in the appropriate container(s).				
15. ✦ Remove and dispose of gloves. Wash your hands.				
16. ✦ Transport the specimen to the testing area.				
17. ★ Perform the required charting or laboratory documentation relating to specimen collection.				

Name: _____

Date: _____

Document: Enter the appropriate information in the chart below.

Grading

Points Earned	_____		
Points Possible	_____	111	111
Percent Grade (Points Earned/Points Possible)	_____		
PASS:	_____	❏ YES ❏ NO ❏ N/A	❏ YES ❏ NO ❏ N/A

Instructor Sign-Off

Instructor: _____ Date: _____

CHAPTER 14
Hematology and Chemistry

CHAPTER OUTLINE

Review the Chapter Outline. If any content area is unclear, review that area before beginning workbook exercises.

A. The Medical Assistant's Role in Hematology and Chemistry

B. The Anatomy and Physiology of Blood

C. Blood Collection Equipment and Procedures

D. Performing Basic Laboratory Testing

E. Blood Chemistry Testing

CHAPTER REVIEW

The following is a summary of the chapter. If any of this material is unclear, review it in the textbook.

There are many procedures for the medical assistant in this specialty area of patient care. Understanding the anatomy and physiology of the hematology system and the chemical components of blood are the building blocks to performing venipuncture using various methods and veins. The proper preparation, collection, and transport of specimens are vital to the reliability of test results in such areas as RBC and WBC counts, differential smears, hematocrit, and erythrocyte sedimentation rates (ESR). Chemical tests that may be performed include glucose and cholesterol.

LEARNING ACTIVITIES AND STUDY AIDS

Review the following study aids and/or complete the activities to ensure that you have achieved the learning objectives for this chapter.

1. Review the chapter to discuss the medical assistant's role in blood specimen collection in the POL.

_____

_____

_____

_____

_____

_____

_____

_____

2. List the three formed (or cellular) components of blood, then explain the difference between serum and plasma.

_____

_____

_____

_____

_____

_____

3. In your own words, describe how blood cells are formed and what the term for blood cell formation is?

_____

_____

_____

_____

_____

_____

4. What is immunohematology and how does it differ from hematology?

_____

_____

_____

_____

_____

_____

_____

5. List each item of equipment and supplies used in blood collection through the following methods.
   butterfly method

_____

_____

_____

   evacuation system

_____

_____

_____

6. When drawing more than one tube of blood from a patient, you must follow the correct order of draw to ensure valid test results. Why?

_____

_____

_____

_____

_____

_____

_____

_____

_____

7. Describe the differences between venipuncture and capillary puncture.

_____

_____

_____

_____

_____

_____

_____

8. List important considerations in the transport of blood specimens.

_____

_____

_____

_____

_____

_____

_____

9. For the following blood tests that the MA typically performs, briefly describe what the test result will tell the doctor that will assist him or her with determining the diagnosis and treatment.

   a. hemoglobin and hematocrit

   _____

   _____

   b. WBC differential

   _____

   _____

   c. ESR (erythrocyte sedimentation rate)

   _____

   _____

10. Since the MA often uses chemistry analyzers in the POL, state the common blood chemistry tests that analyzers can be utilized for as stated in your textbook.

   _____

   _____

_____

_____

_____

_____

_____

_____

11. Discuss the basics of blood typing.

_____

_____

_____

_____

_____

_____

_____

_____

MEDICAL TERMINOLOGY REVIEW

Use a dictionary and highlighted terms in the textbook to define the following terms.

Terms

agglutination _____

_____

anticoagulant _____

_____

coagulation _____

_____

diluent _____

_____

dyscrasia _____

_____

erythrocytes _____

_____

hematology _____

_____

hemostasis _____

_____

immunohematology _____

_____

leukocytes _____

_____

phagocytic _____

_____

phlebotomist _____

_____

phlebotomy _____

_____

plasma _____

_____

serum _____

_____

spectrophotometric _____

_____

thrombocytes _____

_____

venipuncture _____

_____

Abbreviations

FBS _____

_____

HGB _____

_____

MCH _____

_____

MCHC _____

_____

MCV _____

_____

NCCLS _____

_____

PMN _____

_____

CRITICAL THINKING

1. A patient needs to have blood drawn for an ESR and a glucose level. The patient is extremely nervous and worried about the pain she will experience with a blood draw and asks if you can "stick her finger" instead. Will that work in this scenario? Tell why or why not.

_____

_____

_____

_____

2. You have drawn three tubes of blood in a gray top, a lavender top, and a green top. You filled the lavender top first, then the gray top, then the green top. Is this the correct order of draw? If not, what could possibly happen because of this?

_____

_____

_____

_____

3. A patient has come in today for a blood draw to check her cholesterol level. She is 78 years old, has fragile skin, and her veins are impossible to see. Which method of phlebotomy would you use on this patient and why?

_____

_____

_____

_____

4. A patient needs a blood draw today but presents with a rash on both antecubital fossas, and you do not want to draw in this compromised area of skin. What would be your next choice of site and why?

_____

_____

_____

_____

5. Your next patient for phlebotomy today is a 6-year-old child. What special considerations are appropriate for this patient?

_____

_____

_____

_____

CHAPTER REVIEW TEST

MULTIPLE CHOICE

Circle the letter of the correct answer.

1. Which two of the following terms mean the same thing? (circle both terms)

   a. venipuncture
   b. phlebotomy
   c. capillary puncture
   d. antecubital

2. The tourniquet in a hand draw should be about _____ above the wrist.

   a. 2 inches
   b. 3 inches
   c. 4 inches
   d. 5 inches

3. Quality control assessment in basic laboratory testing includes all of the following except:

   a. check of supplies.
   b. check of reagents.
   c. reporting needlesticks.
   d. test performance.

4. A blood hematocrit is defined as the volume of _____ in a given volume of blood and is usually measured as a percentage of the total blood volume.
   a. WBCs
   b. RBCs
   c. platelets
   d. serum

5. The most common site for a blood draw is _____.
   a. wrist.
   b. hand.
   c. foot.
   d. antecubital fossa.

6. A blood draw should be done with the needle bevel up and at a _____ degree angle.
   a. 10
   b. 20
   c. 30
   d. 40

7. Which of the following blood types is known as the universal recipient?
   a. A
   b. B
   c. AB
   d. O

8. Which of the following is not a reason to use a capillary puncture?
   a. The patient is too young for a draw in the antecubital area.
   b. Adults have difficult veins to find.
   c. The patient is too nervous about the pain of an antecubital draw.
   d. A small amount of blood is required.

9. Which three of the following are methods of measuring an ESR.
   a. Zeta
   b. Peta
   c. Westergren
   d. Wintrobe

10. When performing a WBC and platelet count, you will use two of the items listed below. (circle both terms)
    a. Unopette
    b. Accu-Check
    c. glucometer
    d. hemacytometer

TRUE/FALSE

Indicate whether the statement is true (T) or false (F).

_____ 1. A large red top glass tube has no additive but only a clot activator in it.

_____ 2. In relation to blood, agglutination means clumping.

_____ 3. Capillary puncture is also called dermal puncture.

_____ 4. Sometimes charting may not be required for phlebotomy because laboratory processing documentation is sufficient.

_____ 5. Wait until all blood tubes have been collected before asking the patient to release his or her fist.

_____ 6. The National Committee for Clinical Laboratory Standards (NCCLS) has instituted a recommended order of draw to minimize the effects of additive carryover.

_____ 7. MCV, MVHV, and MCV are used to differentiate specific types of anemia.

_____ 8. When drawing blood, you should not promise the patient that the procedure will not hurt.

_____ 9. Always ask the patient if he or she has an allergy to latex when preparing to put on a tourniquet as many are made of latex.

_____ 10. Type O blood is known as the universal donor.

FILL-IN THE BLANK

Using words from the list below, fill in the blanks to complete the following statements.

adhesive-free	electrolytes	skin
ankle or lower extremity	emotionally needy	skin may tear easily
blood glucose	followed instructions	special consideration
butterfly needle (winged infusion)	lancets	special preparation
capillary	leakproof container	transporting
cell counter or analyzer	manual methods	trigger
creatinine	metabolic panel	venous
diabetics	oils from the skin	weak or compromised veins
elderly	permission	
	sealed biohazard bag	

1. Make sure the patient has _____ for the tests ordered as some laboratory tests require _____ beforehand.

2. When _____ blood specimens, place them in an approved _____, such as a _____, before transporting.

3. When an automated _____ is not available, you may nave to rely on _____ to do the cell counts and hematocrits.

4. For patients with _____, or veins that are not easily seen or felt, _____ blood specimens can be drawn more easily with a _____ system.

5. When measuring _____ using a glucomoeter, do not touch the strip to the patient's _____ because _____ may affect the test results.

6. Coban is an _____, self-adhering wrap or bandage that is used for patients allergic to adhesive or whose _____ with adhesive bandaids.

7. The physician's _____ may be required when the MA determines that an _____ vein is the only site to use on a particular patient.

8. The following are those patients who will need _____ or adaption of the procedure of blood drawing: _____, children, the _____, bleeders, and difficult or _____ patients.

9. _____ puncture is performed with special _____ that are usually disposable and have a _____ that releases the actual puncturing device.

10. A basic _____ is a group of chemistry tests that includes glucose, _____, BUN, and _____.

Procedure 14-1

Perform a Butterfly Draw Using a Hand Vein

Objective: The student, using the supplies and equipment listed below, will demonstrate how to obtain a venous blood specimen from the back of the hand using a butterfly system.

Supplies: gloves; sterile butterfly package; cotton balls; tourniquet; vacutainer or syringe; bandage, Coban, or paper tape; alcohol; sharps container; permanent pen for marking lab sample; patient chart

Notes to the Student:

_____

_____

_____

_____

_____

_____

Skills Assessment Requirements

Read and familiarize yourself with the procedure; complete the minimum practice requirements. Document each MPR using proper charting technique. Complete each procedure within a reasonable amount of time, with a minimum of 85% accuracy.

POINT VALUE ✦ = 3-6 points ⋆ = 7-9 points		PRACTICE TRIAL	GRADED TRIAL #1	GRADED TRIAL #2	NOTES:
1. ✦	Wash your hands and gather the equipment.				
2. ⋆	Identify the patient and escort him or her to the treatment area.				
3. ✦	Select the appropriate hand site. Put on gloves.				
4. ✦	Cleanse the skin with alcohol.				
5. ✦	Open the sterile butterfly package and stretch the tubing slightly to prevent it from recoiling when you begin the blood draw.				
6. ✦	Apply the tourniquet to the patient's wrist area, proximal to the wrist bone, at least 3 inches above the venipuncture site.				
7. ✦	Have the patient make a fist or hold a stress ball or roll of gauze to slightly elevate the hand.				
8. ⋆	Enter the vein with the needle. The bevel should face upward, at a 30-degree angle to the skin. Advance the needle into the vein. Some people prefer to pinch the wings upward to hold the needle, while others prefer to hold just one wing from the side. If you enter the vein correctly, you will see blood "flash" into the hub of the needle, occasionally into the tubing. Hand veins have a tendency to "roll," so you may want to do a single-finger or double-finger anchor.				

		PRACTICE TRIAL	GRADED TRIAL # 1	GRADED TRIAL # 2	NOTES:
9. ✦	*Single-finger anchor:* With your thumb, pull the skin taut toward the patient's knuckles to hold the vein in place. Do not put excessive pressure on the vein, as it will collapse and be difficult to enter.				
10. ✦	*Double-finger anchor:* Place your thumb below the puncture site and pull the skin toward the knuckles. Place the index finger of the same hand above the puncture site with slight pressure . You will insert the needle between your two fingers, so take great care to avoid an accidental needle stick.				
11. ✦	When blood appears in the tubing, release the tourniquet.				
12. ⋆	With the needle secured in the vein, pull back on the plunger to obtain the necessary amount of blood for testing. If you are taking blood from the anetcubital space with a vacutainer, advance the tube onto the collection hub with your other hand, using the wings for support.				
13. ✦	When you have obtained the correct amount of blood, break the suction of the vacutainer by removing the tube. (If you are using a syringe, there is no suction.)				

	PRACTICE TRIAL	GRADED TRIAL # 1	GRADED TRIAL # 2	NOTES:
14. ✦ Place a cotton ball or gauze pad over the puncture site without pressure and remove the needle.				
15. ✦ Discard the needle and butterfly collection tubing into a sharps container.				
16. ✦ Bandage as necessary.				
17. ⋆ Label the blood specimen and fill out the laboratory paperwork.				

Name: _____

Date: _____

Document: Enter the appropriate information in the chart below.

Grading

Points Earned	_____		
Points Possible	_____	114	114
Percent Grade (Points Earned/Points Possible)	_____		
PASS:	_____	❑ YES ❑ NO ❑ N/A	❑ YES ❑ NO ❑ N/A

Instructor Sign-Off

Instructor: _____ **Date:** _____

Procedure 14-2

Demonstrate a Venipuncture Using the Evacuation System

Objective: The student will be able to perform a venipuncture using an evacuation system.

Supplies: phlebotomy tray *or* individual items (antiseptic pads, appropriate vacutainers, holder, and needle), tourniquet, handwritten or preprinted specimen order or requisition, appropriate labels, disposable gloves, sharps container

Notes to the Student:

_____

_____

_____

_____

_____

Skills Assessment Requirements

Read and familiarize yourself with the procedure; complete the minimum practice requirements. Document each MPR using proper charting technique. Complete each procedure within a reasonable amount of time, with a minimum of 85% accuracy.

Name: _____

Date: _____

POINT VALUE ✦ = 3-6 points ⋆ = 7-9 points		PRACTICE TRIAL	GRADED TRIAL #1	GRADED TRIAL #2	NOTES:
1. ⋆	Review the physician's order. Verify that the order is legible, includes a diagnosis and other necessary information, and is signed by the physician or his or her assigned person. If any test order is not legible, or if there is any confusion about which test has been ordered, contact the physician or the office nurse for confirmation. Document the correct tests and the name of the person who confirmed the order on the physician's order.				
2. ✦	Wash your hands.				
3. ✦	Prepare the laboratory requisition from the physician's order.				
4. ✦	Make sure all routine and special supplies are available for venipuncture and transporting the specimen.				
5 ⋆	Identify the patient and escort him or her to the treatment area.				
6. ✦	Verify that the patient has been properly prepared.				
7 ✦	Position and reassure the patient.				
8. ✦	Wash your hands and put on disposable gloves.				
9. ✦	Prepare the needle. **For evacuated tubes and holder:** Thread the appropriate needle into the holder until it is secured, using the needle sheath as a wrench.				

		PRACTICE TRIAL	GRADED TRIAL # 1	GRADED TRIAL # 2	NOTES:
10. ✦	**For a syringe:** Insert the needle into the syringe. Move the plunger within the barrel to check movement.				
11. ✦	Apply the tourniquet. Wrap it around the patient's upper arm 3 to 4 inches above the antecubital fossa. Cross the ends of the tourniquet and pull them snugly against the patient's arm. With your thumb and forefinger, hold the tourniquet in place while pulling a loop of one end behind the joined area.				
12. ✦	Select the venipuncture site.				
13. ✦	Ask the patient to make a fist.				
14. ✦	Palpate the antecubital area with your index finger to determine the exact vein location and needle entry site.				
15. ✦	Clean the antecubital area (or other selected site) with an antiseptic wipe, cotton ball soaked in antiseptic, or alcohol wipe. Use a circular motion from the venipuncture site outward.				
16. ✦	Insert the blood collection tube into the holder and onto the needle up to the recessed guideline on the needle holder. Avoid pushing the tube beyond the guideline to prevent loss of vacuum.				

		PRACTICE TRIAL	GRADED TRIAL # 1	GRADED TRIAL # 2	NOTES:
17. ✦	**To perform the venipuncture:** Make sure the patient's arm (or other venipuncture site) is in a downward position to prevent reflux or "backflow."				
18. ✦	Grasp the patient's arm firmly but gently.				
19. ✦	Draw the patient's skin taut with your thumb to anchor the vein.				
20. *	Line the needle bevel-up with the vein. With a single, direct puncture, enter the vein at a 15- to 30-degree angle.				
21. ✦	Hold the needle holder firmly and steadily, and then push the tube forward in the holder until the stopper is punctured with the rear of the needle.				
22. *	As soon as blood is flowing freely, release the tourniquet by pulling on the free end above the loop.				
23. ✦	Ask the patient to release his or her fist. Fill the tubes in the correct order of draw. Invert any tubes containing anticoagulant.				
24. ✦	Remove the last tube from the holder.				
25. ✦	Withdraw the needle from the patient's arm.				
26. ✦	Immediately place a clean gauze pad over the site. Apply pressure or instruct the patient to apply pressure.				

	PRACTICE TRIAL	GRADED TRIAL #1	GRADED TRIAL #2	NOTES:
27. ✦ Remove the needle from the hub and discard the needle in an approved container. Or, if using a syringe, after filling the tubes in the correct order of draw, discard the syringe in an approved container.				
28. ∗ Label each tube with the patient's first and last name, identification number, date and time of collection, and your initials or identifying code. Or, if preprinted computer labels are available, initial each label and attach the labels to the appropriate tubes.				
29. ✦ Check the venipuncture site to make sure bleeding has stopped, and bandage it. Instruct the patient to leave the bandage on for at least 15 minutes.				
30. ✦ Remove and dispose of your gloves. Wash your hands.				
31. ✦ Evaluate the patient for signs of faintness or color loss. If the patient appears stable, thank the patient for cooperating and escort him or her back to the waiting room.				

Document: Enter the appropriate information in the chart below.

Grading

Points Earned	_____		
Points Possible	_____	201	201
Percent Grade (Points Earned/Points Possible)	_____		
PASS:	_____	❏ YES ❏ NO ❏ N/A	❏ YES ❏ NO ❏ N/A

Instructor Sign-Off

Instructor: _____   **Date:** _____

Name: _____

Date: _____

Procedure 14-3

Perform a Capillary Puncture with Microcollection Tubes

Objective: The student, using the supplies and equipment listed below, will demonstrate a capillary puncture.

Supplies: phlebotomy tray or individual items (antiseptic pads and capillary puncture and collection devices), handwritten or preprinted specimen labels, disposable gloves, sharps container

Notes to the Student:

_____

_____

_____

_____

_____

_____

Skills Assessment Requirements

Read and familiarize yourself with the procedure; complete the minimum practice requirements. Document each MPR using proper charting technique. Complete each procedure within a reasonable amount of time, with a minimum of 85% accuracy.

Name: _____

Date: _____

POINT VALUE ✦ = 3-6 points ⋆ = 7-9 points		PRACTICE TRIAL	GRADED TRIAL # 1	GRADED TRIAL # 2	NOTES:
1. ⋆	Review the physician's order and prepare the laboratory requisition.				
2. ✦	Gather the supplies for capillary puncture and specimen transport.				
3. ✦	Wash your hands.				
4. ⋆	Ask the patient to state his or her name. Ask the parents or guardian of babies or young children for identification information. Escort the patient or the parent/guardian with the child to the treatment area.				
5. ✦	Verify that the patient has followed test preparation instructions such as changing the diet or taking special medications and is not allergic to latex.				
6. ✦	Position and reassure the patient.				
7. ✦	Select an age-appropriate dermal puncture site where there is no danger of contact with bone. If possible, warm the site with a warming device or a warm, moist cloth (no warmer than 40°C/105°F) for three minutes.				
8. ✦	Wash your hands and put on disposable gloves.				
9. ✦	Clean the site with an antiseptic wipe, usually 70 percent isopropyl alcohol. Allow the area to thoroughly air-dry, or dry it with clean gauze.				

		PRACTICE TRIAL	GRADED TRIAL # 1	GRADED TRIAL # 2	NOTES:
10. ✦	Choose a puncturing device of the appropriate size. Remove the safety indicator and discard it in the appropriate biohazardous waste container.				
11. ⋆	Place the puncturing device firmly on the prepared skin surface, so that the lancet cuts across the grooves of the finger or heel print. Press the safety trigger to release the puncturing lancet.				
12. ✦	For a finger stick, massage gently from the hand to near the puncture site, keeping the hand below elbow level to obtain the required blood sample.				
13. ⋆	Wipe away the first drop of blood with clean gauze. The first drop contains tissue fluids and may contaminate the blood sample.				
14. ✦	Follow the correct order of draw for capillary puncture specimens to fill the tubes to the fill line: lavender, the other additive tubes, then red.				

		PRACTICE TRIAL	GRADED TRIAL # 1	GRADED TRIAL # 2	NOTES:
15. ★	Collect the specimen by holding the scoop of the microcollection tube directly beneath the puncture site. Apply gentle pressure at the puncture site ends, opening the puncture slightly to maximize blood flow. (For a finger stick, apply gentle, intermittent pressure on the entire finger to allow the capillaries to refill with blood and to help ensure continuous blood flow.)				
16. ✦	Lightly touch the collection scoop to the underside of the drop of blood so that the blood flows through the scoop and into the collection tube.				
17. ✦	Gently tap each tube containing anticoagulant after the addition of each drop of blood to ensure that the blood falls to the anticoagulant/blood mixture.				
18. ✦	After filling the tube, invert it back and forth eight to ten times.				
19. ✦	When the blood collection is complete, wipe the site dry and apply pressure with clean gauze until the bleeding stops.				
20. ✦	Apply a cloth tape bandage to the puncture site.				
21. ✦	Dispose of all used sharps and biohazardous waste in the appropriate containers.				

		PRACTICE TRIAL	GRADED TRIAL # 1	GRADED TRIAL # 2	NOTES:
22. ★	Label each tube with the patient's first and last name, identification number, date and time of collection, and your initials or identifying code. Or, if preprinted computer labels are available, initial each label and attach the labels to the appropriate tubes.				
23. ✦	Remove the disposable gloves and discard appropriately. Wash your hands.				
24. ✦	Instruct the patient, or the patient's parent or guardian, to remove the bandage after at least 15 minutes. Thank the patient or parent/guardian for cooperating or assisting.				
25. ✦	Escort the patient to the waiting room for further instructions.				

Document: Enter the appropriate information in the chart below.

Grading

Points Earned	_____		
Points Possible	_____	168	168
Percent Grade (Points Earned/Points Possible)	_____		
PASS:	_____	❏ YES ❏ NO ❏ N/A	❏ YES ❏ NO ❏ N/A

Instructor Sign-Off

Instructor: _____   Date: _____

Name: _____

Date: _____

Procedure 14-4

Perform a WBC and Platelet Count with a Unopette Vial and Hemacytometer

Objective: The student will be able to perform a WBC and platelet count with a Unopette vial and hemacytometer.

Supplies: Unopette vial and pipette unit, hemacytometer with Neubauer ruling, petri dish, sterile gauze squares, disposable gloves, sharps container, biohazardous waste container

Notes to the Student:

_____

_____

_____

_____

_____

_____

Skills Assessment Requirements

Read and familiarize yourself with the procedure; complete the minimum practice requirements. Document each MPR using proper charting technique. Complete each procedure within a reasonable amount of time, with a minimum of 85% accuracy.

POINT VALUE ✦ = 3-6 points * = 7-9 points	PRACTICE TRIAL	GRADED TRIAL # 1	GRADED TRIAL # 2	NOTES:
1. ✦ Wash your hands.				
2. ✦ Gather equipment and supplies.				
3. ✦ Place the Unopette vial on a flat surface. Push the pipette shield through the diaphragm into the neck of the vial.				
4. ✦ Remove the pipette assembly from the vial, then remove the pipette shield.				
5. * Holding the pipette horizontally, touch the tip to the blood sample—venous, mixed EDTA anticoagulated, or capillary. The capillary action filling the pipette will stop when the blood reaches the capillary bore end in the pipette neck.				
6. ✦ Clean any blood from the outside of the pipette, being careful not to remove any blood from the pipette bore.				
7. * Squeeze and maintain a slight pressure on the Unopette vial to force out the air but not the liquid.				
8. ✦ With your index finger, cover the opening of the pipette overflow chamber. Insert the pipette into the punctured neck opening of the Unopette vial.				
9. ✦ Remove your index finger from the pipette opening. The resulting negative pressure draws blood into the diluent.				

		PRACTICE TRIAL	GRADED TRIAL #1	GRADED TRIAL #2	NOTES:
10. ✦	Rinse the capillary pipette bore by gently squeezing the vial two or three times. Thoroughly mix the blood and diluent by swirling the vial.				
11. ✦	Leave the vial standing for 10 minutes to hemolyze the red blood cells.				
12. ✦	Invert the vial to thoroughly remix and suspend the cells in the fluid.				
13. ⋆	Convert to a dropper assembly by withdrawing the pipette from the reservoir and reseating it in the reverse position.				
14. ✦	Gently squeeze the sides of the vial and discard the first three or four drops. Fill the chamber of the Neubauer hemacytometer with the diluted blood.				
15. ✦	Place the hemacytometer on moistened paper in a petri dish. Cover the petri dish and leave it standing for 10 minutes to allow the cells to settle.				
16. ⋆	**Count and calculate for WBCs and platelets:** *For WBCs,* examine under 40X microscope power with lower light. Count all the white blood cells in the nine large squares of the counting chamber. Count the opposite side in the same manner. Add both sides and divide by two to obtain the average.				

		PRACTICE TRIAL	GRADED TRIAL #1	GRADED TRIAL #2	NOTES:
	Calculation formula: average count × 10/9 × 100 = WBC/mm^3				
17. ⋆	*For platelets,* examine under 40X microscope power with lower light.				
	Count all the platelets in center secondary square of the Neubauer ruling of the counting chamber.				
	Count the opposite side in the same manner. Add both sides and divide by two for the average.				
	Calculation formula: average count × 9 × 10/9 × 100 = PLT/mm^3				
18. ✦	Dispose of all used sharps and biohazardous waste in the appropriate containers.				
19. ✦	Remove the disposable gloves and discard appropriately. Wash your hands.				

Name: _____

Date: _____

Document: Enter the appropriate information in the chart below.

Grading

Points Earned	_____		
Points Possible	_____	129	129
Percent Grade (Points Earned/Points Possible)	_____		
PASS:	_____	❏ YES ❏ NO ❏ N/A	❏ YES ❏ NO ❏ N/A

Instructor Sign-Off

Instructor: _____ **Date:** _____

Procedure 14-5

Prepare a Blood Smear for a Differentiated Cell Count

Objective: The student, using the supplies and equipment listed below, will demonstrate how to prepare a blood smear for a differentiated cell count.

Supplies: materials for venipuncture or capillary puncture, microscope, two glass slides, gauze squares, disposable gloves, sharps container, biohazardous waste container

Notes to the Student:

_____

_____

_____

_____

_____

_____

Skills Assessment Requirements

Read and familiarize yourself with the procedure; complete the minimum practice requirements. Document each MPR using proper charting technique. Complete each procedure within a reasonable amount of time, with a minimum of 85% accuracy.

POINT VALUE ✦ = 3-6 points ⋆ = 7-9 points		PRACTICE TRIAL	GRADED TRIAL # 1	GRADED TRIAL # 2	NOTES:
1. ✦	Wash your hands. Gather equipment and supplies.				
2. ✦	Ensure that the microscope is clean and working properly.				
3. ⋆	Greet and the identify patient and escort him or her to the laboratory draw area.				
4. ✦	Wash your hands and put on disposable gloves.				
5. ⋆	Obtain a drop of blood by any one of the following methods. Place the blood drop 1/2 to 1 inch from the label end of the slide. *For a capillary puncture:* • Puncture the skin per the capillary puncture method. • Wipe the first drop of blood away with a sterile gauze square. Lightly touch the second drop of blood to a slide. *For a fresh venous specimen:* • After you withdraw the needle from the venipuncture site, immediately touch the drop of blood lightly to a slide. *For a venous specimen from a vacutainer:* • Place a capillary tube in the vacutainer. It will automatically draw the correct amount of blood.				

		PRACTICE TRIAL	GRADED TRIAL # 1	GRADED TRIAL # 2	NOTES:
	• With sterile gauze, wipe away any blood from the outside of the tube, being careful not to remove the blood from the tip. • Lightly touch the drop of blood from the capillary tube to a slide.				
6. ✦	Place the second slide lengthwise, in front of, and in contact with the drop of blood. Allow the blood to spread along the edge of the slide by capillary action.				
7. ⋆	At a 30° angle and applying only light pressure, pull the second slide toward the opposite edge of the first slide After sliding approximately 1 inch and as the specimen is feathering, lift the second slide in a sliding arch away from the first slide.				
8. ✦	Allow the slide to air-dry.				
9. ⋆	Label the slide and place it next to the microscope for examination.				
10. ✦	Follow institutional procedure for the cell count, which is performed by a designated individual.				
11. ✦	Dispose of all used sharps and biohazardous waste in the appropriate containers.				
12. ✦	Remove the disposable gloves and discard appropriately. Wash your hands.				
13. ⋆	Document the procedure in the chart or log per institutional procedure.				

Document: Enter the correct information in the chart below.

Grading

Points Earned	_____		
Points Possible	_____	93	93
Percent Grade (Points Earned/Points Possible)	_____		
PASS:	_____	❏ YES ❏ NO ❏ N/A	❏ YES ❏ NO ❏ N/A

Instructor Sign-Off

Instructor: _____ **Date:** _____

Procedure 14-6

Prepare a Smear Stained with Wright's Stain

Objective: The student, using the supplies and equipment listed below, will demonstrate how to prepare a blood smear stained with Wright's stain.

Supplies: clean glass slides (more than needed, in case of a break); transfer device, either a pipette or a capillary tube; blood specimen; Wright's stain; disposable gloves.

Notes to the Student:

_____

_____

_____

_____

_____

_____

Skills Assessment Requirements

Read and familiarize yourself with the procedure; complete the minimum practice requirements. Document each MPR using proper charting technique. Complete each procedure within a reasonable amount of time, with a minimum of 85% accuracy.

Name: ____________________

Date: ____________________

POINT VALUE
✦ = 3-6 points
⋆ = 7-9 points

		PRACTICE TRIAL	GRADED TRIAL # 1	GRADED TRIAL # 2	NOTES:
1. ✦	Have all the necessary materials in your laboratory work station.				
2. ✦	Wash your hands and put on the gloves.				
3. ✦	Mix the blood sample. If it has separated, gently swirl it in the tube.				
4. ✦	With a pipette, take a small sample of the blood and drop it on the slide, approximately 1/4 inch from the end of the slide.				
5. ✦	Hold the end of the slide with one hand. With your other hand, place the other slide directly in front of the blood specimen at a 30-degree angle.				
6. ✦	Pull the spreader slide back into the drop of blood, just until contact is made. This will cause the blood to spread out along the edge of the slide in a thin line. You should be pulling the blood back toward the closer end of the slide.				
7. ✦	To avoid air bubbles, push the spreader slide back toward the opposite end of the slide in a quick, smooth motion, being careful to maintain the 30-degree angle.				

		PRACTICE TRIAL	GRADED TRIAL # 1	GRADED TRIAL # 2	NOTES:
8. ✦	Allow the slide to dry.				
9. ✦	When the slide is dry, label the thick end of the smear with a pencil.				
10. ✦	Place the slide on a staining rack with the blood side up. Flood the smear with Wright's stain.				
11. ✦	Follow the instructions for the waiting time, generally 1 to 3 minutes.				
12. ✦	Add a buffer in an amount equivalent to the Wright's stain. Mix the stain and buffer and blow gently on the mixture for several minutes until a green, metallic sheen appears.				
13. ✦	Rinse the slide completely with distilled water.				
14. ✦	Allow the excess water to drain off the slide and stand it on end to allow it to dry.				

Document: Enter the appropriate information in the chart below.

Grading

Points Earned	_____		
Points Possible	_____	84	84
Percent Grade (Points Earned/Points Possible)	_____		
PASS:	_____	❏ YES ❏ NO ❏ N/A	❏ YES ❏ NO ❏ N/A

Instructor Sign-Off

Instructor: _____ Date: _____

Procedure 14-7

Perform a Microhematocrit by Capillary Tube

Objective: The student, using the supplies and equipment listed below, will demonstrate how to perform a microhematocrit.

Supplies: heparinized capillary tubes, microhematocrit centrifuge, microhematocrit reader, tube sealer or sealing clay, gauze squares, disposable gloves, sharps container, biohazardous waste container

Notes to the Student:

_____

_____

_____

_____

_____

_____

Skills Assessment Requirements

Read and familiarize yourself with the procedure; complete the minimum practice requirements. Document each MPR using proper charting technique. Complete each procedure within a reasonable amount of time, with a minimum of 85% accuracy.

Name: _____

Date: _____

POINT VALUE ✦ = 3-6 points ⋆ = 7-9 points		PRACTICE TRIAL	GRADED TRIAL # 1	GRADED TRIAL # 2	NOTES:
1. ✦	Wash your hands.				
2. ✦	Gather equipment and supplies.				
3. ⋆	Greet and identify the patient and escort him or her to the laboratory draw area. Explain the procedure.				
4. ✦	Wash your hands and put on disposable gloves.				
5. ✦	Perform a capillary puncture or venipuncture.				
6. ✦	Fill a capillary tube with capillary or well-mixed anticoagulated blood approximately 3/4 full.				
7. ✦	Wipe excess blood off the outside of the tube.				
8. ✦	Repeat steps 6 and 7. You will use the second tube as a counterbalance weight in the centrifuge or as a second test to confirm the accuracy of the results.				
9. ✦	Holding each capillary tube by its sides, place the blood-filled end in the sealing clay to form a plug. Pull the tube straight up and out of the sealing clay.				
10. ⋆	Place the capillary tubes in the microhematocrit head grooves opposite each other. Make sure the sealed ends of the tubes face away from the center of the centrifuge and are touching the outside rim of the centrifuge head.				

		PRACTICE TRIAL	GRADED TRIAL # 1	GRADED TRIAL # 2	NOTES:
11. ✦	Attach and secure the lid of the centrifuge.				
12. ✦	Centrifuge the capillary tubes at 12,000 RPM for the optimum time stated on the instrument, usually 2 to 5 minutes.				
13. ✦	Remove the capillary tubes after the centrifuge has stopped spinning.				
14. ✦	Place one centrifuged capillary tube into the groove on the clear plastic piece of the microhematocrit reader with the plug end toward the reader bottom center. The reference line near the top of the groove should be under the separation line in the capillary tube where the clay plug and the RBCs meet.				
15. ✦	Rotate the bottom of the reader plate so that the metal stop on the outer rim makes contact with the left edge of the grooved piece.				
16. ✦	Holding the bottom plate steady, rotate the top plate to align the outer edge of the spiral line with the outer edge of the plasma meniscus.				
17. ✦	Rotate the entire bottom portion of the reader clockwise until the spiral line intersects the line separating the buffy coat and plasma layer.				

	PRACTICE TRIAL	GRADED TRIAL #1	GRADED TRIAL #2	NOTES:
18. ★ Read the results on the ruled scale where the red line intersects it.				
19. ✦ Dispose of all used sharps and biohazardous waste in the appropriate containers.				
20. ✦ Remove the disposable gloves and discard appropriately. Wash your hands.				
21. ★ Document the percentage results on the laboratory requisition or other designated area of the chart.				

Document: Enter the appropriate information in the chart below.

Grading

Points Earned	_____		
Points Possible	_____	138	138
Percent Grade (Points Earned/Points Possible)	_____		
PASS:	_____	❏ YES ❏ NO ❏ N/A	❏ YES ❏ NO ❏ N/A

Instructor Sign-Off

Instructor: _____ Date: _____

Procedure 14-8

Perform an ESR Using the Wintrobe Method

Objective: The student, using the supplies and equipment listed below, will demonstrate performing an ESR using the Wintrobe method.

Supplies: Wintrobe tube (calibrated in millimeters), Wintrobe pipette rack, pipette bulb, DTA-anticoagulated patient blood sample, gauze squares, disposable gloves, sharps container, biohazardous waste container

Notes to the Student:

_____

_____

_____

_____

_____

_____

Skills Assessment Requirements

Read and familiarize yourself with the procedure; complete the minimum practice requirements. Document each MPR using proper charting technique. Complete each procedure within a reasonable amount of time, with a minimum of 85% accuracy.

Name: _____

Date: _____

		PRACTICE TRIAL	GRADED TRIAL # 1	GRADED TRIAL # 2	NOTES:
POINT VALUE ✦ = 3-6 points ⋆ = 7-9 points					
1. ✦	Wash your hands.				
2. ✦	Gather equipment and supplies.				
3. ⋆	Greet and identify the patient and escort him or her to the laboratory draw area. Explain the procedure.				
4. ✦	Wash your hands and put on disposable gloves.				
5. ✦	Perform a capillary puncture or venipuncture.				
6. ✦	Mix thoroughly an EDTA-anticoagulated tube of patient blood.				
7. ✦	Attach a disposable pipette bulb to the top of the Wintrobe tube.				
8. ✦	Place the tip of the Wintrobe tube in the blood specimen. With the pipette bulb, draw a blood sample to the 0 mark.				
9. ✦	Place the filled Wintrobe tube in an exactly vertical position in the rack. Set a timer for 60 minutes.				
10. ⋆	At the end of 60 minutes, record the number of mm the red blood cells have fallen. This result is the sed rate in mm/hr.				
11. ✦	Dispose of all used sharps and biohazardous waste in the appropriate containers.				
12. ✦	Remove the disposable gloves and discard appropriately. Wash your hands.				
13. ⋆	Document the sed rate in mm/hr on the laboratory requisition or other designated area of the chart.				

Name: _____

Date: _____

Document: Enter the appropriate information in the chart below.

Grading

Points Earned	_____		
Points Possible	_____	87	87
Percent Grade (Points Earned/Points Possible)	_____		
PASS:	_____	❑ YES ❑ NO ❑ N/A	❑ YES ❑ NO ❑ N/A

Instructor Sign-Off

Instructor: _____ Date: _____

Procedure 14-9

Measure Blood Glucose Using Accu-Chek™ Glucometer

Objective: The student, using the supplies and equipment listed below, will demonstrate how to measure blood glucose with a glucometer and record patient results.

Supplies: Accu-Chek™ glucometer, Accu-Chek™ test strips, glucose control solutions, puncture device, sterile 2 × 2 gauze, disposable gloves, sharps container, biohazardous waste container

Notes to the Student:

_____

_____

_____

_____

_____

_____

Skills Assessment Requirements

Read and familiarize yourself with the procedure; complete the minimum practice requirements. Document each MPR using proper charting technique. Complete each procedure within a reasonable amount of time, with a minimum of 85% accuracy.

POINT VALUE ✦ = 3-6 points ⋆ = 7-9 points		PRACTICE TRIAL	GRADED TRIAL # 1	GRADED TRIAL # 2	NOTES:
1. ✦	Wash your hands.				
2. ✦	Gather equipment and supplies.				
3. ✦	Verify that calibration and quality control have been performed and are acceptable.				
4. ⋆	Greet and identify the patient and escort him or her to the laboratory draw area. Explain the procedure.				
5. ✦	Wash your hands and put on disposable gloves.				
6. ✦	Check the expiration date on the test strip bottle. Obtain a different bottle if the expiration date has passed.				
7. ✦	Turn on the glucometer by pressing the ON button.				
8. ✦	Follow the manufacturer's directions for entering the 3-digit test-strip code in the display if the glucometer code does not match the code on the test strip bottle.				
9. ✦	Enter the patient identification number. (Home glucometers may not require this information.)				
10. ✦	Wait for the indicator that the monitor is ready for a test strip. Within the short time frame specified by the glucometer model, insert one test strip as directed into the monitor.				

		PRACTICE TRIAL	GRADED TRIAL # 1	GRADED TRIAL # 2	NOTES:
11. ✦	Remove the monitor from the charging station.				
12. ✦	Obtain a capillary blood specimen from the patient following standard procedure for capillary blood collections. Venous or arterial specimens may also be used.				
13. ∗	Touch the edge of the test strip to the drop of blood. The blood will be pulled into the strip. Fill the target area of the strip completely.				
14. ✦	The glucose result will appear in the time frame specified by the manufacturer, usually within 30 seconds.				
15. ✦	Remove the test strip and discard in a biohazard container. Dispose of the lancet or blade in the sharps container.				
16. ✦	Return the monitor to the charging/storage unit.				
17. ✦	Remove the disposable gloves and discard appropriately. Wash your hands.				
18. ∗	Document the date, time, finger used, patient's tolerance of the procedure, and results in the designated area of the chart.				

Hematology and Chemistry **383**

Document: Enter the appropriate information in the chart below.

Grading

Points Earned	_____		
Points Possible	_____	117	117
Percent Grade (Points Earned/Points Possible)	_____		
PASS:	_____	❑ YES ❑ NO ❑ N/A	❑ YES ❑ NO ❑ N/A

Instructor Sign-Off

Procedure 14-10

Determine Cholesterol Level with the ProAct Testing Device

Objective: The student, using the supplies and equipment listed below, will demonstrate how to measure cholesterol level using a ProAct testing device.

Supplies: ProAct testing device, capillary tube containing lithium heparin, lancet device, 2 X 2 gauze pads, sterile, alcohol pads, disposable gloves, patient's chart

Notes to the Student:

_____

_____

_____

_____

_____

_____

Skills Assessment Requirements

Read and familiarize yourself with the procedure; complete the minimum practice requirements. Document each MPR using proper charting technique. Complete each procedure within a reasonable amount of time, with a minimum of 85% accuracy.

POINT VALUE ✦ = 3-6 points ∗ = 7-9 points		PRACTICE TRIAL	GRADED TRIAL # 1	GRADED TRIAL # 2	NOTES:
1. ✦	Wash your hands and put on the gloves.				
2. ∗	Verify the physician's order and the patient's identity. Explain the procedure to the patient.				
3. ✦	Load the lancet device according to the directions.				
4. ✦	Choose a puncture site free of broken skin or bruising.				
5. ✦	Wipe the patient's finger with an alcohol wipe and allow to dry.				
6. ∗	Puncture the finger and wipe away the first drop of blood that forms with the sterile gauze.				
7. ✦	Hold the capillary tube horizontal to the patient's finger, making sure no air bubbles enter the tube. If air bubbles enter, you must throw away the tube and start over again.				
8. ✦	When the tube has filled, remove it and have the patient put pressure on the puncture site with a sterile gauze square.				
9. ✦	Remove a testing strip from the container and peel away the protective foil. Place the strip on a hard work surface.				
10. ✦	Attach the filled capillary tube to the pipette.				

		PRACTICE TRIAL	GRADED TRIAL # 1	GRADED TRIAL # 2	NOTES:
11. ✦	Without touching the tip of the capillary tube to the testing strip, place one drop in the center of the application zone.				
12. ∗	Allow the blood droplet to soak into the testing mesh for 15 to 20 seconds.				
13. ✦	Place the strip in the ProAct device port. The device will start to count down approximately 160 seconds.				
14. ✦	While the machine is running, clean the test area. Throw the pipette and capillary tube into a sharps container.				
15. ✦	When the LED screen indicates, remove the test strip and observe it for uneven color development. (If the color is uneven, you will need to perform the entire test again.)				
16. ✦	Discard the test strip into a biohazardous container.				
17. ∗	Record the test results as displayed in the patient's chart.				

Document: Enter the appropriate information in the chart below.

Grading

Points Earned	_____		
Points Possible	_____	114	114
Percent Grade (Points Earned/Points Possible)	_____		
PASS:	_____	❏ YES ❏ NO ❏ N/A	❏ YES ❏ NO ❏ N/A

Instructor Sign-Off

Instructor: _____ Date: _____

Procedure 14-11

Perform a Mononucleosis Test

Objective: The student, using the supplies and equipment listed below, will demonstrate how to test for infectious mononucleosis.

Supplies: Mono-Test kit, nonsterile disposable gloves, blood serum or plasma, disposable capillary tube

Notes to the Student:

_____

_____

_____

_____

_____

_____

Skills Assessment Requirements

Read and familiarize yourself with the procedure; complete the minimum practice requirements. Document each MPR using proper charting technique. Complete each procedure within a reasonable amount of time, with a minimum of 85% accuracy.

POINT VALUE ✦ = 3-6 points ✱ = 7-9 points		PRACTICE TRIAL	GRADED TRIAL #1	GRADED TRIAL #2	NOTES:
1. ✱	Bring all liquid reagents to room temperature. Check the expiration date of all reagents in the kit.				
2. ✦	Wash and dry your hands and put on disposable gloves.				
3. ✦	After obtaining a blood sample from the patient and processing it to separate the serum, fill the capillary tube to the marked line with the serum.				
4. ✦	Using the glass slide and rubber bulb in the kit, place a small drop of the specimen serum in the first of the three circles on the slide.				
5. ✦	Place a single drop of the negative control in the second circle on the slide.				
6. ✦	Place a single drop of the positive control in the third circle.				
7. ✦	Holding the bottle of Mono-Test reagent upright between your palms, gently roll it back and forth, making certain that the reagent RBCs that have settled in the tube are mixed thoroughly.				
8. ✦	Hold the dropper 1 inch above the slide and place one drop of reagent into each of the three circles. Make certain the dropper does not come into contact with the slide and become contaminated.				

		PRACTICE TRIAL	GRADED TRIAL # 1	GRADED TRIAL # 2	NOTES:
9. ✦	Using the enclosed stirrers, one for each circle, quickly and thoroughly mix each area and spread it out to the full 1-inch diameter of the circle.				
10. ✦	Observe the slide as you rock it back and forth gently for exactly 2 minutes.				
11. ⋆	Agglutination is a positive test result; no agglutination is negative. Verify the test results by comparing them to the positive and negative controls on the slide.				
12. ✦	Clean the work area, disposing of the test in a biohazardous container. Wash your hands.				
13. ⋆	Record the test results.				

Document: Enter the appropriate information in the chart below.

Grading

Points Earned	_____		
Points Possible	_____	87	87
Percent Grade (Points Earned/ Points Possible)	_____		
PASS:	_____	❑ YES ❑ NO ❑ N/A	❑ YES ❑ NO ❑ N/A

Instructor Sign-Off

Instructor: _____ Date: _____

CHAPTER 15
Urology and Nephrology

CHAPTER OUTLINE

Review the Chapter Outline. If any content area is unclear, review that area before beginning workbook exercises.

- A. The Medical Assistant's Role in Urology and Nephrology
- B. The Anatomy and Physiology of the Urinary System
- C. Renal Diseases
- D. Diagnostic Procedures
- E. Urinalysis
- F. The Male Reproductive System

CHAPTER REVIEW

The following is a summary of the chapter. If any of this material is unclear, review it in the textbook.

As in all body systems and specialties, the medical assistant must know the anatomy and physiology of the system. In this chapter, the urinary system and the male reproductive system are discussed. Knowledge of the functions and diseases of both systems, including infertility, is required. The medical assistant will collect specimens; perform urinalysis, including physical and chemical and setup of microscopic examination of urine; perform patient teaching such as how to do a testicular self-exam; and assist the physician with procedures.

LEARNING ACTIVITIES AND STUDY AIDS

Review the following study aids and/or complete the activities to ensure that you have achieved the learning objectives for this chapter.

1. After reading the chapter in your textbook, state what is included in the medical assistant's role in urology and nephrology.

   _____

   _____

   _____

   _____

   _____

   _____

   _____

   _____

2. List the four primary structures of the urinary system and state the function of each one.

_____

_____

_____

_____

_____

_____

_____

3. Review the appropriate section in this chapter of your textbook and make a flash card about how urine is formed in the kidneys. List the nephron, the glomerulus, proximal tubule, loop of nephron (Henle), the distal tubule, and the collecting ducts and include the functions of each part on the flash card.

_____

_____

_____

_____

_____

_____

_____

_____

4. Review the narrative information in your textbook to make flash cards of the common renal diseases or conditions listed below. State the name of the disease and a brief description on each card.

a. chronic renal failure _____

_____

_____

b. acute renal failure _____

_____

c. pyelonephritis _____

_____

d. neurogenic bladder _____

_____

e. hydronephrosis _____

_____

f. renal calculi _____

_____

_____

5. When a patient is in end stage renal disease, there are two types of dialysis used for treatment. Review the information in your textbook and then, using your own words, briefly describe both types of dialysis.

_____

_____

_____

_____

_____

_____

_____

6. Urinary system infections originate in the urethra and bladder. Answer the following questions regarding these UTIs:

   a. When the infections migrate to the kidney, what is the name of the condition?

   _____

   _____

   b. What are two reasons that females get cystitis?

   _____

   _____

   c. How should a female cleanse the area of the urethra to avoid this?

   _____

   _____

   d. Why are females more prone to UTIs than males?

   _____

   _____

7. What causes neurogenic bladder? What does the term *incontinence* mean? What are three causes of incontinence (one is in females only)?

_____

_____

_____

_____

_____

_____

_____

8. List two common obstructive disorders of the urinary system. What are the two types of treatments for renal calculi discussed in the textbook? Check a medical dictionary or medical terminology textbook for the meanings of the following word *parts*: calcul/o, extra, litho, tripsy.

_____

_____

_____

_____

_____

9. State one noninvasive diagnostic test and three invasive procedures used in the diagnosis of urinary diseases and disorders.

_____

_____

_____

_____

_____

_____

10. Make flashcards of the nine points of urine specimens and their testing goals—make them as brief as possible and in your own words. Note only what you may not remember or just enough to jog your memory if you are on extern or on the job and do not have time to read through the material in the textbook.

_____

_____

_____

_____

_____

_____

_____

11. Physical characteristics of urine indicate various conditions, both normal and abnormal. State the normal values of appearance—color, odor, pH, specific gravity, blood, and leukocytes.

_____

_____

_____

_____

_____

_____

12. What is the purpose of using chemical test strips in urinalysis?

_____

_____

_____

_____

_____

_____

13. State the formed elements that can be viewed in a microscopic examination of urine.

_____
_____
_____
_____
_____
_____
_____

14. State the external structures and the internal structures of the male reproductive system.

_____
_____
_____
_____
_____
_____

15. List and describe the diseases and disorders of the male reproductive system. List the three conditions/diseases of the prostate gland and those of the male reproductive system.

_____
_____
_____
_____
_____
_____
_____

MEDICAL TERMINOLOGY REVIEW

Use a dictionary and highlighted terms in the textbook to define the following terms.

Terms

aliquot _____
_____

anuria _____
_____

bilirubin _____
_____

crescentic _____

_____

cryptorchism _____

_____

cystitis _____

_____

dialysis _____

_____

distal tubule _____

_____

electrolytes _____

_____

fistula _____

_____

flank _____

_____

glomerulonephritis _____

_____

glomerulus _____

_____

hematuria _____

_____

hydronephrosis _____

_____

incontinence _____

_____

jaundice _____

_____

kidney _____

_____

lithotripsy _____

_____

loop of nephron _____

_____

nephrologist _____

_____

nephrology _____

_____

nephrons _____

_____

nocturia _____

oliguria _____

periorbital edema _____

plasmapheresis _____

polyuria _____

prodromal _____

prostatitis _____

proteinuria _____

proximal tubule _____

pyelonephritis _____

pyuria _____

renal _____

renal calculus (plural: calculi) _____

sequela (plural: sequelae) _____

testis (plural testes, also called testicle) _____

trigone _____

turbidity _____

ureter _____

urethra _____

urinalysis _____

urinary bladder _____

_____

urinary meatus _____

_____

urobilinogen _____

_____

urologist _____

_____

urology _____

_____

Abbreviations

BPH _____

_____

DRE _____

_____

ESRD _____

_____

UA _____

_____

UTI _____

_____

CRITICAL THINKING

1. You drew blood for a PSA after your patient has been examined by the physician. What is wrong with this?

_____

_____

_____

_____

2. If you were working in a fertility clinic within a urology practice, you would undoubtedly have preprinted history forms specifically designed to elicit reproductive and fertility-related information. When the patient has the initial evaluation, the MA would go over the form with the patient after he or she has completed it, or would ask the questions and complete the form with the patient. Although this is not discussed in your textbook specifically, think of five questions that might be on that form.

_____

_____

_____

_____

3. Imagine this scenario: You are a female. You have completed your externship and have been hired by a urology clinic in your first full-time medical assistant position. You are directed by the physician to instruct a patient in performing a testicular self-exam. You are suddenly nervous about doing this to a real patient even though you have practiced this in your medical assisting program with other students. Describe in one or two paragraphs how you would feel and what you would do or tell yourself to bolster your own comfort and confidence.

_____

_____

_____

_____

4. You are to instruct a 68-year-old female patient in the collection of a 24-hour urine specimen. Explain this, in your own words, as if you were speaking to the patient. Avoid medical terms that the patient may not understand very well but avoid treating the patient as if she is a child.

_____

_____

_____

_____

5. You have collected a clean-catch urine specimen from Mrs. Gonzalez, a long-time patient, and you have already performed the physical assessment of the color, odor, and clarity. Following are the results of your chemical testing. Fill in the normal value for each, circle those that are abnormal as if flagging them for the physician, and then state the possible reasons for the abnormal results.

	Your Results on Mrs. Gonzalez	Normal Value	Possible Causes
Color	orange-red		
Clarity	cloudy		
pH	7.8		
Specific gravity	1.026		
Protein	++ or positive		
Glucose	0		
Ketones	0		
Bilirubin	0		
Urobilinogen	4		
Blood	+		
Leukocytes	++++		
Nitrite	0		

CHAPTER REVIEW TEST

MULTIPLE CHOICE

Circle the letter of the correct answer.

1. Which of the following is not an electrolyte?

    a. calcium

    b. potassium

    c. sodium

    d. nucleic acid

2. Circle the tests that are invasive.

    a. cystoscopy

    b. urinalysis

    c. IVP

    d. voiding cystogram

3. Circle the three answers that apply to complete the following statement: In an IVP, the contrast media is used to enhance details of the _____ and _____.

    a. prostate

    b. kidneys

    c. urethra

    d. bladder

4. Certain aspects of three functions of the kidney can be tested with a urinalysis. Choose those three from the following list.

    a. water balance

    b. waste excretion

    c. endocrine regulatory activity

    d. acid-base balance

5. Changes in pH can:

    a. break down or alter chemical constituents.

    b. precipitate crystals or dissolve crystals already present.

    c. affect urine color.

    d. disintegrate cells and casts that were present.

6. A 24-hour urine specimen is collected to measure specific urine components. Circle those in the list below that are affected by hydration, activity and exercise, and metabolic rate, and which vary throughout the day.

    a. cancer

    b. creatinine

    c. calcium

    d. ketones

    e. potassium

    f. specific gravity

    g. protein

    h. glucose

    i. urea nitrogen

    j. lead levels

    k. drug levels

7. Which of the following techniques are appropriate when testing urine with a chemical test strip? (circle all those that apply)

    a. Do not touch the reactive reagent materials on the strips.

    b. Tighten the lid of the bottle immediately after removing a strip.

    c. Dry the strips immediately if any moisture falls into or collects in the bottle.

    d. Check the expiration date of the strips.

8. Which of the following is *not* a true statement about male reproductive/fertility disorders based on the material in your textbook?
   a. A urologist may be the one to diagnose and treat male infertility problems.
   b. Previous infectious diseases of the system can lead to infertility.
   c. African American males are at greater risk for prostate and bladder cancers.
   d. Cryptorchism is a testicular disorder.
   e. All of the above are true.

9. Which of the following is a formed element in urine that can be viewed under a microscope? (circle all that apply)
   a. parasites
   b. sperm cells
   c. creatinine
   d. epithelial cells
   e. platelets
   f. yeast

10. Sexually active couples who do not conceive after _____ of unprotected sex are considered to have a fertility problem.
    a. one year
    b. two years
    c. six months
    d. nine months

TRUE/FALSE

Indicate whether the statement is true (T) or false (F).

_____ 1. The loop of Henle is an instrument used in cystoscopy.

_____ 2. DRE stands for digital rectal examination.

_____ 3. Peritoneal analysis is the term for peritoneal analysis.

_____ 4. Females are more prone to UTIs than males due to a longer urethra.

_____ 5. An IVP is used to diagnosis renal calculus.

_____ 6. The urologist specializes in treating urinary system diseases and conditions, and the fertility specialist treats male reproductive diseases and conditions.

_____ 7. Sperm cells are also called spermatogens.

_____ 8. A thin tube that is inserted into the urinary bladder to withdraw urine is called a catheter.

_____ 9. A male can contract an STD through blood and body fluids.

_____ 10. Each region of the nephron plays a major role in the kidney formation of urine.

FILL IN THE BLANK

Using words from the list below, fill in the blanks to complete the following statements.

15 and 40	color change	specific gravity
20 and 35	discomfort or pain	STDs
abnormal	genitals	sterility
bladder and urethra	life-threatening	testicular self-exam
cancer	pathogens	urethra and meatus
catheter	physical	urinalysis
catheterization	physiological	urine components
cleaned	reagent pad	water
color	red or red-brown	water balance

1. Although the _____ are normally sterile, a urine specimen can be contaminated with microorganisms from the lower portion of the _____.

2. The patient should feel no _____ after the _____ is removed.

3. Each _____ on a chemical test strip is saturated with chemicals that react with _____ to produce a predictable _____.

4. _____ is the measurement of a specific volume of urine to an equal volume of _____.

5. As with a female patient, it is imperative that the male patient's _____ be appropriately and thoroughly _____ before _____ to prevent the introduction of _____.

6. A refractometer is used to determine the _____ of urine in the _____ portion of a _____.

7. The most common set of _____ shades of color of urine is _____.

8. One of the _____ functions of the kidneys is maintaining the body's _____ by adjusting the amount or water in the urine.

9. Untreated _____ are spread unknowingly, can cause _____, and may even become _____.

10. Testicular _____ is relatively common between the ages of _____, although males between the ages of _____ should perform a monthly _____.

Procedure 15-1

Demonstrate Patient Instruction for a Clean-Catch Urine Specimen

Objective: The student, using the supplies and equipment listed below, will demonstrate how to instruct the patient on obtaining a clean-catch specimen.

Supplies: sterile specimen container, label, antiseptic wipes, chart, requisition slip (if necessary)

Notes to the Student:

_____

_____

_____

_____

_____

_____

Skills Assessment Requirements

Read and familiarize yourself with the procedure; complete the minimum practice requirements. Document each MPR using proper charting technique. Complete each procedure within a reasonable amount of time, with a minimum of 85% accuracy.

POINT VALUE ✦ = 3-6 points * = 7-9 points		PRACTICE TRIAL	GRADED TRIAL # 1	GRADED TRIAL # 2	NOTES:
1. ✦	Wash your hands. Gather equipment and supplies.				
2. *	Identify the patient and guide him or her to the treatment area.				
	Instruct the patient to:				
3. ✦	Wash the hands.				
4. ✦	Open the sterile urine container and place the lid on a flat area with the inside facing up.				
5. ✦	Open the antiseptic wipes and place them on top of their packaging.				
6. *	*If male:* Retract the foreskin, if present. Cleanse the glans penis with the antiseptic wipes with a circular motion from the meateal opening and proceeding outward. Repeat, using all the antiseptic wipes.				
7. *	*If female:* Spread the labia apart with one hand. Wipe from front to back. Use one wipe to cleanse one side, then discard the wipe. Cleanse the other side with a new wipe and discard it. Finally, with a new wipe, cleanse down the middle across the meatus, and discard the wipe.				

		PRACTICE TRIAL	GRADED TRIAL # 1	GRADED TRIAL # 2	NOTES:
8. ★	After cleansing, the patient should: • Discard all the used wipes in an appropriate waste container. • Void some urine into the toilet and stop (an uncircumcised male should also bring the foreskin forward). • Restart voiding to half-fill the sterile container. • Finish voiding into the toilet. • Wash the hands. • Put the lid on the container without touching the inside of the lid. • Place it in the designated receiving site.				
9. ✦	Wash your hands.				
10. ★	Chart your observations of the urine specimen as well as the date, time collected, and tests ordered.				
11. ✦	If the specimen is to be tested at another laboratory, complete a laboratory requisition slip. Take the specimen to the lab or refrigerator or add preservative.				

Document: Enter the appropriate information in the chart below.

Grading

Points Earned	_____		
Points Possible	_____	81	81
Percent Grade (Points Earned/Points Possible)	_____		
PASS:	_____	❏ YES ❏ NO ❏ N/A	❏ YES ❏ NO ❏ N/A

Instructor Sign-Off

Instructor: _____   **Date:** _____

Procedure 15-2

Demonstrate Patient Instruction for Collection
of a 24-Hour Specimen

Objective: The student, using the supplies and equipment listed below, will demonstrate the ability to instruct the patient to obtain a quality 24-hour specimen for accurate testing, diagnosis, and treatment.

Supplies: 24-hour specimen container, smaller collection container, patient instruction sheet, chart, requisition slip

Notes to the Student:

_____

_____

_____

_____

_____

_____

Skills Assessment Requirements

Read and familiarize yourself with the procedure; complete the minimum practice requirements. Document each MPR using proper charting technique. Complete each procedure within a reasonable amount of time, with a minimum of 85% accuracy.

POINT VALUE ✦ = 3-6 points ∗ = 7-9 points		PRACTICE TRIAL	GRADED TRIAL # 1	GRADED TRIAL # 2	NOTES:
1. ✦	Wash your hands. Gather equipment and supplies.				
2. ∗	Identify the patient and guide him or her to the treatment area.				
	Instruct the patient to:				
3. ✦	Wash the hands.				
4. ✦	Void into the toilet upon arising record the time (from this time and for the next 24 hours, all urine will go into the 24-hour collection container).				
5. ∗	Void all urine into the smaller collection container to pour into the larger container. Each time wash, rinse, and air-dry the smaller container. After each specimen is placed in the larger specimen container, screw the lid tightly and put it in the refrigerator or portable cooler.				

		PRACTICE TRIAL	GRADED TRIAL #1	GRADED TRIAL #2	NOTES:
6. ✦	At the end of the 24-hour period, bring the large container to the medical office or laboratory. (The first voided specimen of the second morning is the last specimen to be added to the container, ending the collecting period.)				
7. ✦	Ask the patient if any problems occurred during the specimen collection. If too much urine was collected or if some was spilled during collection, tell the patient a new collection must be started.				
8. ✦	Fill out a lab requisition slip for the specimen when it is brought to the office or taken directly to an outside laboratory.				
9. ⋆	Chart your observations of the urine specimen, the date, time collected, tests ordered, and any other pertinent information.				

Document: Enter the appropriate information in the chart below.

Grading

Points Earned	_____		
Points Possible	_____	63	63
Percent Grade (Points Earned/Points Possible)	_____		
PASS:	_____	❏ YES ❏ NO ❏ N/A	❏ YES ❏ NO ❏ N/A

Instructor Sign-Off

Instructor: _____ Date: _____

Procedure 15-3

Perform Catheterization of a Female Patient

Objective: The student, using the supplies and equipment listed below, will demonstrate how to perform catheterization of a female patient.

Supplies: lighting source, preferably a gooseneck lamp, sterile specimen container, sterile drapes, sterile catheterization kit or straight catheter, sterile K-Y gel or other lubricant, sterilized Mayo stand, sterile gloves, nonsterile latex gloves, biohazardous waste receptacle, several 2 × 2 sterile gauze squares (minimum of 6), Betadine or other iodine solution, maxipad or pantyliner, patient chart, lab order forms

Notes to the Student:

_____

_____

_____

_____

_____

_____

Skills Assessment Requirements

Read and familiarize yourself with the procedure; complete the minimum practice requirements. Document each MPR using proper charting technique. Complete each procedure within a reasonable amount of time, with a minimum of 85% accuracy.

Name: _____

Date: _____

POINT VALUE ✦ = 3-6 points ⋆ = 7-9 points		PRACTICE TRIAL	GRADED TRIAL # 1	GRADED TRIAL # 2	NOTES:
1. ✦	Gather all needed supplies to bring into the room. Generally, the patient will already be disrobed and covered with a drape. Bringing all supplies into the room on one trip avoid opening the door more than once while your patient is in a potentially embarrassing position.				
2. ✦	Explain the procedure to the patient and obtain verbal permission to begin touching her.				
3. ✦	If the patient is not unclothed, explain the correct dorsal recumbent position and draping.				
4. ✦	Position the gooseneck lamp to so that it is directed at the genital area, but do not turn it on, as it may heat up quickly and make the patient uncomfortable.				
5. ✦	Wash your hands and put on nonsterile gloves. Open the catheterization kit.				
6. ✦	Ask the patient to keep her knees apart and take slow deep breaths while lifting her hips off the table surface.				
7. ✦	When her hips have cleared the surface, slide a sterile drape beneath her by encircling the corners with your hands. Avoid touching the patient or the table with your hands.				

		PRACTICE TRIAL	GRADED TRIAL #1	GRADED TRIAL #2	NOTES:
8. ✦	Open a second sterile drape and place it over the patient's genital area, making sure that the vulvar area is exposed.				
9. ✦	Place the insertion portion of the kit on the sterile drape you placed under the patient's hips, between her knees.				
10. ✦	Remove the gloves and wash your hands.				
11. ✦	Following sterile technique, put on sterile gloves.				
12. ✦	Soak the 2 x 2 gauze pads in Betadine or other iodine solution.				
13. ✦	Open the sterile lubricant and place it on the sterile field on the Mayo stand. Open the remaining items, including the sterile container, and place them on the tray.				
14. ★	Cleanse the patient with the Betadine-soaked gauze squares. Separate the labia with the thumb and index finger of your nondominant hand. With your other hand, take a gauze square and wipe one side of the labia from top to bottom in one pass. Throw the square away. Take another square, repeat on the other side, and discard. Do not let the hand that is separating the labia touch and thereby contaminate your other hand.				

		PRACTICE TRIAL	GRADED TRIAL #1	GRADED TRIAL #2	NOTES:
15. ★	With a third gauze square, cleanse the urinary meatus with a circular motion, working from the inside to the outside. Discard the square.				
16. ★	With your dominant hand, pick up the catheter, your thumb and index finger approximately 3 inches from the end to be inserted.				
17. ✦	Dip the insertion end of the catheter into the sterile lubricant. Make sure the opposite end of the catheter is in the collection portion of the kit's tray.				
18. ✦	Thread the catheter into the urinary meatus approximately 2 to 3 inches, until urine begins to flow into the collection tray.				
19. ★	If you meet resistance when threading the catheter, do not force it in. Resistance can be an indication of a problem. Remove the catheter and notify the physician.				
20. ✦	After a small amount of the urine has flowed into the collection tray, move the end of the catheter into the sterile collection container.				

		PRACTICE TRIAL	GRADED TRIAL #1	GRADED TRIAL #2	NOTES:
21. ✦	Measure the urine that has flowed from the bladder. Emptying more than 500 ml at one time may cause the bladder to spasm. If more than 500 ml has been released, clamp the catheter, wait 10 to 15 minutes, and release the remainder of the urine.				
22. ✦	When the bladder is completely empty, gently remove the catheter.				
23. ✦	Secure the collection container's lid in place and prepare the paperwork for laboratory testing.				
24. ✦	Remove all supplies and dispose of them in a biohazardous container.				
25. ✦	Assist the patient in sitting up and dressing if necessary.				
26. ✦	Inform the patient that the Betadine used to cleanse the labia may stain her undergarments, and offer her a maxipad or pantyliner to protect her clothing.				
27. ∗	Document the procedure in the patient's chart.				

Document: Enter the appropriate information in the chart below.

Grading

Points Earned	_____		
Points Possible	_____	177	177
Percent Grade (Points Earned/ Points Possible)	_____		
PASS:	_____	❏ YES ❏ NO ❏ N/A	❏ YES ❏ NO ❏ N/A

Instructor Sign-Off

Instructor: _____ Date: _____

Procedure 15-4

Perform Catheterization of a Male Patient

Objective: The student, using the supplies and equipment listed below, will demonstrate how to perform catheterization of a male patient.

Supplies: lighting source, preferably a gooseneck lamp, waterproof underpad, sterile specimen container, sterile catheterization kit or straight catheter, sterile drapes, sterile K-Y gel or other lubricant, sterilized Mayo stand, sterile gloves, nonsterile latex gloves, biohazardous waste receptacle, several 2 × 2 sterile gauze squares (minimum of 6), Betadine or other iodine solution, fenestrated drape, patient chart, lab order forms

Notes to the Student:

_____

_____

_____

_____

_____

_____

Skills Assessment Requirements

Read and familiarize yourself with the procedure; complete the minimum practice requirements. Document each MPR using proper charting technique. Complete each procedure within a reasonable amount of time, with a minimum of 85% accuracy.

POINT VALUE ✦ = 3-6 points ∗ = 7-9 points		PRACTICE TRIAL	GRADED TRIAL # 1	GRADED TRIAL # 2	NOTES:
1. ✦	Wash your hands. Collect all the needed supplies and bring into patient's room.				
2. ✦	Explain the procedure to the patient and explain that it will be necessary to remove all articles of clothing from the waist down.				
3. ✦	Assist the patient, if needed, into the supine position.				
4. ✦	Wash your hands and put on nonsterile gloves.				
5. ✦	Following sterile technique, open the catheterization kit and place the items on the sterile field on the Mayo stand.				
6. ✦	Wrap the corners of the sterile underpad over your hands and place it over the patient's thighs, sliding it under the penis.				
7. ✦	Remove the gloves, wash your hands, and put on sterile gloves.				
8. ✦	Being careful not to touch the patient or the table, place a fenestrated drape over the genital area so that the penis is exposed.				
9. ✦	Soak the 2 x 2 gauze pads in Betadine and place them on the patient's thighs for easy access.				

		PRACTICE TRIAL	GRADED TRIAL # 1	GRADED TRIAL # 2	NOTES:
10. ★	With your nondominant hand, grasp the penis below the glans and hold it upright. If the patient is uncircumcised, retract the foreskin to expose the meatus.				
11. ★	With your dominant hand, cleanse the meatus with a gauze square in a circular motion, working from the inside to the outside. Discard the gauze.				
12. ✦	Repeat step 11 a total of three times, using a fresh gauze square each time you cleanse.				
13. ✦	Dip the insertion tip of the catheter into lubricant to cover the 7 or 8 inches that will be inserted into the penis. Place the opposite end of the catheter in the collection tray.				
14. ★	Hold the penis firmly at a straight, upward angle to straighten the urethra for easier insertion.				
15. ✦	Ask the patient to constrict the penis muscles in the same manner as when trying to urinate. While he is doing this, gently thread the catheter into the penis until urine begins to flow, generally 6 to 8 inches.				
16. ★	Never force the catheter. If you meet resistance, discontinue the procedure and notify the physician.				

		PRACTICE TRIAL	GRADED TRIAL # 1	GRADED TRIAL # 2	NOTES:
17. ✦	After a small amount of the urine has flowed into the collection tray, move the end of the catheter into the sterile collection container.				
18. ★	Measure the urine that has flowed from the bladder. Emptying more than 500 ml at one time may cause the bladder to spasm. If more than 500 ml has been released, clamp the catheter, wait 10 to 15 minutes, and release the remainder of the urine.				
19. ✦	When the bladder is completely empty, gently remove the catheter.				
20. ✦	Secure the collection container's lid in place and prepare the paperwork for laboratory testing.				
21. ✦	Remove all supplies and dispose of them in a biohazardous container.				
22. ✦	Assist the patient in sitting up and dressing if necessary.				
23. ✦	Inform the patient that the Betadine used to cleanse the glans may transfer to his undergarments and stain them.				
24. ★	Document the procedure in the patient's chart.				

Name: _____

Date: _____

Document: Enter the appropriate information in the chart below.

Grading

Points Earned	_____		
Points Possible	_____	162	162
Percent Grade (Points Earned/ Points Possible)	_____		
PASS:	_____	❏ YES ❏ NO ❏ N/A	❏ YES ❏ NO ❏ N/A

Instructor Sign-Off

Instructor: _____ **Date:** _____

Procedure 15-5

Perform a Urinalysis with a Chemical Test Strip and Prepare the Specimen for Microscopic Examination

Objective: The student, using the supplies and equipment listed below, will demonstrate how to perform a urinalysis with chemical test strips.

Supplies: chemical reagent urine test strips, blotting paper, urine container, centrifuge and test tubes, microscope, slide and cover slip, pipette, disposable gloves, biohazardous waste receptacle, urinalysis report form

Notes to the Student:

_____

_____

_____

_____

_____

_____

Skills Assessment Requirements

Read and familiarize yourself with the procedure; complete the minimum practice requirements. Document each MPR using proper charting technique. Complete each procedure within a reasonable amount of time, with a minimum of 85% accuracy.

POINT VALUE ✦ = 3-6 points ⋆ = 7-9 points		PRACTICE TRIAL	GRADED TRIAL # 1	GRADED TRIAL # 2	NOTES:
1. ✦	Wash your hands. Gather equipment and supplies. Check the expiration date on the reagent strip container.				
2. ⋆	Identify the patient and guide him or her to the treatment area.				
3. ✦	Provide the patient with a labeled urine container. Instruct the patient on how to obtain the specimen and where to leave it.				
4. ✦	Wash your hands. Put on disposable gloves.				
5. ✦	After the patient leaves the specimen in the designated area, move it to the testing area.				
6. ⋆	Observe and describe the urine's color, quantity, and odor. Inform the physician that the specimen is ready for testing.				
7. ✦	Remove one reagent strip and recap the bottle tightly and immediately. Do not touch the test area of the strip. If necessary, place the strip temporarily on a dry paper towel while you open the urine specimen container.				

		PRACTICE TRIAL	GRADED TRIAL # 1	GRADED TRIAL # 2	NOTES:
8. ✦	Dip the test strip briefly in the urine, making sure to cover all testing areas. Pull the strip gently back against the inner edge of the container mouth, then place the length of the strip at a right angle to the blotting paper to remove excess urine.				
9. ✦	Hold the reagent test areas of the strip next to, but not touching, the matching areas on the test strip bottle. Note the reaction reading at the time mentioned on the bottle for each square of reagent.				
10. ✦	Dispose of the urine test strip in the biohazardous waste container.				
11. ✶	**Prepare urine for microscopic examination by the physician**: Put approximately 10 cc in a tube on one side of the centrifuge, and on the opposite side an equal amount of liquid in another tube. Run the centrifuge for 5 minutes.				
12. ✦	Pour out most of the liquid (supernatant) from the tube, but keep the sediment.				

		PRACTICE TRIAL	GRADED TRIAL # 1	GRADED TRIAL # 2	NOTES:
13. ✦	Mix the remaining liquid with the sediment and pipette a couple of drops of moistened sediment onto a slide.				
14. ✦	Cover with a cover slip. Position and focus the slide under the lighted microscope.				
15. ✦	Remove the gloves and discard in proper container. Wash your hands.				
16. ⋆	Chart the results on the reporting urine lab slip immediately, including the date, time, and urine test strip brand name. Record the color, odor, volume, and cloudiness or sediment.				
17. ⋆	On the patient's chart, chart the date and time of specimen collection and procedure performance.				
18. ✦	Return to the microscope examination area for cleaning and disposal.				

Name: _____

Date: _____

Document: Enter the appropriate information in the chart below.

Grading

Points Earned	_____		
Points Possible	_____	123	123
Percent Grade (Points Earned/ Points Possible)	_____		
PASS:	_____	❏ YES ❏ NO ❏ N/A	❏ YES ❏ NO ❏ N/A

Instructor Sign-Off

Instructor: _____ Date: _____

Procedure 15-6

Demonstrate Patient Instruction for Testicular Self-Examination

Objective: The student will demonstrate how to instruct the patient on performing a testicular self-examination.

Supplies: none

Notes to the Student:

_____

_____

_____

_____

_____

_____

Skills Assessment Requirements

Read and familiarize yourself with the procedure; complete the minimum practice requirements. Document each MPR using proper charting technique. Complete each procedure within a reasonable amount of time, with a minimum of 85% accuracy.

POINT VALUE ✦ = 3-6 points ✶ = 7-9 points		PRACTICE TRIAL	GRADED TRIAL # 1	GRADED TRIAL # 2	NOTES:
1. ✦	Wash your hands.				
2. ✶	Identify the patient and guide him to the treatment area.				
3. ✦	Instruct the patient to: • Take a warm bath or shower to relax the scrotum. • In the clinical setting, the patient should take several deep breaths.				
4. ✦	Observe the contour of the scrotum. If one testicle is slightly larger or lies somewhat lower than the other, this is considered normal.				
5. ✦	Elevate the right leg to the level of a toilet, chair, or bed to expose the right testicle.				
6. ✦	With the left hand, lightly support the right testicle. With the right hand, palpate the right testicle for hardness, lumps, or anything unusual.				
7. ✦	Reverse the process by elevating the left leg to examine the left testicle. Support the left testicle with the right hand and, with the left hand, palpate the left testicle.				
8. ✦	If the patient finds any abnormalities or has any questions, he should contact the physician.				
9. ✶	Document patient education in the patient's chart.				

Name: _____

Date: _____

Document: Enter the appropriate information in the chart below.

Grading

Points Earned	_____		
Points Possible	_____	60	60
Percent Grade (Points Earned/ Points Possible)	_____		
PASS:	_____	❏ YES ❏ NO ❏ N/A	❏ YES ❏ NO ❏ N/A

Instructor Sign-Off

Instructor: _____ **Date:** _____

CHAPTER 16
Medical Imaging

CHAPTER OUTLINE

Review the Chapter Outline. If any content area is unclear, review that area before beginning workbook exercises.

- A. The Medical Assistant's Role in Medical Imaging
- B. Radiology
- C. Equipment
- D. Safety Precautions and Patient Protection
- E. Limited-Scope Radiography
- F. Scheduling Radiographs
- G. Assisting with an X-ray
- H. Filing and Loaning Radiographic Records

CHAPTER REVIEW

The following is a summary of the chapter. If any of this material is unclear, review it in the textbook.

The field of medical imaging includes radiology, sonography, and magnetic resonance imaging. The medical assistant who works with imaging must be knowledgeable about the various areas of imaging, the equipment, safety precautions, patient protection, and patient preparation. The MA usually works in limited-scope radiology but may prepare for and assist with many imaging procedures. Scheduling x-rays at other facilities, verifying insurance, and obtaining preauthorization as well as postprocedure care or instructions, if any, can all fall within the medical assistant's duties.

LEARNING ACTIVITIES AND STUDY AIDS

Review the following study aids and/or complete the activities to ensure that you have achieved the learning objectives for this chapter.

1. Assuming that you have read this chapter of your textbook at least once already, from memory list the tasks of the MA in medical imaging. Then, go back to the book and check your answers, filling in any that you may have missed.

   _____

   _____

   _____

   _____

2. Tell in your own words what an x-ray is. What purpose do x-rays serve in patient care?

_____

_____

_____

_____

_____

_____

_____

3. Next to each area of medical imaging listed below, state what each method can show or do to help you understand why certain studies are performed.

   a. radiography and contrast studies

   _____

   b. fluoroscopy

   _____

   c. computed tomography

   _____

   d. magnetic resonance imaging

   _____

   _____

   e. sonography

   _____

   _____

   f. nuclear medicine

   _____

   _____

4. Make one list of all the various types of medical imaging equipment that you find mentioned in this chapter of your textbook. Do not include disposable supplies such as pen and paper, cotton balls, etc.

   _____

   _____

   _____

   _____

   _____

   _____

5. Adherence to safety guidelines that protect both patient and technician during radiographic procedures is vital. Knowledge and understanding of those guidelines is required so that you don't have to think about them; they become habit. Make one flash card and list the basic safety guidelines in medical imaging. Make them brief and in your own words; include just enough to help you remember when on the job.

_____

_____

_____

_____

_____

_____

_____

6. State the definition of limited-scope radiography as stated in your textbook. Then utilize the Internet to find information about your state laws/regulations regarding limited-scope radiology. Possible sources of information would be the state board that licenses/certifies radiology technicians and technologists, the American Registry of Radiology Technologists, your state Department of Health, your local chapter of the American Association of Medical Assistants, or a local chapter of radiology techs.

_____

_____

_____

_____

_____

_____

_____

7. The medical assistant is often the person who schedules radiology tests at other locations. Make a list with two columns for onsite and offsite scheduling. Briefly list the important points of each as discussed in your textbook.

_____

_____

_____

_____

_____

_____

8. Explain in your own words what you would do to prepare the x-ray room for a radiographic procedure.

_____

_____

_____

_____

_____

_____

_____

9. Flash cards are excellent learning aids for memorizing information such as the terminology and abbreviations in every chapter and would also work well for most tables in this chapter. Make one card with the possible reactions to contrast media that are discussed in the Tips for Success.

_____

_____

_____

_____

_____

_____

_____

_____

10. Design a chart on one piece of paper that could be a quick reference for patient preparation and instructions for the following imaging studies:

   a. contrast upper GI

_____

_____

   b. lower GI

_____

_____

   c. IVP

_____

_____

   d. cholecystogram

_____

_____

   e. mammography procedures

_____

_____

11. Make flash cards of the proper positions for the following x-ray projections. You can use words to describe each one or use stick figures, drawings, and arrows for a visual reminder. Include AP, PA, and RL.

_____

_____

_____

_____

_____

_____

MEDICAL TERMINOLOGY REVIEW

Use a dictionary and highlighted terms in the textbook to define the following terms.

Terms

angiography _____

_____

arthrography _____

_____

cholecystography _____

_____

echocardiogram _____

_____

fluoroscopy _____

_____

mammogram _____

_____

myelography _____

_____

radiation _____

_____

radiology _____

_____

radiologist _____

_____

radiograph _____

_____

radiography _____

_____

radiolucent _____

_____

radiopaque _____

_____

sonography _____

_____

ultrasound _____

_____

x-rays _____

_____

Abbreviations

ALARA _____

_____

AP _____

_____

CAT _____

_____

CT _____

_____

LL _____

_____

MRI _____

_____

PA _____

_____

PET _____

_____

RL _____

_____

CRITICAL THINKING

1. You have placed a patient on the table for an x-ray and notice that the lead strip around the table has a few very small cracks in it. What should you do?

   _____

   _____

   _____

2. A 22-year-old female patient needs to have an x-ray of her shoulders. What must you remember to ask this particular patient that you may not ask all patients?

   _____

   _____

   _____

3. Mr. Abdul has come in for a cholecystogram. As you put the patient into the room, you verify that he has followed the preparation instructions of taking iodine the day before and then NPO this morning. He looks surprised and then admits he forgot to take the iodine. What would you do?

   _____

   _____

   _____

4. A patient comes to the front desk and does not have an appointment. She wants to get a copy of a mammogram she had at the clinic about twelve years ago. What can you tell this patient?

_____

_____

_____

_____

5. Your next patient has come in for an MRI and answers no to your question of whether he has any metal or a pacemaker implanted in his body. As the patient removes his shirt to put on a gown, you notice he has a bright-colored tattoo on his posterior right flank. What should you say?

_____

_____

_____

CHAPTER REVIEW TEST

MULTIPLE CHOICE

Circle the letter of the correct answer.

1. Which of the following are considered serious reactions to contrast medium? (circle all that apply)
   a. headache
   b. diarrhea
   c. hypotension
   d. wheezing

2. A patient lying face down is in the _____ position.
   a. lateral
   b. recumbent
   c. prone
   d. oblique

3. Which of the following is not a radiation shield containing 1/16 inch of lead?
   a. gonadal shield
   b. gloves
   c. thyroid shield
   d. half apron

4. Which of the following are types of contrast media? (circle all that apply)
   a. gas
   b. normal saline
   c. barium sulfate
   d. iodine

5. Medications with the potential to interact with iodine and cause serious reactions include: (circle all that apply)
   a. glucophage.
   b. beta-blockers.
   c. metformin.
   d. calcium channel blockers.

6. Which of the following are reasons that an MRI could not be performed on a patient? (circle all that apply)

   a. The patient has a pacemaker.
   b. The patient has a metal foreign body in his eye.
   c. The patient has metal staples in the chest.
   d. The patient has body tattoos with dye containing metal.

7. Which two of the following choices are examples of radiographs requiring contrast medium?

   a. intravenous pyelogram
   b. echocardiogram
   c. barium swallow
   d. cleansing enema

8. Adduction is moving a body part

   a. toward the midline.
   b. away from midline.
   c. upward.
   d. toward the outside.

9. Supination is

   a. turning a body part toward the midline.
   b. turning a body part away from midline.
   c. turning the palm of the hand downward.
   d. turning the palm of the hand upward.

10. When a patient takes iodine orally, he or she may have a _____ taste in the mouth.

    a. salty
    b. sour
    c. bitter
    d. metallic

TRUE/FALSE

Indicate whether the statement is true (T) or false (F).

_____ 1. The acronym ALARA stands for as low as reasonably achievable.

_____ 2. A mammogram should be scheduled one week after menses, when the breasts are less tender.

_____ 3. Flexion is increasing the angle between two bones.

_____ 4. The common x-rays in limited-scope radiography include some skull procedures.

_____ 5. Some patients may experience claustrophobia when having a CT scan or an MRI.

_____ 6. To obtain the best radiographic image possible, it is important to understand the use of anatomical landmarks to position the patient properly.

_____ 7. The effects of radiation are cumulative.

_____ 8. You must be aware of medical practice acts in your community and state regarding limited-scope radiography.

_____ 9. Although procedures vary from facility to facility, it is typical that the patient or another facility can check out an x-ray for up to 10 days.

_____ 10. A contrast medium is a radiolucent substance that provides a more accurate visualization of the internal body organs and tissues.

FILL IN THE BLANK

Using words from the list below, fill in the blanks to complete the following statements.

allergic
allowed in your state
childbearing age
computed tomography (CT)
dissecting planes
education
equal or unequal
expose and develop film

front and back
front to back
iodine or shellfish
nuclear medicine
positioning
pregnant
radioactive

safety precautions
sonography
swallows or is injected
target tissue or organ
three-dimensional
training
vertically

1. In nuclear medicine, the patient either _____ with a _____ material called a tracer that is absorbed by the _____.

2. Related to limited-scope radiology: After the appropriate _____ and if it is _____, you may be asked to _____ in addition to preparing the patient.

3. The coronal plane divides the body into _____ portions.

4. The sagittal plane divides the body _____ into _____ right and left sections.

5. In the anteroposterior view (AP), the central ray is directed from _____.

6. Any female of _____ must be asked if she could be _____.

7. Regarding patient preparation and instructions for an IVP: This procedure should not be performed on a patient who is _____ to _____.

8. Medical imaging is a specialty that encompasses radiology, _____, fluoroscopy, _____, magnetic resonance imaging (MRI), and _____.

9. Computed tomography can scan a body part in _____ or "slices," then assembles them to produce a _____, 360-degree image.

10. The medical assistant's role in medical imaging may involve patient _____, preparation, and _____, scheduling, and following _____.

Procedure 16-1

Perform General Procedure for X-Ray Examination

Objective: The student, using the supplies and equipment listed below, will demonstrate how to x-ray a patient.

Supplies: physician's order, patient chart, dosimeter badge, X-ray film, X-ray film holder, X-ray machine, processing machine, lead aprons for MA and patient, paper drapes as needed

Notes to the Student:

_____

_____

_____

_____

_____

_____

Skills Assessment Requirements

Read and familiarize yourself with the procedure; complete the minimum practice requirements. Document each MPR using proper charting technique. Complete each procedure within a reasonable amount of time, with a minimum of 85% accuracy.

POINT VALUE ✦ = 3-6 points ⋆ = 7-9 points		PRACTICE TRIAL	GRADED TRIAL # 1	GRADED TRIAL # 2	NOTES:
1. ⋆	Verify the patient's identity and the physician's order.				
2. ✦	Check the X-ray equipment.				
3. ✦	Explain the procedure to the patient.				
4. ✦	Instruct the patient to remove the appropriate clothing for the X-ray. Provide paper drapes for modesty. For chest and neck X-rays, the patient should remove all jewelry and large hair bands, which may obstruct the view of the structures.				
5. ✦	Position the patient according to the X-ray view(s) required.				
6. ✦	Set the controls with the X-ray tube and cassette at the proper distance.				
7. ✦	If necessary, ask the patient to take a deep breath and hold it.				
8. ⋆	Stand behind the lead wall or shield to take the X-ray. Instruct the patient to adjust to a comfortable position while you develop the X-rays and have them reviewed. The patient should not dress or leave the X-ray suite until the physician has indicated that the X-rays are satisfactory.				
9. ✦	With the physician's approval, assist the patient in dressing, if necessary.				
10. ✦	Label the X-ray and X-ray sleeve according to office procedure.				
11. ⋆	Document the procedure in the patient's chart.				

Document: Enter the appropriate information in the chart below.

Grading

Points Earned	_____		
Points Possible	_____	75	75
Percent Grade (Points Earned/ Points Possible)	_____		
PASS:	_____	❏ YES ❏ NO ❏ N/A	❏ YES ❏ NO ❏ N/A

Instructor Sign-Off

Instructor: _____   Date: _____

Procedure 16-2

File and Loan Radiographic Records

Objective: The student, using the supplies and equipment listed below, will demonstrate how to file and loan X-rays.

Supplies: X-ray films, consent form, larger envelope or film jacket, labels

Notes to the Student:

_____

_____

_____

_____

_____

_____

Skills Assessment Requirements

Read and familiarize yourself with the procedure; complete the minimum practice requirements. Document each MPR using proper charting technique. Complete each procedure within a reasonable amount of time, with a minimum of 85% accuracy.

POINT VALUE ✦ = 3-6 points ⋆ = 7-9 points		PRACTICE TRIAL	GRADED TRIAL #1	GRADED TRIAL #2	NOTES:
1. ✦	Place the films in a large film envelope labeled with the patient's name, DOB, date of procedure, and physician's name. The films will be taken to a radiologist to be read.				
2. ✦	If the films are to be taken by the patient to another facility or physician, note the destination and receiving physician's name on the patient record.				
3. ✦	Record the transfer of all films in a log or file, along with the time, date, patient's name, destination, and receiving physician.				
4. ⋆	Obtain the patient's signed consent for any films the patient takes from the ownership facility to another physician or diagnostic center.				

Name: _____

Date: _____

Document: Enter the appropriate information in the chart below.

Grading

Points Earned	_____		
Points Possible	_____	27	27
Percent Grade (Points Earned/ Points Possible)	_____		
PASS:	_____	❏ YES ❏ NO ❏ N/A	❏ YES ❏ NO ❏ N/A

Instructor Sign-Off

Instructor: _____   Date: _____

CHAPTER 17
Cardiology and Cardiac Testing

CHAPTER OUTLINE

Review the Chapter Outline. If any content area is unclear, review that area before beginning workbook exercises.

    A.   The Medical Assistant's Role in Cardiology

    B.   The Anatomy and Physiology of the Heart

    C.   Diseases and Disorders of the Heart

    D.   Diagnostic Tests

    E.   Identifying Arrhythmias/Dysrhythmias

CHAPTER REVIEW

The following is a summary of the chapter. If any of this material is unclear, review it in the textbook.

The cardiovascular system includes a wide variety of conditions and diseases that require testing, diagnosis, and treatment, often in the outpatient setting where the MA most likely works. As in all body systems, knowledge of the anatomy and physiology and the pathology of the cardiovascular system is vital. The medical assistant may do blood testing, perform EKGs, apply Holter monitors, schedule and possibly assist in tests such as the stress test, echocardiogram, and various scans. An MA may schedule a cardiac catheterization or other treatments, such as insertion of a stent, coronary artery bypass surgery, or a heart transplant. The signs, symptoms, diseases, and conditions the MA must know about include, but are not limited to, angina, myocardial infarction, sudden cardiac arrest, hypertension, congestive heart failure, pulmonary edema, cardiomyopathy, arrhythmias, infective and inflammatory diseases, valvular diseases, phlebitis and thrombophlebitis, embolus, and peripheral vessel conditions such as Raynaud's and Buerger's. Diagnostic tests include, but are not limited to, the EKG, echocardiograms, stress testing, thallium and MUGA scans. The signs and symptoms of an emergency situation must be recognized and acted upon immediately in this type of practice. This specialty is quite varied and offers many opportunities for the medical assistant.

LEARNING ACTIVITIES AND STUDY AIDS

Review the following study aids and/or complete the activities to ensure that you have achieved the learning objectives for this chapter.

1. Review the information in the chapter on the role of the medical assistant in a cardiology practice. State the duties an MA may perform or assist with.

_____

_____

_____

_____
_____
_____
_____

2. List the four basic anatomical parts of the heart and state each one's physiology.

_____
_____
_____
_____
_____
_____

3. Explain the electrical conduction system of the heart by starting with the SA node and listing each part of the heart that the electrical activity travels through. Briefly state what occurs in each part in a statement for each.

_____
_____
_____
_____
_____
_____
_____

4. In your own words explain coronary artery disease.

_____
_____
_____
_____
_____
_____

5. State the symptoms of angina, then explain the treatment.

_____
_____
_____
_____

_____

_____

_____

_____

6. Review myocardial infarction in the chapter. Then make a table that shows the symptoms, causes, and treatment for this disease.

Symptoms	Causes	Treatment

7. Review material in this chapter of the textbook regarding sudden cardiac arrest. Close the book and give a definition of this along with a list of the reasons it may occur. Always go back and check the material after you answer from memory, then study the areas that you may have forgotten.

_____

_____

_____

_____

_____

_____

_____

8. Review hypertension in the chapter. Then make a table that shows the symptoms, causes, diagnosis, and treatment of this silent killer.

Symptoms	Causes	Diagnosis	Treatment

9. After reading the information in your textbook, perform additional research on congestive heart failure. Check a medical dictionary or encyclopedia, the Internet (reputable sites only such as the American Heart Association or a URL ending in .edu), medical journals, medical textbooks as appropriate for the subject, or other resources. Formulate your understanding of what this condition is, not the symptoms or causes. Explain the definition in your own words.

_____

_____

_____

_____

_____

_____

_____

_____

10. Describe pulmonary edema.

_____

_____

_____

_____

_____

_____

11. Make a table of the symptoms, causes, diagnosis, and treatment of both *dilated cardiomyopathy* and *hypertrophic cardiomyopathy*.

Dilated Cardiomyopathy

Symptoms	Causes	Diagnosis	Treatment

Hypertrophic Cardiomyopathy

Symptoms	Causes	Diagnosis	Treatment

12. What are the four major classifications of cardiac arrhythmias?

_____

_____

_____

_____

_____

_____

_____

13. Compare the causes and symptoms of infective heart disorders: endocarditis, myocarditis, pericarditis, rheumatic fever, and rheumatic heart disease by listing them in the following format:

	Causes	Symptoms
Endocarditis		
Myocarditis		
Pericarditis		
Rheumatic Fever		
Rheumatic Heart Disease		

14. Compare the various valvular disorders by listing the diseases for each of the four valves and then fill in the area of physiology of each.

Valve/Condition	Physiology
Mitral	
insufficiency	
stenosis	
prolapse	
Aortic	
insufficiency	
stenosis	
Tricuspid	
insufficiency	
stenosis	
Pulmonic	
insufficiency	
stenosis	

15. Compare the vascular disorders, including embolisms, arteriosclerosis, aneurysms, phlebitis, thrombophlebitis, deep-vein thrombosis, Raynaud's disease, and Buerger's disease by filling in the definitions and symptoms of each in the table format.

	Definition	Symptoms
embolism		
arteriosclerosis		
aneurysm		
phlebitis		
thrombophlebitis		
deep-vein thrombosis		
Raynaud's disease		
Buerger's disease		

16. What is an electrocardiogram and how does it help in diagnosis of cardiac conditions?

_____
_____
_____
_____
_____
_____
_____
_____

17. Describe the Holter monitor and state its importance in diagnosis of cardiac conditions.

_____
_____
_____
_____
_____
_____
_____
_____

18. What is stress testing? What is its function in cardiology?

_____
_____
_____
_____
_____
_____
_____
_____

19. Explain the echocardiogram and its importance in cardiac diagnosis and treatment.

_____

_____

_____

_____

_____

_____

_____

_____

20. Explain the thallium scan in your own words.

_____

_____

_____

_____

_____

_____

_____

21. Describe a MUGA scan.

_____

_____

_____

_____

_____

_____

_____

22. Review the information in the textbook on arrhythmias in cardiology. Review the four aspects of classification: disturbance of impulse formation or origin, disturbance of conduction, consistency of the point of origin, and prognosis. Make four cards—one for each classification. On one side, state in one or two sentences what causes that type of arrhythmia, then on the other side of the card, list the various arrhythmias under the particular classification. Then write one sentence about each arrhythmia.

_____

_____

_____

_____

_____

_____

_____

23. Why is consent for cardiac procedures so important?

_____

_____

_____

_____

_____

_____

_____

_____

MEDICAL TERMINOLOGY REVIEW

Use a dictionary and highlighted terms in the textbook to define the following terms.

Terms

amplitude _____

_____

aneurysm _____

_____

angina _____

_____

angioplasty _____

_____

anterior _____

_____

apex _____

_____

arrhythmia _____

_____

arteriosclerosis _____

_____

artifact _____

_____

asystole _____

_____

atherosclerosis _____

_____

atrium _____

_____

augmented lead _____

_____

automaticity _____

_____

bradycardia _____

_____

cardiac catheterization _____

_____

cardiomegaly _____

_____

cardiomyopathy _____

_____

conduction system _____

_____

conductivity _____

_____

contractility _____

_____

coronary artery bypass _____

_____

coronary artery disease _____

_____

depolarization _____

_____

diastole _____

_____

dysrhythmia _____

_____

ejection fraction _____

_____

embolism _____

_____

embolus _____

_____

endocarditis _____

_____

excitability _____

_____

fibrillation _____

_____

focus _____

_____

hemoptysis _____

_____

interatrial septum _____

_____

internodal pathway _____

_____

interventricular septum _____

_____

isoelectric line _____

_____

mitral valve prolapse _____

_____

multifocal _____

_____

myocardial infarction _____

_____

myocarditis _____

_____

palpitations _____

_____

pericarditis _____

_____

precordical lead _____

_____

premature ventricular contraction (PVC) _____

_____

repolarization _____

_____

sinoatrial (SA) node _____

_____

stenosis _____

_____

stent _____

_____

systole _____

_____

tachycardia _____

_____

thromboembolism _____

_____

thrombosis _____

_____

thrombus _____

_____

unifocal _____

_____

ventricle _____

_____

Abbreviations

A-fib _____

_____

AV _____

_____

BBB _____

_____

CAB _____

_____

CABG _____

_____

CAD _____

_____

CHF _____

_____

DVT _____

_____

ECG/EKG _____

_____

EF _____

_____

MI _____

_____

MVP _____

_____

NSR _____

_____

PR _____

_____

PVC _____

_____

QRS _____

_____

SA _____

_____

ST _____

_____

V-fib _____

_____

V-tach _____

_____

CRITICAL THINKING

1. You are working at the front desk and looking out at the patients who have been waiting for their appointments. One man appears to be holding his left hand in front of his chest, he seems to be SOB, and his face looks sweaty or clammy. What is your first thought about this patient? Describe what the danger signs are to you even though the patient has not come up to the desk to voice a complaint about how is feeling. What might you ask the patient and how would you handle that?

_____

_____

_____

2. You are performing an EKG. As it is printing, you notice that there is a normal waveform and complex but the beats per minute are over 100 bpm. What do you think the problem could be? Use the information from Table 17-10, Cardiac Rhythms, to speculate on what the doctor might diagnose.

_____

_____

_____

_____

3. You are doing a history on a new patient and the patient states that she often feels that her heart has "skipped a beat." Review the information on identifying arrhythmias and dysrhythmias, then state what this may be. Then define what this condition is.

_____

_____

_____

_____

4. What would you do if a patient fell in the waiting room and had no pulse? Explain in detail.

_____

_____

_____

_____

5. You need to perform an EKG on an elderly female patient, but she seems to be nervous or fearful. What are some of the signs the patient might exhibit that lead you to the conclusion she is fearful of the EKG? How would that fear affect the EKG?

_____

_____

_____

_____

CHAPTER REVIEW TEST

MULTIPLE CHOICE

Circle the letter of the correct answer.

1. The type of hypertension that results when a prolonged state of elevated blood pressure develops without apparent cause is
   a. malignant.
   b. essential.
   c. insidious.
   d. congestive.

2. Which heart disease/condition has the following symptoms: shortness of breath, weight gain, edema, exhaustion, fluid retention possibly with swollen feet and hands and facial puffiness?
   a. pulmonary edema
   b. cardiomyopathy
   c. congestive heart failure
   d. arrhythmia

3. Which of the following is a characteristic of cardiac muscle cells? (circle all that apply)
   a. contractility
   b. excitability
   c. conductivity
   d. none of the above are characteristics

4. The pericardium is the outer surface of the sac around the heart, and inflammation of this is called
   a. pericarditis.
   b. pericardiumosis.
   c. pericardiumitis.
   d. pericardosis.

5. Which of the following is not one of the heart valves?
   a. mitral
   b. bicuspid
   c. aortic
   d. valvular

6. Myocarditis is an inflammation of the cardiac muscle caused by a (circle all that apply)
   a. bacteria.
   b. dyspnea.
   c. parasite.
   d. virus.

7. An _____ is a diagnostic test for the patency and structure of blood vessels.
   a. stress test
   b. echocardiogram
   c. angiogram
   d. cardiac catheterization

8. Sinus _____ is a normal waveform and complex but has fewer than 60 beats per minute.
   a. rhythm
   b. tachycardia
   c. bradycardia
   d. atrial fibrillation

9. The outermost layer of the heart is the
   a. endocardium.
   b. intracardium.
   c. pericardium.
   d. myocardium.

10. Which of the following are electrolytes? (circle all that apply)
    a. potassium
    b. magnesium
    c. iron
    d. sodium

TRUE/FALSE

Indicate whether the statement is true (T) or false (F).

_____ 1. Pulmonic insufficiency is when blood flow into the pulmonary artery is obstructed.

_____ 2. Myocardial infarction is often referred to as the silent killer because so many people who have it are unaware of it.

_____ 3. Rhythms originating in the SA node with normal conduction through the heart are called sinus rhythms.

_____ 4. "The heart is autorhythmic" means there is a disturbance of impulse formation.

_____ 5. Thrombophlebitis is an inflammatory condition that occurs in a vein where a thrombus has formed on the wall.

_____ 6. An electrical conduction system within the myocardium regulates the pumping action of the heart.

_____ 7. Atherosclerosis is the result of plaque buildup in the arteries over a period of years.

_____ 8. Hypertension occurs when blood pressure readings are consistently over 140/90.

_____ 9. The cardiac cycle begins with the firing of the AV node and is characterized by the T wave on the EKG.

_____ 10. Palpitations are irregular and often erratic heartbeats felt by the patient.

FILL IN THE BLANK

Using words from the list below, fill in the blanks to complete the following statements.

24-hour period	CHF	noninvasive
abnormal EKG	conduction path	pacemaker
angina-type pain	conduction system	portable
aorta and the coronary vessels	contractility	reduced blood flow
arm or groin	electrical activity	sinoatrial (SA) node
arrest	heart structures	standstill
arrhythmia	hemorrhage	surfaces
bacterial infection	inflammation	trauma
cardiac condition	interstitial fluid	visual
catheter	life-threatening situation	workload
chambers	massive insult	

1. An echocardiogram provides a _____ concept of the _____ coordinated with the _____ and the _____ of the myocardium.

2. Myocardial ischemia is the result of _____ to the myocardium, which causes _____.

3. Pulmonary edema follows _____ as the lungs fill with _____ and pressure builds in the lung tissue, increasing the _____ of the heart.

4. An electrocardiogram is a recording of the _____ of the heart.

5. The medical assistant performing EKGs must know when to alert the physician to an _____ or a _____.

6. The conduction system originates in the _____, also known as the
    _____.

7. Sudden cardiac arrest occurs when the conduction system of the myocardium sustains a
    _____, such as ischemia in the area of the essential cardiac _____,
    a lethal _____ that causes cardiac _____, electrocution, major
    _____to the chest and heart, massive _____, drug overdose, respi-
    ratory _____, and drowning.

8. Endocarditis, an _____ of the lining of the heart _____and valve
    _____, is usually the result of a _____.

9. During a cardiac catheterization, a _____ is threaded through an artery in the
    _____to the _____ and dye is injected into the vessels.

10. A Holter monitor is a _____ form of monitoring that allows _____
    recording of the patient's _____ over a _____.

Procedure 17-1

Perform an Electrocardiogram

Objective: The student, using the supplies and equipment listed below, will demonstrate how to perform a 12-lead ECG.

Supplies: Electrocardiograph with wires, electrodes, and ECG paper, patient gown and drape as necessary for privacy and warmth, alcohol pads, supplies for shaving if needed

Notes to the Student:

_____

_____

_____

_____

_____

_____

Skills Assessment Requirements

Read and familiarize yourself with the procedure; complete the minimum practice requirements. Document each MPR using proper charting technique. Complete each procedure within a reasonable amount of time, with a minimum of 85% accuracy.

POINT VALUE ✦ = 3–6 points ⋆ = 7– 9 points		PRACTICE TRIAL	GRADED TRIAL # 1	GRADED TRIAL # 2	NOTES:
1. ✦	Wash your hands. Assemble the equipment and supplies.				
2. ⋆	Identify the patient and escort him or her to the patient examination room.				
3. ✦	Explain the procedure to relieve the patient's apprehension.				
4. ✦	Ask the patient to disrobe from the waist up. Assist the patient into a gown, with the opening in front. Assure the patient that his or her privacy will be respected.				
5. ✦	Help the patient recline on the examination table or bed where the procedure will be performed.				
6. ✦	Cover the patient with the drape, leaving the arms and legs exposed. You may need to raise pants legs to expose the calves of the lower legs.				
7. ✦	Cleanse the skin with alcohol pads where the electrodes will be applied. If chest hair will interfere with contact between the electrodes and the skin, remove the hair with soap and/or shaving cream and a disposable razor.				
8. ⋆	Apply the electrodes in the correct positions, making sure the wires do not touch the cart or examination table and that they follow the normal contours of the body. The power cord should not cross under the examination table or bed.				

		PRACTICE TRIAL	GRADED TRIAL # 1	GRADED TRIAL # 2	NOTES:
9. ✦	Explain to the patient that the electrocardiograph is a sensitive machine and that he or she must remain as still as possible during the procedure.				
10. ⋆	Calibrate the electrocardiograph and run the ECG. Mark the leads if necessary.				
11. ✦	When the ECG is complete, remove the electrodes and cleanse any residual conduction gel from the patient's skin.				
12. ✦	Assist the patient in dressing. Discard the gown, if it is disposable; otherwise place it in a laundry hamper.				
13. ✦	Cleanse the equipment. Sanitize the leads by wiping them with antiseptic solution, then store them in the appropriate compartment of the electrocardiograph cart. Replace any necessary supplies. Wash your hands.				
14. ⋆	Label the electrocardiograph paper with the patient's name, DOB, and the date and time. Document the patient's tolerance of the procedure.				
15. ✦	Per physician preference, instruct the patient to wait to discuss the test with the physician or make a follow-up appointment.				

Document: Enter the appropriate information in the chart below.

Grading

Points Earned	_____		
Points Possible	_____	102	102
Percent Grade (Points Earned/Points Possible)	_____		
PASS:	_____	❏ YES ❏ NO ❏ N/A	❏ YES ❏ NO ❏ N/A

Instructor Sign-Off

Instructor: _____ Date: _____

Procedure 17-2

Applying a Holter Monitor

Objective: The student, using the supplies and equipment listed below, will demonstrate how to apply a Holter monitor.

Supplies: medical order for the Holter monitor, Holter monitor, ECG electrodes, ECG recording cassette, fresh batteries (or recharged batteries), patient gown and drape as necessary for privacy and warmth, supplies for shaving if needed, alcohol pads, 4 × 4 gauze pad, liquid abrasive, adhesive tape, patient diary, patient chart, gloves

Notes to the Student:

_____

_____

_____

_____

_____

_____

Skills Assessment Requirements

Read and familiarize yourself with the procedure; complete the minimum practice requirements. Document each MPR using proper charting technique. Complete each procedure within a reasonable amount of time, with a minimum of 85% accuracy.

Name: _____

Date: _____

		PRACTICE TRIAL	GRADED TRIAL # 1	GRADED TRIAL # 2	NOTES:
POINT VALUE ✦ = 3-6 points ★ = 7-9 points					
1. ✦	Run a test of the equipment to make sure it is functioning properly and that the batteries are fresh.				
2. ★	With the patient sitting on the exam table, explain the procedure while showing the patient the equipment.				
3. ✦	Instruct the patient to remove all clothing from the waist up. If the exam room is cool, offer the patient a blanket.				
4. ✦	Because the electrodes of the Holter monitor must be in constant contact with the skin, you may have to shave the electrode sites. If so, explain the reason for shaving before you begin.				
5. ✦	Wash your hands and put on gloves.				
6. ✦	Cleanse the skin with alcohol wipes to remove all lotions, cologne or perfume, and body oil.				
7. ✦	Moisten a 4 × 4 gauze with liquid abrasive and abrade the skin at the electrode sites until it is slightly red to ensure the electrodes adhere.				
8. ✦	Take the electrodes from their packaging and remove the adhesive covering from each one.				

		PRACTICE TRIAL	GRADED TRIAL # 1	GRADED TRIAL # 2	NOTES:
9. ✦	Check for moist gel on each electrode and apply the adhesive side to the skin site, using circular pressure from the center outward.				
10. ✦	Attach the lead wires to the electrodes and tape a loop to the electrode wires to the skin.				
11. ✦	Cover each electrode site with nonallergenic tape, which will remain in place over the next 24 hours.				
12. ✦	Verify the correct electrode placement by connecting the electrodes to the ECG machine and obtaining a test strip.				
13. ✦	Help the patient to dress, if necessary, being careful not to disturb any of leads.				
14. ★	Test the Holter monitor by placing a cassette into it and making certain it runs smoothly. Plug the electrode cable into the recorder, and note the starting time in the patient diary and patient chart.				
15. ✦	Make an appointment for 24 hours later to review the monitor and remove the electrodes.				
16. ★	Document the procedure in the patient's chart.				

Name: _____

Date: _____

Document: Enter the appropriate information in the chart below.

Grading

Points Earned	_____		
Points Possible	_____	105	105
Percent Grade (Points Earned/Points Possible)	_____		
PASS:	_____	❑ YES ❑ NO ❑ N/A	❑ YES ❑ NO ❑ N/A

Instructor Sign-Off

Instructor: _____ Date: _____

CHAPTER 18
Pulmonology and Pulmonary Testing

CHAPTER OUTLINE

Review the Chapter Outline. If any content area is unclear, review that area before beginning workbook exercises.

    A.   The Medical Assistant's Role in Pulmonology

    B.   The Anatomy and Physiology of the Pulmonary System

    C.   Diseases and Disorders of the Pulmonary System

    D.   Pulmonary Assessment and Diagnosis

    E.   Inhalers and Nebulizers

    F.   Oxygen Therapy

CHAPTER REVIEW

The following is a summary of the chapter. If any of this material is unclear, review it in the textbook.

The specialty of pulmonology provides many areas for the medical assistant to assist patients and the physician. Upper respiratory infections are most often treated in ENT, whereas problems with the lower repiratory tract fall under the specialty of pulmonology. A knowledge of the anatomy and physiology and breathing patterns is needed as well as of the various obstructive diseases, infectious/inflammatory conditions, and the mechanical insults that can affect the patient's adequate respiration. The MA may perform a variety of pulmonary testing measures and pulse oximetry as well as provide instruction in treatments such as the use of inhalers and nebulizers.

LEARNING ACTIVITIES AND STUDY AIDS

Review the following study aids and/or complete the activities to ensure that you have achieved the learning objectives for this chapter.

1. State in your own words the medical assistant's role in a pulmonology practice.

_____

_____

_____

_____

_____

_____

_____

2. Draw a picture of the airway structures, label the parts, and briefly state their basic functions.

3. After reviewing lung and chest mechanics and the gas mechanics of respiration in your textbook, close the book and formulate your explanation of these mechanics. You have been asked by the physician to write a short paragraph on each topic in layman's terms and to mail it to Mrs. McCarty, an established patient. Write those two paragraphs in your own words from memory. Check the textbook and determine whether you included the basic information in the right terms for a patient.

_____

_____

_____

_____

_____

_____

_____

_____

4. Describe the causes for obstructive respiratory conditions, infectious and inflammatory pulmonary conditions, pulmonary malignancies, and mechanical insults. Include signs and symptoms when stated in your textbook. Complete the chart below with the information needed for a quick reference tool.

Disease	Causes	Signs/Symptoms
COLD/COPD		
Infectious/ Inflammatory		
Pulmonary Malignancies		
Mechanical Insults		

5. List breathing patterns on one side of a flash card and the definitions on the other.

_____

_____

_____

6. Make a flash card that lists the pulmonary function tests discussed in your textbook on one side and the basic information about them on the other. As in question 5 above, this should be brief with only enough information to jog your memory.

_____

_____

_____

_____

_____

_____

_____

7. Discuss the role of inhalers and nebulizers in pulmonary treatment. What is the purpose of inhaler and nebulizer treatments? You have a 24-year-old male patient with asthma. Describe the symptoms or condition in which this patient would use an inhaler and when he would use a nebulizer.

_____

_____

_____

_____

_____

_____

_____

8. State the reasons that oxygen therapy would be ordered. Briefly state how it would be administered in the outpatient setting.

_____

_____

_____

_____

_____

_____

_____

MEDICAL TERMINOLOGY REVIEW

Use a dictionary and highlighted terms in the textbook to define the following terms.

Terms

alveolus (plural: alveoli) _____

_____

apnea _____

_____

asthma _____

_____

bronchiole _____

_____

bronchitis _____

_____

bronchodilator _____

_____

bronchus (plural: bronchi) _____

_____

diaphragm _____

_____

dyspnea _____

_____

emphysema _____

_____

eupnea _____

_____

hemoptysis _____

_____

hypoxemia _____

_____

immunocompetence _____

_____

intradermal _____

_____

noninvasive _____

_____

orthopnea _____

_____

pulmonary function testing _____

_____

tachypnea _____

_____

Abbreviations

AFB _____

_____

COLD _____

_____

ENT _____

_____

O_2 sat _____

_____

$PaCO_2$ _____

_____

PaO_2 _____

_____

PEF _____

_____

PFT _____

_____

PPD _____

_____

TB _____

_____

CRITICAL THINKING

1. You have prepared an intradermal Mantoux test for a patient who is elderly. You check both anterior forearms to select a site for the injection but find that both of her arms are covered in a heat rash. Where else could this test be administered? The Internet, medical dictionaries and encyclopedias, and various patient care and/or clinical books are good sources to research this if you need help.

_____

_____

_____

_____

2. You have been asked to help a young patient and her mother with a nebulizer treatment for the child. The child is in such respiratory distress that you work quickly to get it prepared and started. About five minutes into the treatment, you realize you did not perform a PFT on the patient for a baseline prior to starting the nebulizer and medication. Although this is not covered in the textbook,

use critical thinking skills to determine what you would do. You may even offer more than one possible course of action.

_____

_____

_____

_____

3. A patient has been put on home oxygen therapy, and you have set up the delivery of the equipment. You have instructed the patient on the use and maintenance of the equipment. Instruct the patient about safety around oxygen; write your answer as if speaking to the patient.

_____

_____

_____

_____

4. A patient needs to start using an inhaler at home on a daily basis. The patient has rheumatoid arthritis and cannot hold the inhaler the usual way. What would you do or how would you teach this patient to use the inhaler?

_____

_____

_____

_____

5. You have a patient with obstructive lung disease who wants to know why he has a hard time breathing. This person has a form of COLD that doesn't allow him to exhale very much. Explain briefly here, as if explaining to the patient, why he feels so short of breath.

_____

_____

_____

_____

CHAPTER REVIEW TEST

MULTIPLE CHOICE

Circle the letter of the correct answer.

1. The beginning of the lower airway is the
   a. bronchi.
   b. trachea.
   c. alveoli.
   d. bronchioles.

2. In an arterial blood gas, the normal range for the pH level of the arteries is
   a. between 7.35 – 7.45.
   b. between 1.35 – 1.45.
   c. between 35 – 45.
   d. >7.45.

3. Peak flow testing measures a patient's ability to
   a. inhale
   b. exhale
   c. breathe.
   d. utilize oxygen

4. Because the medication's composition may be affected by_____, prepare the medication syringe immediately prior to administration.
   a. coming to room temperature
   b. the medication crystals settling in the syringe
   c. exposure to light
   d. the short life of the PPD

5. Influenza vaccinations are recommended yearly for: (circle all that apply)
   a. patients with chronic illnesses.
   b. children over 5 years of age.
   c. healthcare workers.
   d. patients with pneumonia.

6. Orthopnea means
   a. rapid breathing.
   b. difficult breathing.
   c. congested breathing.
   d. breathing in an upright position.

7. Which of the following are sounds associated with pulmonary conditions? (circle all that apply)
   a. rales
   b. eupnea
   c. clubbing
   d. wheezing
   e. barrel chest

8. Sputum that is blood tinged is called
   a. hemostasis.
   b. hemoptysis.
   c. hematocrit.
   d. hemolysis.

9. Which of the following are the major points of instructing a patient in the use of an inhaler?
   a. Shake the canister thoroughly to mix the medication particles evenly.
   b. Hold the canister at an angle for correct delivery.
   c. Note any physical problems the patient may have that may prevent him or her correctly handling the inhaler.
   d. The patient must inhale slowly and as deeply as possible then hold it.

10. Oxygen therapy is administered for three primary reasons. What are the three primary reasons?
    a. decrease the work of the heart
    b. to lower oxygen levels
    c. increase the work of breathing
    d. reverse or prevent low blood oxygen levels

TRUE/FALSE

Indicate whether the statement is true (T) or false (F).

_____ 1. Oxygen is a prescription drug that is administered only with a physician's order.

_____ 2. The upper airway consists of the nose and the adjacent zone of the pharynx.

_____ 3. Mucous is a thick fluid secreted by membranes.

_____ 4. Saliva begins digestion in the mouth.

_____ 5. The Mantoux test is used to screen patients for contact with or presence of the active disease state of TB.

_____ 6. Acute rhinitis is the most common URI.

_____ 7. The pulse oximeter uses an infrared light to measure oxygen in the tissues.

_____ 8. The acronym ABCD stands for airway, breathing, cardiovascular, defibrillation.

_____ 9. A peak flow meter can detect an asthma attack before symptoms occur.

_____ 10. The Mantoux test is administered by intradermal injection of petrified protein derivative (PPD).

FILL IN THE BLANK

Using words from the list below, fill in the blanks to complete the following statements. Note: Some terms are used in more than one statement.

atelectasis	infections
baseline	inhalation capacity
blockage	inhaling
blood gas	lung diseases
breathing	mechanics
continuous musical	nasal cannula
crackles	noninvasive
diagnosing or screening	normal
elasticity	oxygen
emboli	oxygen saturation
exchange	respiratory distress
exhaling	steadily worsening
hemoptysis	tumors
high-pitched	

1. In an outpatient setting, _____ is usually delivered by way of a _____.

2. When referring to the lungs, *compliance* means the _____ of the lungs for _____.

3. There are a variety of abnormal respiratory sounds such as wheezing, which has a _____ sound, rales, which sound like _____, and stridor, which is a _____, harsh sound.

4. Chest x-rays are noninvasive tools for _____ for respiratory _____, lung _____, or sudden _____.

5. Pulse oximetry is a _____ screening test of _____ status or _____ of tissues.

6. Lung volume testing measures the _____ of the lungs such as in emphysema.

7. With spirometry PFT, _____ information can be obtained about a patient's _____ breathing, deep _____, or _____.

8. Mechanical insults to the pulmonary system include pulmonary _____, _____ and the symptoms of _____.

9. Chronic obstructive lung disease (COLD) is the collective name for _____ characterized by long-term, _____ airway _____.

10. Pulmonary physiology can be separated into lung tissue _____, chest _____ and gas _____.

Procedure 18-1

Demonstrate Performance of Spirometry

Objective: The student, using the supplies and equipment listed below, will demonstrate how to assist the patient in the performance of spirometry testing.

Supplies: spirometer, disposable mouthpiece and tubing, nose clip, chart, forms and lab slips for documentation and testing

Notes to the Student:

_____

_____

_____

_____

_____

_____

Skills Assessment Requirements

Read and familiarize yourself with the procedure; complete the minimum practice requirements. Document each MPR using proper charting technique. Complete each procedure within a reasonable amount of time, with a minimum of 85% accuracy.

POINT VALUE ✦ = 3-6 points ✱ = 7-9 points		PRACTICE TRIAL	GRADED TRIAL # 1	GRADED TRIAL # 2	NOTES:
1. ✦	Wash your hands. Gather equipment and supplies.				
2. ✱	Identify the patient and guide him or her to the treatment area.				
3. ✦	Record the patient's history and main complaint. Explain the entire procedure.				
4. ✦	If the patient is chewing gum, ask him or her to dispose of it (to prevent choking during the test). If a female patient is wearing lipstick, ask her to remove it to create a tight seal.				
5. ✦	Ask the patient to place the mouthpiece in his or her mouth and to close the lips tightly around the mouthpiece to make a good seal.				
6. ✦	Place the nose clips on the patient's nose, sealing the nostrils closed.				
7. ✱	Ask the patient to inhale as deeply as he or she possibly can and hold the breath for a short time. Then tell the patient to blow the air out into the mouthpiece as hard and as fast as possible— until he or she cannot blow out any more air.				

		PRACTICE TRIAL	GRADED TRIAL #1	GRADED TRIAL #2	NOTES:
8. ✦	Repeat this procedure two more times, giving the patient a few minutes in between.				
9. ✦	The electronic equipment will usually "select" the best of the three breathing tests.				
10. ∗	Document patient compliance with and tolerance of the testing procedure.				
11. ✦	Follow cleaning procedures to prepare the equipment and the area for the next patient.				
12. ✦	Wash your hands.				

Document: Enter the appropriate information in the chart below.

Grading

Points Earned	_____		
Points Possible	_____	81	81
Percent Grade (Points Earned/ Points Possible)	_____		
PASS:	_____	❑ YES ❑ NO ❑ N/A	❑ YES ❑ NO ❑ N/A

Instructor Sign-Off

Instructor: _____ Date: _____

Procedure 18-2

Demonstrate Performance of Peak Flow Testing

Objective: The student, using the supplies and equipment listed below, will demonstrate how to assist the patient in the performance of peak flow testing.

Supplies: peak flow meter, patient log or diary of peak flow readings, patient chart

Notes to the Student:

_____

_____

_____

_____

_____

_____

Skills Assessment Requirements

Read and familiarize yourself with the procedure; complete the minimum practice requirements. Document each MPR using proper charting technique. Complete each procedure within a reasonable amount of time, with a minimum of 85% accuracy.

POINT VALUE ✦ = 3-6 points * = 7-9 points		PRACTICE TRIAL	GRADED TRIAL # 1	GRADED TRIAL # 2	NOTES:
1. ✦	Wash your hands. Gather equipment and supplies.				
2. *	Identify the patient and guide him or her to the treatment area.				
3. *	Instruct the patient to take as deep a breath as possible, place the mouthpiece just in front of the teeth, then use his or her lips to make a complete seal. Ask the patient to exhale as hard and as fast as possible.				
4. ✦	Have the patient repeat step 3 three times.				
5. ✦	If test results also need to be taken after medication, allow the patient to rest. Administer the medication, then repeat the test.				
6. ✦	Clean the equipment and dispose of contaminated materials appropriately.				
7. ✦	Wash your hands.				
8. *	Record the results. Compare the results with previous readings.				

Name: _____

Date: _____

Document: Enter the appropriate information in the chart below.

Grading

Points Earned	_____		
Points Possible	_____	57	57
Percent Grade (Points Earned/ Points Possible)	_____		
PASS:	_____	❏ YES ❏ NO ❏ N/A	❏ YES ❏ NO ❏ N/A

Instructor Sign-Off

Instructor: _____ Date: _____

Procedure 18-3

Demonstrate the Performance of the Mantoux Test by Intradermal Injection

Objective: The student, using the supplies and equipment listed below, will demonstrate how to perform the Mantoux test.

Supplies: patient chart, disposable gloves, alcohol wipes, sharps container, tuberculin syringe with needle, vial of medication, bandage strips

Notes to the Student:

_____

_____

_____

_____

_____

_____

Skills Assessment Requirements

Read and familiarize yourself with the procedure; complete the minimum practice requirements. Document each MPR using proper charting technique. Complete each procedure within a reasonable amount of time, with a minimum of 85% accuracy.

POINT VALUE ✦ = 3-6 points ✶ = 7-9 points		PRACTICE TRIAL	GRADED TRIAL # 1	GRADED TRIAL # 2	NOTES:
1. ✦	Wash your hands and gather the equipment.				
2. ✶	Identify the patient and guide him or her to the treatment area.				
3. ✦	Wash your hands again and put on disposable gloves.				
4. ✦	Ask the patient to reach out with one hand and turn the palm upward. Find a site without hair or blemishes on the forearm.				
5. ✦	Cleanse the skin with an alcohol wipe and allow it to thoroughly air-dry.				
6. ✦	Cleanse the top of the PPD vial with an alcohol wipe and allow it to air-dry. Withdraw 0.1 cc from the vial and hold it in your dominant hand.				
7. ✦	Place your nondominant hand under the patient's forearm and gently pull the skin tight. Ask the patient to keep the arm still. Insert the needle bevel just into and under the skin at a 10- to 15-degree angle.				
8. ✶	Inject the medication slowly to create a raised blister, or wheal.				
9. ✦	Release the skin, then withdraw the needle and blot the area gently with an alcohol wipe.				

		PRACTICE TRIAL	GRADED TRIAL #1	GRADED TRIAL #2	NOTES:
10. ✦	Discard the syringe in the sharps container.				
11. ✦	Make an appointment for the patient to return and have the injection site checked after 48 to 72 hours.				
12. ★	Document the procedure, including a description of the Mantoux test site.				
13. ★	When the patient returns, measure only the induration, not the redness. For positive results, measure in millimeters (mm) and follow local public health guidelines for reporting.				

Name: _____

Date: _____

Document: Enter the appropriate information in the chart below.

Grading

Points Earned	_____		
Points Possible	_____	90	90
Percent Grade (Points Earned/ Points Possible)	_____		
PASS:	_____	❑ YES ❑ NO ❑ N/A	❑ YES ❑ NO ❑ N/A

Instructor Sign-Off

Instructor: _____ Date: _____

Procedure 18-4

Demonstrate Patient Instruction in the Use of an Inhaler

Objective: The student, using the supplies and equipment listed below, will demonstrate how to instruct and/or help the patient use an inhaler for the first time.

Supplies: patient's prescription inhaler, patient's chart

Notes to the Student:

_____

_____

_____

_____

_____

_____

Skills Assessment Requirements

Read and familiarize yourself with the procedure; complete the minimum practice requirements. Document each MPR using proper charting technique. Complete each procedure within a reasonable amount of time, with a minimum of 85% accuracy.

Name: _____

Date: _____

POINT VALUE ✦ = 3-6 points ⋆ = 7-9 points		PRACTICE TRIAL	GRADED TRIAL # 1	GRADED TRIAL # 2	NOTES:
1. ✦	Wash your hands and gather the equipment.				
2. ⋆	Identify and guide the patient to the treatment area.				
3. ⋆	Give the patient the following instructions:				
	• Shake the canister thoroughly. • Hold the canister upright within 2 inches of the mouth. Place the mouthpiece in your mouth, sealing the opening with your lips. • Activate the inhaler (usually by pressing the canister down) to spray. Breathe slowly but deeply after the medication is delivered. • Hold your breath for as long as possible, up to 10 seconds. • Begin breathing normally again.				
4. ✦	Follow the physician's instructions for immediate repeat use.				
5. ⋆	Document the patient's ability to follow instructions. Inform the physician if the patient has any problems with self-administration. Give the patient backup written instructions.				

Name: _____

Date: _____

Document: Enter the appropriate information in the chart below.

<table>
<tr><td></td><td></td></tr>
<tr><td></td><td></td></tr>
<tr><td></td><td></td></tr>
<tr><td></td><td></td></tr>
<tr><td></td><td></td></tr>
</table>

Grading

Points Earned	_____		
Points Possible	_____	39	39
Percent Grade (Points Earned/ Points Possible)	_____		
PASS:	_____	❏ YES ❏ NO ❏ N/A	❏ YES ❏ NO ❏ N/A

Instructor Sign-Off

Instructor: _____ **Date:** _____

Procedure 18-5

Demonstrate Patient Assistance in the Use of a Nebulizer

Objective: The student, using the supplies and equipment listed below, will demonstrate how to assist the patient in the use of a nebulizer.

Supplies: compressor, nebulizer with mask and tubing, medications, patient's chart

Notes to the Student:

_____

_____

_____

_____

_____

_____

Skills Assessment Requirements

Read and familiarize yourself with the procedure; complete the minimum practice requirements. Document each MPR using proper charting technique. Complete each procedure within a reasonable amount of time, with a minimum of 85% accuracy.

POINT VALUE ✦ = 3-6 points ⋆ = 7-9 points		PRACTICE TRIAL	GRADED TRIAL #1	GRADED TRIAL #2	NOTES:
1. ✦	Wash your hands. Gather equipment and supplies.				
2. ⋆	Identify the patient and guide him or her to the treatment area.				
3. ✦	Obtain vital signs.				
4. ✦	Wash your hands again.				
5. ✦	Prepare the nebulizer cup with medication(s) as ordered and/or prescribed.				
6. ✦	Turn on the compressor.				
7. ✦	Instruct, or help, the patient to hold the mask while the medication is being delivered.				
8. ⋆	Continue treatment until no medication remains in the nebulizer. Monitor the patient's pulse every 5 minutes throughout the treatment. If the pulse rises to 120 beats per minute or the patient's condition worsens, stop the treatment and tell the physician.				
9. ✦	Dispose of used materials in the appropriate containers.				
10. ✦	Wash your hands.				
11. ⋆	Document the patient's vital signs at the beginning, middle, and end of the treatment. Also describe patient signs and symptoms at beginning and end of treatment.				

Document: Enter the appropriate information in the chart below.

Grading

Points Earned	_____		
Points Possible	_____	75	75
Percent Grade (Points Earned/ Points Possible)	_____		
PASS:	_____	❏ YES ❏ NO ❏ N/A	❏ YES ❏ NO ❏ N/A

Instructor Sign-Off

Instructor: _____ Date: _____

CHAPTER 19
EENT

CHAPTER OUTLINE

Review the Chapter Outline. If any content area is unclear, review that area before beginning workbook exercises.

  A. The Medical Assistant's Role in an EENT Practice
  B. The Anatomy and Physiology of the Eye
  C. The Anatomy and Physiology of the Ear
  D. The Anatomy and Physiology of the Nose
  E. The Anatomy and Physiology of the Throat

CHAPTER REVIEW

The following is a summary of the chapter. If any of this material is unclear, review it in the textbook.

An EENT practice covers a wide variety of subspecialties and duties for a medical assistant. In addition to the anatomy and physiology of the eyes, ears, nose, and throat, this specialty includes refractive, infectious, and degenerative disorders of the eye as well as foreign bodies; ear, nose, and throat disorders; diagnostic procedures; irrigations and the instillation of medications. Examples of the procedures and tests the MA may perform in an EENT office include visual acuity and color vision testing, audiometry, eye and ear irrigations, and applying medications to the ear and eye by instillation of drops or ointments. The medical assistant may work with a number of various healthcare providers such as otologists, rhinologists, otolaryngologists, audiologists, and ophthalmologists.

LEARNING ACTIVITIES AND STUDY AIDS

Review the following study aids and/or complete the activities to ensure that you have achieved the learning objectives for this chapter.

1. List the typical duties of a medical assistant in the EENT office.

_____

_____

_____

_____

_____

_____

_____

2. There are various EENT healthcare providers. Make a list with a brief description of each role.

_____

_____

_____

_____

_____

_____

_____

_____

_____

3. Make flash cards of the anatomy of the eye and state the physiology of each part. There are three major layers with other related parts—be sure to include the additional parts in your list.

_____

_____

_____

_____

_____

_____

_____

_____

4. Make a master list of the diseases and disorders of the eye. State each one with a brief description. You will be adding diseases and disorders of the ear, nose, and throat to this list in later activities.

_____

_____

_____

_____

_____

_____

_____

_____

5. Discuss diagnostic procedures and assessments related to the eyes.

_____

_____

_____

_____

_____

_____

_____

_____

6. Make flash cards of the anatomy of the ear and state the physiology of each part. There are three areas of the ear under which to list the anatomy.

_____

_____

7. Add the diseases and disorders of the ear to the master list created in question 4. List these under the three zones mentioned in the textbook.

8. Discuss diagnostic procedures and assessments related to the ears.

9. Make flash cards of the anatomy of the nose and nasal passages and state the physiology of each part. State these under the three zones listed in the textbook.

10. Add the diseases of the nasal passages and sinuses to the master list created in question 4.

_____

_____

11. Make flash cards of the anatomy of the throat and state the physiology of each part. There are three regions of the throat.

_____

_____

_____

_____

_____

_____

12. Add the diseases of the throat to the master list created in question 4.

_____

_____

_____

_____

_____

_____

_____

MEDICAL TERMINOLOGY REVIEW

Use a dictionary and highlighted terms in the textbook to define the following terms.

Terms

acuity _____

_____

audiologist _____

_____

audiometry _____

_____

cerumen _____

_____

decibel _____

_____

degenerative _____

_____

intraocular _____

laryngologist _____

nasal septum _____

ophthalmologist _____

optician _____

optometrist _____

otic _____

otologist _____

otolaryngologist _____

otorhinolaryngologist _____

purulent _____

rhinologist _____

Abbreviations

dB _____

EENT _____

FB _____

OD _____

OS _____

CRITICAL THINKING

1. You need to perform a Snellen visual acuity test and an Ishihara color vision test per the physician's orders. You do not have an occluder or the Ishihara plates. Which of the tests, if any, could you still perform using a different item and what replacement item(s) can you use?

   _____

   _____

   _____

2. If a patient called in for an appointment for possible hearing loss, which specialist would be most appropriate?

   _____

   _____

   _____

3. In the case study for this chapter, answer the following questions:

   a. What is the likely treatment the physician will order for the 4-year-old girl with sand in her eye?

   _____

   _____

   b. Who would likely perform the Snellen visual acuity test on the college student?

   _____

   _____

   c. What specialist would be most appropriate to see the 3-year-old boy with a toy stuck in his nose?

   _____

   _____

4. You work for an optometrist in the optical department of a large medical center. The provider sees a patient and performs tonometry only to find the intraocular pressure reading is very high. What specialist would the optometrist refer this patient to for the IOP?

   _____

   _____

   _____

5. You are asked by the physician to perform an ear irrigation on a 12-year-old patient because the tympanic membrane cannot be seen due to a large amount of cerumen. How will you know when the irrigation is completed?

   _____

   _____

   _____

CHAPTER REVIEW TEST

MULTIPLE CHOICE

Circle the letter of the correct answer.

1. Which physician would prescribe adaptive lenses?
   a. ophthalmologist
   b. otologist
   c. optometrist
   d. rhinologists

2. Which instrument measures intraocular pressure?
   a. ophthalmoscope
   b. tonometer
   c. slit lamp
   d. otoscope

3. Bright light reduces pupil size as the circular muscle of the _____ contracts.
   a. choroid
   b. cornea
   c. retina
   d. iris

4. Items used to cover one eye while testing the other eye during a Snellen visual acuity test include: (circle all that apply)
   a. card.
   b. occluder.
   c. spud.
   d. spatula.

5. The outer or external ear is comprised of the: (circle all that apply)
   a. auricle.
   b. pinna.
   c. external auditory canal.
   d. cerumen.

6. Which tasks does the medical assistant perform in an EENT practice? (circle all that apply)
   a. performing audiometry
   b. performing tonometry
   c. performing eye and ear irrigations
   d. testing visual acuity

7. The chonchae are the nasal bones located in the most interior portion of the nose; their purpose is to: (circle all that apply)
   a. warm the air.
   b. soften the palate.
   c. filter air inhaled by trapping particles.
   d. humidify air before it reaches the respiratory zone.

8. One of the three types of color *deficiency* is
   a. protanopia.
   b. myopia.
   c. Daltonism.
   d. Ishihara.

9. Which of the following reduce functions of the sinuses? (circle all that apply)
   a. to reduce the weight of the eyeballs.
   b. to reduce the weight of the skull.
   c. to enhance phonation.
   d. to produce vocal sounds.

10. The three tiny bones or ossicles in the middle ear are:
    a. otosclerosis.
    b. malleus.
    c. stapes.
    d. incus.

TRUE/FALSE

Indicate whether the statement is true (T) or false (F).

_____ 1. Humors of the eye are watery fluids that help maintain the eye's internal pressure.

_____ 2. The laryngopharanyx is just above the soft palate.

_____ 3. The two types of color blindness are achromatic vision and Daltonism.

_____ 4. Drops used to stain the eyes for an ophthalmological exam are called fluorescein.

_____ 5. Cerumen can block the passage of sound waves to the external ear.

_____ 6. An eye patch may be ordered to keep the eyelid from passing back and forth over the cornea.

_____ 7. Hearing tests include tuning fork testing.

_____ 8. The holes in the nose are known as nares.

_____ 9. Labyrinthitis is also known as otitis media.

_____ 10. An eye spud is used to remove a foreign particle or rust ring from the retina.

FILL IN THE BLANK

Using words from the list below, fill in the blanks to complete the following statements.

20 feet	insult	sedation
30 feet	interior	sense of smell
acoustic stimuli	iris	sensory receptors
breath	light refraction	septum
ciliary muscle	normal vision	sinusitis
cold	patient	straight path
eardrum	polyps	topical anesthetic
fogging	rhinitis	Vienna speculum
frequencies	rods and cones	warmed

1. A _____ is a device used to examine the external auditory canal and _____.

2. The olfactory zone is the most _____ portion of the nose where the _____ is located.

3. The intrinsic muscles within the eye are the _____ and the _____.

4. The laryngeal mirror is usually _____ under running water to prevent _____ by the patient's _____.

5. The retina is the innermost layer of the eye and contains _____ called _____.

6. The audiometer measures the patient's response to _____ of specific _____.

7. A score on the Snellen visual acuity test of 20/30 means that the _____ is able to read at _____ what a person with _____ can read at _____.

8. Disorders of the nose or nasal passages include the inflammatory conditions of _____ and paranasal _____, structural conditions of the _____, nasal _____, epistaxis, traumatic _____, the common _____, and foreign bodies.

9. Use of a laryngoscope requires _____ of the patient and application of a _____.

10. Vision is the result of _____ (bending from a _____).

Name: _____
Date: _____

Procedure 19-1

Measure Distance Visual Acuity with a Snellen Chart

Objective: The student, using the supplies and equipment listed below, will demonstrate how to assist the patient in testing the visual acuity of both eyes.

Supplies: Snellen chart; occluder, spatula, or card; patient chart

Notes to the Student:

_____

_____

_____

_____

_____

_____

Skills Assessment Requirements

Read and familiarize yourself with the procedure; complete the minimum practice requirements. Document each MPR using proper charting technique. Complete each procedure within a reasonable amount of time, with a minimum of 85% accuracy.

POINT VALUE ✦ = 3-6 points ★ = 7-9 points		PRACTICE TRIAL	GRADED TRIAL #1	GRADED TRIAL #2	NOTES:
1. ✦	Wash your hands. Gather equipment and supplies.				
2. ★	Identify the patient and guide him or her to the treatment area.				
3. ✦	Record the patient's history and main complaint. Explain the entire procedure to the patient.				
4. ✦	Position the patient, standing or sitting, at the 20-foot line. Give the patient the occluder. Observe patient during the procedure for head tilting, squinting, and tearing.				
5. ✦	Ask the patient to cover the left eye, keeping it open, and to read aloud from the top line to the smallest line of readable letters.				
6. ★	Record the right-eye vision with the number of errors. For one or two errors, record the vision fraction and minus one or two. For more than two errors, record the vision fraction as noted one line above on the Snellen chart. For example, if the patient reads the 20/40 line with the right eye and two errors, the result is recorded as OD 20/40-2. If the patient reads the 20/40 line with the right eye and three errors, the result is OD 20/50, or one line above the 20/40 line.				

	PRACTICE TRIAL	GRADED TRIAL #1	GRADED TRIAL #2	NOTES:
7. ✦ Next, ask the patient to repeat the procedure, covering the right eye and reading with the left.				
8. ⋆ Record the left-eye vision with the number of errors.				
9. ✦ Wash your hands and report the results to the physician.				

Document: Enter the appropriate information in the chart below.

Grading

Points Earned	_____		
Points Possible	_____	63	63
Percent Grade (Points Earned/Points Possible)	_____		
PASS:	_____	❑ YES ❑ NO ❑ N/A	❑ YES ❑ NO ❑ N/A

Instructor Sign-Off

Instructor: _____ Date: _____

Procedure 19-2

Performing the Ishihara Color Vision Test

Objective: The student, using the supplies and equipment listed below, will demonstrate how to determine color vision acuity using Ishihara color plates.

Supplies: Ishihara color plates book, pen, patient chart

Notes to the Student:

_____

_____

_____

_____

_____

_____

Skills Assessment Requirements

Read and familiarize yourself with the procedure; complete the minimum practice requirements. Document each MPR using proper charting technique. Complete each procedure within a reasonable amount of time, with a minimum of 85% accuracy.

Name: _____

Date: _____

POINT VALUE ✦ = 3-6 points ⋆ = 7-9 points		PRACTICE TRIAL	GRADED TRIAL #1	GRADED TRIAL #2	NOTES:
1. ✦	Explain the procedure to the patient.				
2. ⋆	Follow the physician's directions for administering the total book or in sections.				
3. ✦	Ask the patient to identify the number in each plate with both eyes.				
4. ✦	Have the patient cover the left eye and read the book again, then the right eye. Write down the page number of any plates the patient misses. (The correct answer is on the back of each page.)				
5. ✦	Follow the directions on the last page of the book to determine the level of color blindness, if any.				
6. ⋆	Document the procedure in the patient's chart.				

Name: _____

Date: _____

Document: Enter the appropriate information in the chart below.

Grading

Points Earned	_____		
Points Possible	_____	42	42
Percent Grade (Points Earned/Points Possible)	_____		
PASS:	_____	❏ YES ❏ NO ❏ N/A	❏ YES ❏ NO ❏ N/A

Instructor Sign-Off

Instructor: _____ **Date:** _____

Procedure 19-3

Perform Eye Irrigation

Objective: The student, using the supplies and equipment listed below, will demonstrate how to irrigate the patient's eye.

Supplies: irrigating solution, sterile basin, irrigating syringe, protective gear (gown, face shield, disposable gloves), towels, kidney-shaped basin, tissues, patient chart

Notes to the Student:

_____

_____

_____

_____

_____

_____

Skills Assessment Requirements

Read and familiarize yourself with the procedure; complete the minimum practice requirements. Document each MPR using proper charting technique. Complete each procedure within a reasonable amount of time, with a minimum of 85% accuracy.

POINT VALUE ✦ = 3-6 points ✶ = 7-9 points		PRACTICE TRIAL	GRADED TRIAL # 1	GRADED TRIAL # 2	NOTES:
1. ✦	Wash your hands. Gather equipment and supplies.				
2. ✶	Identify the patient and guide him or her to the treatment area.				
3. ✦	Record the patient's history and main complaint.				
4. ✦	Review the physician's order for the patient's name, the volume and name of the irrigating solution, and which eye to irrigate.				
5. ✶	Ask the patient about medication allergies. Explain the entire procedure.				
6. ✶	Check the label of the irrigating solution against the physician's order before pouring it into the sterile basin for irrigation.				
7. ✦	Wash your hands.				
8. ✦	Put on the gown, face shield, and gloves before proceeding with irrigation.				
9. ✦	Ask the patient to lie or sit down with the head tilted toward the eye to be irrigated. Place a towel and the kidney-shaped basin next to the patient's face to catch irrigating fluid.				
10. ✦	With your dominant hand, fill the irrigating syringe with the prescribed irrigating solution.				

		PRACTICE TRIAL	GRADED TRIAL # 1	GRADED TRIAL # 2	NOTES:
11. ✦	With your nondominant hand, press with a tissue against the patient's cheekbone beneath the eye to expose more of the eye surface.				
12. ★	While holding the syringe approximately 1/2 inch from the eye, gently direct the fluid toward the inside surface of the lower conjunctiva and from the inner to outer corner of the eye.				
13. ✦	Continue irrigating until the prescribed volume is used. Depending on the cause and symptoms, the physician may order further irrigation.				
14. ✦	When irrigation is complete, dry the area around the affected eye with tissues.				
15. ✦	Remove your protective clothing and place it in the proper laundry and waste containers.				
16. ✦	Wash your hands.				
17. ★	Document the patient's tolerance of the procedure, the amount and kind of irrigating solution, and the irrigated.				

Name: _____

Date: _____

Document: Enter the appropriate information in the chart below.

Grading

Points Earned	_____		
Points Possible	_____	123	123
Percent Grade (Points Earned/ Points Possible)	_____		
PASS:	_____	❏ YES ❏ NO ❏ N/A	❏ YES ❏ NO ❏ N/A

Instructor Sign-Off

Instructor: _____ Date: _____

Procedure 19-4

Perform Instillation of Eye Medication

Objective: The student, using the supplies and equipment listed below, will perform eye medication instillation.

Supplies: prescription medication (drops or ointment), disposable gloves, tissues, patient chart

Notes to the Student:

_____

_____

_____

_____

_____

_____

Skills Assessment Requirements

Read and familiarize yourself with the procedure; complete the minimum practice requirements. Document each MPR using proper charting technique. Complete each procedure within a reasonable amount of time, with a minimum of 85% accuracy.

POINT VALUE ✦ = 3-6 points ∗ = 7-9 points		PRACTICE TRIAL	GRADED TRIAL # 1	GRADED TRIAL # 2	NOTES:
1. ✦	Wash your hands. Gather equipment and supplies.				
2. ✦	Take the medication from the storage shelf. Check the label against the physician's order.				
3. ∗	Identify the patient and guide him or her to the treatment area. Check the patient's identification against the physician's order and medication name.				
4. ✦	Note the medication dosage to be administered.				
5. ∗	Ask the patient about allergies. Explain the entire procedure.				
6. ✦	Wash your hands and put on disposable gloves.				
7. ✦	Ask the patient to lie down or sit with the head tilted back with both eyes open. (It may be necessary to ask the sitting patient to look at the ceiling.) If the patient is wearing an eye patch, remove it.				
8. ✦	Give the patient a tissue to hold in each hand until after the procedure. With your nondominant hand and a tissue, press on the lower cheekbone and gently pull the lower eyelid down to expose the cornea and conjunctival sac.				

	PRACTICE TRIAL	GRADED TRIAL #1	GRADED TRIAL #2	NOTES:
9. ★ *To administer eye drops:* Fill the eyedropper with your dominant hand. Hold the dropper approximate 1/2 inch away from the patient's eye, and administer the prescribed dose into the conjunctival sac. *To administer the ointment:* Rest your dominant hand on the patient's forehead, hold the tube, and lightly squeeze ointment into the conjunctival sac from the inner to outer corner of the patient's eye.				
10. ✦ Release the patient's lower eyelid and tell the patient to close the eye.				
11. ✦ Repeat the procedure in the other eye, if ordered by the physician.				
12. ✦ Instruct the patient to use a separate tissue for each eye to wipe away excess medication.				
13. ✦ Apply an eye patch, if ordered by the physician.				
14. ✦ Provide a waste container for the patient to discard the used tissue into. Dispose of the gloves and tissue.				
15. ✦ Wash your hands.				
16. ★ Document the patient's tolerance of the procedure, the amount and kind of medication administered, and the eye(s) treated.				

Document: Enter the correct information in the chart below.

Grading

Points Earned	_____		
Points Possible	_____	108	108
Percent Grade (Points Earned/Points Possible)	_____		
PASS:	_____	❏ YES ❏ NO ❏ N/A	❏ YES ❏ NO ❏ N/A

Instructor Sign-Off

Instructor: _____ **Date:** _____

Procedure 19-5

Performing Simple Audiometry

Objective: The student, using the supplies and equipment listed below, will demonstrate how to perform bilateral audiology testing.

Supplies: audiometer, earphones, audiometric test report form, patient chart

Notes to the Student:

_____

_____

_____

_____

_____

_____

Skills Assessment Requirements

Read and familiarize yourself with the procedure; complete the minimum practice requirements. Document each MPR using proper charting technique. Complete each procedure within a reasonable amount of time, with a minimum of 85% accuracy.

POINT VALUE ✦ = 3-6 points ⋆ = 7-9 points	PRACTICE TRIAL	GRADED TRIAL #1	GRADED TRIAL #2	NOTES:
1. ✦ Wash your hands. Gather equipment and supplies.				
2. ✦ Prepare the testing area to ensure quiet during the procedure.				
3. ⋆ Identify the patient and guide him or her to the testing area.				
4. ✦ Inform the patient that only one ear at a time will be tested. Instruct the patient to raise one finger or nod when he or she first hears the sound.				
5. ✦ Place earphones on the patient.				
6. ✦ Administer low-frequency sounds to one ear to determine the patient's baseline hearing measurements and ability to follow test instructions.				
7. ⋆ Plot the results from each tone on the graph immediately.				
8. ✦ Continue raising the tone frequency by 10 dB (decibels) and recording the results until the patient can no longer hear in the first ear.				

		PRACTICE TRIAL	GRADED TRIAL # 1	GRADED TRIAL # 2	NOTES:
9. ✦	Lower the tone by 5 dB until the patient signals, to confirm the lowest frequency the patient can hear in that ear.				
10. ✦	Repeat the procedure with the other ear.				
11. ⋆	Give the audiometric test results to the physician.				
12. ✦	Prepare the audiometric equipment and room for next the patient.				

Document: Enter the appropriate information in the chart below.

Grading

Points Earned	_____		
Points Possible	_____	81	81
Percent Grade (Points Earned/Points Possible)	_____		
PASS:	_____	❏ YES ❏ NO ❏ N/A	❏ YES ❏ NO ❏ N/A

Instructor Sign-Off

Instructor: _____ Date: _____

Procedure 19-6

Perform Ear Irrigation

Objective: The student, using the supplies and equipment listed below, will demonstrate how to irrigate the patient's ear.

Supplies: irrigating solution, sterile basin, irrigating syringe, collection cup or basin, towels, cotton ball(s), patient chart

Notes to the Student:

_____

_____

_____

_____

_____

_____

Skills Assessment Requirements

Read and familiarize yourself with the procedure; complete the minimum practice requirements. Document each MPR using proper charting technique. Complete each procedure within a reasonable amount of time, with a minimum of 85% accuracy.

POINT VALUE ✦ = 3-6 points ∗ = 7-9 points		PRACTICE TRIAL	GRADED TRIAL #1	GRADED TRIAL #2	NOTES:
1. ✦	Wash your hands. Gather equipment and supplies.				
2. ∗	Identify the patient and guide him or her to the treatment area. Explain the entire procedure.				
3. ∗	Check the label of the irrigating solution when you take it from the shelf and against the physician's order.				
4. ✦	Position the patient in a sitting position and instruct him or her to lean the head toward the side to be irrigated.				
5. ✦	Check the condition of the external auditory canal with the otoscope.				
6. ✦	Drape a towel across the patient's shoulder, under the ear.				
7. ✦	Fill the irrigating syringe with prescribed solution from the sterile basin.				
8. ✦	Place the collection basin under the ear and against the skin. Instruct the patient or other office personnel to hold the basin in place.				
9. ∗	For a child under three years, gently pull the auricle down and back. For a child over 3 years or an adult, gently pull the auricle ear up and back.				
10. ✦	Gently place the tip of the irrigating syringe into the external auditory canal and point to the side or top. Do not point directly toward the tympanic membrane.				

		PRACTICE TRIAL	GRADED TRIAL # 1	GRADED TRIAL # 2	NOTES:
11. *	Instill the irrigating solution with gentle pressure on the plunger of the syringe.				
12. ✦	Place the irrigation basin aside.				
13. ✦	Use the otoscope to determine if more irrigation is needed.				
14. ✦	Repeat the procedure until the desired results are obtained. If the patient experiences discomfort or other difficulties, report to the physician.				
15. ✦	After irrigation, instruct and/or assist the patient to lie down with the head tilted toward the irrigated ear.				
16. ✦	Place a towel under the head to catch the drainage				
17. ✦	Help the patient to a sitting, then standing position. Assess the patient for light-headedness or dizziness. Escort the patient to the waiting room.				
18. ✦	Clean the treatment area and remove reusable equipment to the utility cleaning area.				
19. ✦	Wash your hands.				
20. *	Document the patient's tolerance and the results of the procedure.				

Document: Enter the appropriate information in the chart below.

Grading

Points Earned	_____		
Points Possible	_____	135	135
Percent Grade (Points Earned/ Points Possible)	_____		
PASS:	_____	❏ YES ❏ NO ❏ N/A	❏ YES ❏ NO ❏ N/A

Instructor Sign-Off

Instructor: _____ **Date:** _____

Procedure 19-7

Perform Instillation of Ear Medication

Objective: The student, using the supplies and equipment listed below, will demonstrate how to instill medication into the patient's ear.

Supplies: medication, disposable gloves, cotton balls, patient chart

Notes to the Student:

_____

_____

_____

_____

_____

_____

Skills Assessment Requirements

Read and familiarize yourself with the procedure; complete the minimum practice requirements. Document each MPR using proper charting technique. Complete each procedure within a reasonable amount of time, with a minimum of 85% accuracy.

POINT VALUE ✦ = 3-6 points ✶ = 7-9 points		PRACTICE TRIAL	GRADED TRIAL # 1	GRADED TRIAL # 2	NOTES:
1. ✦	Wash your hands. Gather equipment and supplies.				
2. ✶	Check the label when removing the medication from the shelf and against the physician's order.				
3. ✦	Do not administer the medication unless it is at room temperature.				
4. ✶	Identify the patient and guide him or her to the treatment area. Check the patient name against the physician's order and against the medication.				
5. ✦	Explain the entire procedure to the patient. Ask about any allergies.				
6. ✦	Instruct the patient to lie on the side opposite the ear to be treated.				
7. ✦	Position the auricle as in Procedure 19-6.				
8. ✶	Hold the ear dropper or bottle tip about 1/2 inch above the external auditory canal and gently squeeze the bulb to administer the prescribed number of drops.				
9. ✦	Instruct the patient to lie still for 10 minutes.				

		PRACTICE TRIAL	GRADED TRIAL #1	GRADED TRIAL #2	NOTES:
10. ✦	Loosely place a small cotton ball, if the physician orders it, at the opening to the canal				
11. ✦	Repeat the procedure for the other ear, if ordered. Recap the medication bottle and dispose of waste materials.				
12. ✦	Remove and dispose of the gloves. Wash your hands.				
13. ✦	Escort the patient back to the waiting room.				
14. ✶	Document the patient's tolerance of the procedure, the medication, the dosage administered, and which ear received treatment.				

Document: Enter the appropriate information in the chart below.

Grading

Points Earned	_____		
Points Possible	_____	96	96
Percent Grade (Points Earned/Points Possible)	_____		
PASS:	_____	❑ YES ❑ NO ❑ N/A	❑ YES ❑ NO ❑ N/A

Instructor Sign-Off

Instructor: _____ Date: _____

CHAPTER 20
Immunology and Allergies

CHAPTER OUTLINE

Review the Chapter Outline. If any content area is unclear, review that area before beginning workbook exercises.

    A. The Medical Assistant's Role in Immunology and Allergy

    B. The Anatomy and Physiology of the Immune System

    C. Diseases and Disorders of the Immune System

CHAPTER REVIEW

The following is a summary of the chapter. If any of this material is unclear, review it in the textbook.

An immunology and allergy clinic can be a busy and challenging specialty to work in. Efficiently and correctly taking a patient's history and vital signs, performing allergy testing, and assisting a physician in this area requires a thorough understanding of the immune and allergy responses. There are also autoimmune disorders and hypersensitivity that fall within this specialty, and a medical assistant's skill in performing intradermal injections will be utilized.

LEARNING ACTIVITIES AND STUDY AIDS

Review the following study aids and/or complete the activities to ensure that you have achieved the learning objectives for this chapter.

1. What are the medical assistant's duties in the immunology office?

_____

_____

_____

_____

_____

_____

_____

_____

2. Answer the following questions regarding the immune system:
   a. List the body's barriers to bacterial and viral infection and foreign bodies.

   _____

   _____

   _____

   b. What is the purpose of the lymphatic vessel system?

   _____

   _____

   _____

   c. What are the primary organs and the secondary organs of this system?

   _____

   _____

3. In your own words, describe each of the following:
   a. acquired immunity _____

   _____

   b. active immunity _____

   _____

   c. cell-mediated immunity_____

   _____

   d. humoral immunity _____

   _____

4. Review the section of this chapter that discusses immunodeficiency diseases, then define immunodeficiency disease in your own words.

   _____

   _____

   _____

   _____

   _____

   _____

   _____

   _____

5. Review the section in this chapter on autoimmune diseases. Close the book and make a list of the common autoimmune disorders. Go back to the textbook and add any that you may have forgotten.

   _____

   _____

   _____

   _____

_____
_____
_____

6. Look at a medical dictionary or medical encyclopedia and read the definitions of hypersensitivity and allergic reactions. Check the Internet by searching for the terms "hypersensitivity" and "allergic reactions." Review the textbook's definitions of these terms. Write a short summary of the definitions you found at each source and list your sources (include the URLs of websites you visit).

_____
_____
_____
_____
_____
_____
_____
_____

MEDICAL TERMINOLOGY REVIEW

Use a dictionary and highlighted terms in the textbook to define the following terms.

Terms

ankylosis _____
_____

antibody _____
_____

antigen _____
_____

antipyretic _____
_____

autoimmunity _____
_____

carditis _____
_____

dysfunction _____
_____

dysphagia _____
_____

dysphasia _____
_____

ecchymosis _____

electromyography _____

hematopoietic _____

hemolytic _____

immunodeficiency _____

interphalangeal _____

intrinsic factor _____

megakaryocytes _____

neuritis _____

petechiae _____

reactive _____

subcutaneous _____

Abbreviations

CSF _____

EMG _____

LE _____

N & V _____

RA _____

SCID _____

CRITICAL THINKING

1. Review and recall Standard Precautions (discussed in another chapter—look this up if necessary). Would you do any additional preparation when drawing blood from an AIDS patient than you would from another patient? Explain your answer.

_____

_____

_____

_____

2. You are in the clinic and two patients come to the front desk without appointments. Both are having breathing difficulties. One patient has just mowed his lawn and is extremely congested in both nose and airways. The other patient has just come from lunch at a Thai restaurant next door. She had taken about three bites of her food and then her tongue and throat became itchy. It progressed quickly and now her tongue is starting to swell. Which patient has the most emergent problem and why?

_____

_____

_____

_____

3. Make a list with a column for the following people if they are living and within your contact: your children, yourself, your parents, and each of their parents. If this is not possible in your family, try to use at least three people you know who are related to each other. Fill in the any allergies that each person has. It is common for allergies to run in families. When illustrated visually on paper, using your own family or friends can sometimes show patterns that were not apparent otherwise.

_____

_____

_____

_____

4. A patient has been coming in weekly for allergy injections. You have just administered her dose as prescribed by the physician, and you have asked her to wait in the office for about 20 minutes for observation before she leaves. Answer the following questions:

   a. Why would you want the patient to wait for a while before leaving?

   _____

   _____

   b. What symptoms might the patient exhibit in that 20 minutes?

   _____

   _____

5. A patient has just been diagnosed with several allergies, and you are giving her patient education and instructions at the end of her first visit. Explain in your own words, as if you were telling the patient (you need to use laymen's terms), what allergens and antigens are.

_____

_____

_____

_____

CHAPTER REVIEW TEST

MULTIPLE CHOICE

Circle the letter of the correct answer.

1. Which of the following are part of the four components of the body's immune system? (circle all that apply)
   a. humoral
   b. cell-mediated
   c. specific
   d. nonspecific

2. Aspirin has three actions, while acetaminophen has only two of those same actions. Which of the following choices is the action that aspirin has but acetaminophen does not?
   a. antipyretic
   b. analgesic
   c. hemopoietic
   d. anti-inflammatory

3. Which of the following are methods of diagnostic allergy testing? (circle all that apply)
   a. skin patch
   b. scratch testing
   c. ESR
   d. intradermal

4. A severe and prolonged form of asthma that can be life threatening is called
   a. asthma anaphylaxis
   b. anaphylaxis asthmaticus
   c. status asthmaticus
   d. status anaphylaxis

5. Which of the following are common food allergies as listed in your textbook? (circle all that apply)
   a. fish
   b. peanut butter
   c. lobster
   d. walnuts

6. Which statement is false in relation to HIV/AIDS transmission prevention strategies?
   a. Maintain a monogamous relationship.
   b. Avoid food that has been touched or prepared by someone with AIDS.
   c. If you get a tattoo, be sure a new needle is used.
   d. Use condoms.

7. Which of the following is not one of the five types of leukocytes discussed in this chapter of your textbook?
   a. monocytes
   b. eosinophils
   c. macrophages
   d. polymorphonuclear

8. Which of the following is not one of the three general categories of immune system diseases and disorders?
   a. hypersentivity and allergy reactions
   b. genetic disorders
   c. autoimmune disorders
   d. immunodeficiency diseases

9. The thymus gland decreases in size and function from _____ and on.
   a. birth
   b. early childhood
   c. mid adulthood
   d. puberty

10. The primary set of organs in the immune system are: (circle all that apply)
   a. bone marrow
   b. liver
   c. thymus gland
   d. tonsils

TRUE/FALSE

Indicate whether the statement is true (T) or false (F).

_____ 1. Kaposi's sarcoma is an infectious opportunistic condition common in AIDS.

_____ 2. All lymphocytes form in the bone marrow.

_____ 3. Food allergies can be severe but not life threatening.

_____ 4. Immunity is the ability to resist a particular disease or condition.

_____ 5. Hashimoto's thyroiditis is a condition of the GI system.

_____ 6. An allergist is a physician who specializes in diagnosing and treating the immune system and its functions.

_____ 7. Active immunity is short-term immunity.

_____ 8. The medical assistant must watch for signs of allergic reactions when allergy desensitization injections are given.

_____ 9. An autoimmune disease could result from unknown causes, genetic weaknesses, or in combination with other disease processes.

_____ 10. Hay fever is an allergic reaction.

FILL IN THE BLANK

Using words from the list below, fill in the blanks to complete the following statements.

aggressive

antigen-antibody
    reactions

antigens

cell-mediated

defense

desensitization

fight and protect

gastric mucosa

immune system

infectious
    microorganisms

inflammatory

inflammation

itself

laboratory testing

medication

nonspecific

phagocytosis

plasma

RBCs

repeated exposure

T-cell

testing

tissue rejection

transplant recipient

vitamin B_{12}

1. Immunodeficiency diseases result when the _____ is unable or becomes unable to _____ the body from disease.

2. Anaphylactic reactions are increasingly severe _____ to _____ to an allergen.

3. The intrinsic factor is a substance secreted by the _____ that is necessary for the absorption of _____ and the development of _____.

4. Body tissues respond to injury with _____, also known as a _____ immune response.

5. The lymphatic vessel system filters _____ from the lymph system and uses substances within _____ to activate the _____ response.

6. Suppression of the inflammatory response to prevent _____ is accomplished with _____ for the remainder of a _____'s life.

7. Autoimmune diseases result from _____ that develop from _____ activity by the body's immune system against _____.

8. Immunology and allergy are often combined within one practice, where allergy _____, allergy _____, and _____ are performed.

9. Monocytes are the first line of _____ in _____.

10. The _____ response is responsible for the production of _____ lymphocytes.

Chapter 21
Dermatology

CHAPTER OUTLINE

Review the Chapter Outline. If any content area is unclear, review that area before beginning workbook exercises.

    A.   The Medical Assistant's Role in Dermatology

    B.   The Anatomy and Physiology of the Skin

    C.   Diseases and Disorders of the Skin

    D.   Cosmetic Treatment for Skin Conditions

CHAPTER REVIEW

The following is a summary of the chapter. If any of this material is unclear, review it in the textbook.

A dermatology practice sees patients with a variety of skin and appendage issues. These include dermatitis, congenital disorders, infectious disorders, fungal and parasitic diseases, pigmentation and benign disorders, and skin cancer. The medical assistant may do a variety of tasks from taking the patient's medical history and vital signs to assisting with various examinations and procedures. As in all systems, the MA would prepare the patient and provide instructions. Knowledge of the anatomy and physiology and the various types of disorders and treatments are important for the medical assistant working with a dermatologist.

LEARNING ACTIVITIES AND STUDY AIDS

Review the following study aids and/or complete the activities to ensure that you have achieved the learning objectives for this chapter.

1. Explain in your own words the medical assistant's role in the dermatology office.

_____

_____

_____

_____

_____

_____

_____

_____

2. Make a list of the common types of dermatitis.

   _____

   _____

   _____

   _____

   _____

   _____

3. Provide a definition of a congenital disorder and then offer an example of a common type of congenital skin disorder.

   _____

   _____

   _____

   _____

   _____

   _____

   _____

4. Make a list of the common types of infectious skin disorders.

   _____

   _____

   _____

   _____

   _____

   _____

   _____

5. Give a definition of dermatophytoses and give an example of a common fungal skin disease.

   _____

   _____

   _____

   _____

   _____

   _____

   _____

6. Give two examples of common types of parasitic skin diseases, as discussed in the textbook.

   _____

   _____

   _____

_____
_____
_____
_____
_____

7. Define pigmentation and list three examples of pigmentation disorders that are stated in the textbook.

_____
_____
_____
_____
_____
_____
_____

8. Differentiate between benign and malignant neoplasms. List the common types of benign skin disorders.

_____
_____
_____
_____
_____
_____
_____

9. List the three types of skin cancer and state briefly what the letters stand for in the "ABCD rule."

_____
_____
_____
_____
_____
_____
_____
_____

MEDICAL TERMINOLOGY REVIEW

Use a dictionary and highlighted terms in the textbook to define the following terms.

Terms

appendage _____
_____

cauterization _____

collagen _____

cryosurgery _____

dermatitis _____

dermatology _____

dermatologist _____

dermatophytoses _____

integumentary system _____

keratin _____

lesion _____

melanin _____

melanocytes _____

neuralgia _____

sebaceous glands _____

Abbreviations

AK _____

BCC _____

SCC _____

UV _____

CRITICAL THINKING

1. As you are assisting an elderly patient get into a gown for an examination, you notice she has a dime-sized mole with an irregular border on her back. You realize the patient likely cannot see it and may be unaware of it. Would you mention it to the patient or only to the physician? State the reason for your answer.

_____

_____

_____

_____

2. Go to the Internet and locate a reputable site that provides pictures of various skin conditions, including lice. Draw a picture of head lice and state how this condition is treated.

3. What possible advice could you give to a patient who has had a skin cancer removed today and works daily as a lifeguard in the sun?

_____

_____

_____

_____

4. A female patient comes in for an examination for excessive dark hair she has developed in the last six months or so. She asks you what it is and what can be done for it, but she has not seen the physician yet. What would you say to this patient at this time? Hint: The answer is not specifically in the book and will require your current knowledge and critical thinking skills regarding the medical assistant's scope of practice.

_____

_____

_____

_____

5. Although not specifically stated in the text, what precautions would you recommend to a patient who has an infectious skin disorder to prevent it from spreading?

_____

_____

_____

_____

CHAPTER REVIEW TEST

MULTIPLE CHOICE

Circle the letter of the correct answer.

1. Which of the following two tasks may be the responsibility of the medical assistant as stated in the textbook?
   a. cryosurgery
   b. suture removal
   c. biopsy
   d. dressing application

2. Which of the following are infectious skin diseases? (circle all that apply)
   a. carbuncles
   b. leprosy
   c. herpes zoster
   d. chloasma

3. The three cosmetic treatments discussed in this chapter of the textbook are: (circle all that apply)

   a. laser resurfacing
   b. chemical peel
   c. plastic surgery
   d. dermabrasion

4. Which of the following is not a parasitic skin condition?
   a. pediculus humanus dermatitis
   b. pediculus humanus corporis
   c. pediculus humanus pubis
   d. pediculus humanus capitis

5. Psoriasis is characterized by: (circle all that apply)
   a. silvery scales.
   b. pus-filled lesions.
   c. pale, moist patches of skin
   d. itching and soreness

6. Lyme disease is transmitted
   a. by deer ticks.
   b. by sun exposure.
   c. by droplets.
   d. from one person to another by fluid in the lesions.

7. Which of the following is not an appendage of the skin?
   a. hair
   b. keratin
   c. sweat glands
   d. nails

8. Which of the following are signs of rosacea? (circle all that apply)
   a. pustules
   b. swelling
   c. rhinopyema
   d. scarring

9. Which of the following statements about dermatitis are false? (circle all that apply)
   a. It is an inflammatory condition.
   b. Eczema is one form of it.
   c. Psoriasis is one form of it.
   d. It can be acute or chronic.

10. Folliculitis is an inflammation and infection: (circle all that apply)
    a. caused by *Staphylococcus*.
    b. caused by iron deficiency.
    c. of a hair follicle.
    d. also known as a carbuncle or furuncle.

TRUE/FALSE

Indicate whether the statement is true (T) or false (F).

_____ 1. A congenital disorder is one that is inherited.

_____ 2. Alopecia is a medical term for thinning hair.

_____ 3. The largest organ of the body is the skin.

_____ 4. Insults or injuries to the skin may disrupt any of several bodily functions involved with the skin.

_____ 5. Benign neoplasms do not metastasize or spread to distant sites in the body.

_____ 6. The three layers of the skin are the epidermis, dermis, and endodermis.

_____ 7. Skin cells originate in the subcutaneous layer.

_____ 8. Older Americans are at greater risk for BCC and AK as a result of long-term exposure to the sun's UV rays in the days before the link between such exposure and skin cancer was scientifically established.

_____ 9. Basal cell melanoma is a type of skin cancer.

_____ 10. Hair is a living keratin tissue.

FILL IN THE BLANK

Using words from the list below, fill in the blanks to complete the following statements

ABCD rule	fat cells	polycystic
appearance	generalized illness	*Staphylococcus*
blood and lymph	hair growth	subcutaneous
common	heat and cold	subcutaneous tissue
connective tissue	inflammation and infection	support
curable	insulation	sweat and sebaceous
cushions	irritations or lesions	toxins
dehydration	microorganisms	temperature
dermis	nails	tumors
diagnosed early	nerve	vitamin D

1. Skin cancers are initially diagnosed according to their _____. Malignant melanoma is identified by the _____.

2. The integumentary system includes the _____, hair, and _____ glands.

3. Skin cancers are the most _____ type of cancer as well as the most _____ when _____.

4. The skin serves as a barrier to prevent _____ and other foreign bodies from entering; regulate _____; protect against _____; be an environmental sensor, including pain, temperature, and touch; synthesize _____ from sunlight; and excrete _____ in perspiration.

5. The dermis contains _____ vessels, _____ cell endings, and skin _____ organs.

6. Hirsutism is a condition of excessive _____, which may be caused by _____ ovaries or _____ of the adrenal glands and ovaries.

7. A break in the defense system of the skin may result in _____ as well as localized _____.

8. Cellulitis is a condition of _____ of the skin and subcutaneous tissue commonly caused by _____.

9. Sweat glands are located in the _____ and the _____.

10. The innermost layer of skin, the _____ tissue, is made up of _____ and _____ and acts as _____ for the body; provides protection against extreme _____ and against heat loss; and _____ and protects underlying structures.

CHAPTER OUTLINE

Review the Chapter Outline. If any content area is unclear, review that area before beginning workbook exercises.

    A.   The Medical Assistant's Role in the Endocrinology Office

    B.   The Anatomy and Physiology of the Endocrine System

    C.   Endocrine Disorders

CHAPTER REVIEW

The following is a summary of the chapter. If any of this material is unclear, review it in the textbook.

Some of the tasks of the medical assistant in an endocrinology practice include taking vital signs and patient history, obtaining blood and urine specimens, performing blood glucose tests, discuss dietary instructions, diabetic foot care, and glucose self-monitoring. A thorough understanding of the anatomy and physiology of the endocrine system as well as its connection to the nervous system is important along with the various endocrine disorders, the glands, and the role of hormones.

LEARNING ACTIVITIES AND STUDY AIDS

Review the following study aids and/or complete the activities to ensure that you have achieved the learning objectives for this chapter.

1. Define the medical assistant's role in assessment and other tasks in the endocrinology office.

    _____

    _____

    _____

    _____

    _____

    _____

    _____

2. Check your textbook for the anatomy of the endocrine system. Also check two other resources, such as other textbooks or the Internet, for pictures of the glands of the endocrine system. Draw a picture

of each gland and label with the name of the gland, including both names if there is more than one part that secretes hormones.

3. State the physiology of the endocrine system.

_____
_____
_____
_____
_____
_____
_____
_____

4. Review Table 22-2 in the textbook and then list the pituitary gland disorders stated there.

_____
_____
_____
_____
_____
_____
_____
_____

5. Review Table 22-2 in the textbook and then list the thyroid gland disorders stated there.

_____
_____
_____
_____
_____
_____
_____
_____

6. Review Table 22-2 in the textbook and then list the parathyroid gland disorders stated there.

_____
_____
_____

_____

_____

_____

_____

7. Review Table 22-2 in the textbook and then list the adrenal gland disorders stated there.

_____

_____

_____

_____

_____

_____

_____

8. Review Table 22-3: Hypoglycemia and Hyperglycemia, which are glucose metabolism disorders. Make two flash cards, one for each of the disorders. Put the name on one side and the signs and symptoms on the other side.

_____

_____

_____

_____

_____

_____

_____

_____

MEDICAL TERMINOLOGY REVIEW

Use a dictionary and highlighted terms in the textbook to define the following terms.

Terms

endocrine glands _____

_____

exocrine glands _____

_____

gluconeogenesis _____

_____

hormones _____

_____

hypothalamus _____

_____

Abbreviations

ACTH _____

_____

ADH _____

_____

FBS _____

_____

FSH _____

_____

GHB A1c _____

_____

GH _____

_____

IDDM _____

_____

LH _____

_____

MSH _____

_____

NIDDM _____

_____

PTH _____

_____

T_3 _____

_____

T_4 _____

_____

TSH _____

_____

CRITICAL THINKING

1. You have a 28-year-old female patient who is four months pregnant. She has come in stating she has symptoms of diabetes—her OB physician found that her urine glucose was high and sent her to your endocrinology office. Although the physician always diagnoses and orders tests, what do you think the first step will be for this patient? State the two tests that may be ordered by the provider.

_____

_____

_____

_____

2. A pregnant patient who is overdue for going into labor may need a hormone to help stimulate the process of uterine contractions. What hormone may be given? What endocrine gland would produce this hormone naturally? What else does this hormone stimulate?

_____

_____

_____

_____

3. In the case study in your textbook, what are the three things that this patient could control that may help his physical condition?

_____

_____

_____

_____

4. In the case study in the textbook, the patient seems to be in denial or at least resistant to lifestyle changes. Once you have given the patient all the education possible in your office, what are the three resources listed at the end of the chapter that would be most appropriate for him to contact?

_____

_____

_____

_____

5. Consider the same case study and answer this question with your opinion. There are no specific right answers for this, but please give your opinion using your critical thinking skills. If the patient tells you during the patient education that he refuses to change lifestyle, what would you do or say?

_____

_____

_____

_____

CHAPTER REVIEW TEST

MULTIPLE CHOICE

Circle the letter of the correct answer.

1. Which of the following are symptoms of hyperglycemia? (circle all that apply)

   a. fruity odor to breath
   b. moist skin

   c. less urine produced
   d. lowered blood pH level

2. Hypersecretion of _____ by the pituitary gland causes excessive growth.
   a. thymosin
   b. calcitonin

   c. testosterone
   d. growth

3. A simple goiter is caused by which hormone?

   a. adrenocortical

   b. thyroid

   c. growth

   d. melatonin

4. Signs of hypothyroidism include which of the following? (circle all that apply)

   a. pale, cool skin

   b. increased appetite

   c. weight loss

   d. intolerance to cold

5. Epinephrine is secreted by which organ?

   a. pancreas islets

   b. parathyroids

   c. adrenal medulla

   d. posterior pituitary

6. Which of the following is not a role the medical assistant may play in dealing with the diabetic patient?

   a. discussing the importance of foot care

   b. encouraging patients to stop immediately any drugs that may be producing side effects

   c. teaching the patient about insulin administration (depending on state laws and physician direction)

   d. instructing the patient in use of a glucometer

7. Which gland(s) is/are located above the kidneys?

   a. pancreas

   b. thymus

   c. adrenals

   d. pineal

8. Which gland works in concert with the sympathetic nervous system?

   a. adrenal medulla

   b. adrenal cortex

   c. pancreas

   d. thyroid

9. Which of the following glands secretes the thyroid stimulating hormone?

   a. thyroid

   b. parathyroids

   c. pituitary, anterior lobe

   d. thymus

10. Diminished release of vasopressin, or antidiuretic hormone, by the posterior lobe of the pituitary causes

   a. concentrated urine.

   b. delayed sexual maturity.

   c. slowed metabolic rate.

   d. dilute urine.

TRUE/FALSE

Indicate whether the statement is true (T) or false (F).

_____ 1. The hypothalamus controls the activity of the gland by releasing factors to the anterior pituitary gland.

_____ 2. Endocrine disorders are the result of too much or too little of a particular hormone being stimulated or released.

_____ 3. Gestational diabetes is a form of diabetes that has its onset during adult age instead of childhood.

_____ 4. Myxedema is a severe or acute hypothyroid state in adults that may lead to hypoglycemia, among other things.

_____ 5. The pancreas is both an endocrine and an exocrine gland.

_____ 6. Cushing's syndrome is caused by the hyposecretion of adrenocortical secretions.

_____ 7. The opposite of hypoglycemia is insulin shock.

_____ 8. The two control systems of the body are the gastrointestinal and endocrine systems.

_____ 9. The thyroid gland requires iron in the diet in order to function properly.

_____ 10. Hypoparathyroidism causes low serum sodium levels.

FILL IN THE BANK

Using words from the list below, fill in the blanks to complete the following statements. Note: Some terms may be used in more than one statement.

30	ductless	insurance claims
40	electrical system	maturity
abrupt	estrogen	melatonin
anterior and posterior	follicle	messages
autonomic system	four	midbrain
brain	free or low-cost	pharmaceutical
calcium levels	gradual	sperm maturation
chemical substances	hormones	targeted organs
development	hypoglycemia and hyperglycemia	thyroid
	hypothalamus	

1. Two serious glucose metabolism disorders, _____, are complications of diabetes mellitus.

2. A medical assistant can help diabetic patients by researching _____ companies that provide _____ insulin and medical supplies, knowing how to help patients contact local trustee or welfare offices, and providing assistance with filing _____.

3. The pituitary gland is a minute structure located in the _____, in the middle of the skull. It consists of _____ lobes and is controlled by the _____.

4. The pineal gland is located in the central portion of the _____ and is believed to secrete _____.

5. The endocrine system consists of _____ glands that affect the functions of _____ in the body by secreting _____.

6. Hormones are _____ that influence and control body functions such as growth and _____, sexual _____, and metabolism. Hormones send _____ to other glands and _____.

7. The follicle-stimulating hormone stimulates _____ secretion and _____ development in females and _____ in males.

8. The nervous system, including the _____, exerts control over body functions in a way similar to an _____.

9. The parathyroid glands, usually _____ in number, are attached to the surface of the _____ gland and affect _____ in the blood.

10. IDDM often has an _____ onset, usually appears before the age of _____. NIDDM often has a _____ onset, usually appearing in adults over the age of _____.

CHAPTER 23
Emergency Care

CHAPTER OUTLINE

Review the Chapter Outline. If any content area is unclear, review that area before beginning workbook exercises.

    A. The Medical Assistant's Role in Emergencies

    B. Emergency Resources

    C. Medical Office Preparedness

    D. Emergency Intervention

CHAPTER REVIEW

The following is a summary of the chapter. If any of this material is unclear, review it in the textbook.

Regardless of the type of practice or specialty the medical assistant works in, there can always be emergencies in the office, and every medical assistant should know basic first aid, CPR, and use of the AED. Patients may experience a wide variety of emergency symptoms and conditions/injuries that require medical assistance. A few examples include seizures, allergic reactions, heart attack or stroke, animal bites, burns, respiratory distress, and bleeding. Understanding the office protocol for an emergency and knowing where and how to use emergency equipment and supplies is a top priority.

LEARNING ACTIVITIES AND STUDY AIDS

Review the following study aids and/or complete the activities to ensure that you have achieved the learning objectives for this chapter.

1. Define the medical assistant's role in emergency care.

_____

_____

_____

_____

_____

_____

_____

_____

2. Describe the role of the EMS.

_____

_____

_____

_____

_____

_____

3. Make a flash card with a list of the equipment and supplies maintained for emergencies in a medical office. This can be used later for a quick reference.

_____

_____

_____

_____

_____

_____

_____

4. Explain what is meant by early intervention with CPR and AED.

_____

_____

_____

_____

_____

_____

5. State in your own words how chest pain emergencies are handled in the medical office.

_____

_____

_____

_____

_____

_____

_____

6. Read through the section on respiratory distress in this chapter in your textbook. List the types of respiratory distress and then state the appropriate interventions for respiratory distress.

_____

_____

_____

_____

_____

_____

_____

7. Name the different types of shock with a brief definition of each one.

_____

_____

_____

_____

_____

_____

_____

8. On a flash card, list the different types of bleeding on the front and the appropriate treatment on the back. The exact answer may not be stated in the textbook so review the material to compile your best answer on treatments.

_____

_____

_____

_____

_____

_____

_____

9. On flash cards, compare open and closed wounds by stating the type in one column and the treatment next to it in another column.

_____

_____

_____

_____

_____

_____

10. Define the three classifications of burns, three types of frostbite, and the thermal insults of heat stroke, heat exhaustion, and hypothermia stated in your textbook. Include their appropriate treatment briefly, but you do not have to present every type of burn treatment (such as chemical and radiation).

_____

_____

_____

11. What are the appropriate interventions for musculoskeletal injuries? Include fractures, sprains, strains, and dislocations.

_____

_____

_____

_____

_____

_____

12. State the general signs and symptoms of allergic reactions and appropriate treatment.

_____

_____

_____

_____

_____

_____

13. Give six examples of neurological emergencies and the appropriate general interventions for the group of emergencies.

_____

_____

_____

_____

_____

_____

14. Create flash cards listing acute abdominal pain, diabetic crises, poisoning, and foreign bodies in the eyes, ears, and nose. Include the appropriate treatment for each condition.

_____

_____

_____

_____

_____

_____

15. What are the appropriate interventions for psychosocial emergencies?

_____

_____

_____

_____

_____

_____

_____

MEDICAL TERMINOLOGY REVIEW

Use a dictionary and highlighted terms in the textbook to define the following terms.

Terms

abrasion _____

_____

Ambu bag _____

_____

anaphylaxis _____

_____

avulsion _____

_____

cyanosis _____

_____

epistaxis _____

_____

hyperglycemia _____

_____

hypertension _____

_____

hyperthermia _____

_____

hypoglycemia _____

_____

hypothermia _____

_____

incision _____

_____

laceration _____

_____

patent _____

_____

sepsis _____

_____

status epilepticus _____

_____

venous _____

_____

Abbreviations

ABCD _____

_____

AED _____

_____

AHA _____

_____

ARC _____

_____

CPR _____

_____

CVA _____

_____

ED _____

_____

ETA _____

_____

LOC _____

_____

NS _____

_____

SOB _____

_____

TIA _____

_____

CRITICAL THINKING

1. A patient has presented to the front desk without an appointment and is obviously SOB, her lips and fingertips appear a bit cyanotic. She seems weak and needs to be seated somewhere quickly. What would you do?

_____

_____

_____

_____

2. A patient who is sitting in the waiting room comes to the front desk with epistaxis, and the blood flow is very heavy. What would you do?

_____

_____

_____

_____

3. A patient's wife comes up to the front desk with some questions for the MA before her husband is seen. She asks how she could tell if her husband has or is having a stroke. How would you explain a CVA's signs and symptoms? (You are not diagnosing but simply giving the signs and symptoms in general.)

_____

_____

_____

_____

4. Why must you wash your hands after taking off gloves? Won't the gloves keep your skin clean so that you do not have to wash every time? Explain this in your own words.

_____

_____

_____

_____

5. If you come upon an unconscious person that you did not witness collapse, what should you do first? Would your answer be the same or different if the person was a 6-month-old infant?

_____

_____

_____

_____

CHAPTER REVIEW TEST

MULTIPLE CHOICE

Circle the letter of the correct answer.

1. Appendicitis pain would be located in which region or area of the body?

   a. pelvis
   b. back or flank region
   c. lower left quadrant
   d. lower right quadrant

2. Which types of abuse are mandatory to report regardless of the patient's wishes? (circle all that apply)

   a. child
   b. elder
   c. domestic or spousal
   d. rape (unless state law dictates this)

3. In open or compound fractures, what else should be treated in addition to the bone?

   a. soft tissue
   b. cartilage and tendons
   c. joints above and below the break
   d. the patient's fluid needs

4. Which of the following are appropriate questions or statements for a choking victim? (circle all that apply)

   a. Can you speak?
   b. Calm down so I can help you.
   c. What are you choking on?
   d. Are you choking?

5. What is the appropriate order of steps for an unresponsive, nonbreathing adult with an obstructed airway as stated in your textbook?

   a. Sweep the mouth, perform abdominal thrusts, attempt ventilations.
   b. Attempt ventilation, perform abdominal thrusts, sweep mouth.
   c. Perform abdominal thrusts, sweep the mouth, attempt ventilations.
   d. Attempt ventilation, sweep mouth, reattempt ventilation.

6. Which of the following is not one of the three criteria used to classify a burn?

   a. source of burn
   b. depth of burn
   c. when the burn occurred
   d. depth of burn

7. Why is a patient asked to wait in the office for 20 minutes following the administration of a medication, in this case a medication for anaphylactic shock?

   a. To ensure the patient lets the medication take effect before he or she moves around much.
   b. To observe for any potential reactions.
   c. The patient needs to rest.
   d. The patient must have a second dose after 20 minutes.

8. Which of the following is not a pressure point used to help control bleeding?

   a. carotid
   b. femoral
   c. vena cava
   d. brachial

9. What are some possible sources or causes of burns? (circle all that apply)
   a. chemicals
   b. radiation
   c. electricity
   d. hyperthermia

10. A/an _____ type of wound has torn skin and underlying tissue, and the edges are not smooth.
    a. avulsion
    b. incision
    c. abrasion
    d. laceration

TRUE/FALSE

Indicate whether the statement is true (T) or false (F).

_____ 1. An AED is not used on an infant.

_____ 2. Having a crash cart in the facility has legal liability issues for the practice.

_____ 3. Lock jaw is also known as an avulsion.

_____ 4. Establishing a baseline assessment of a head injury patient is often done using the Glasgow Coma Scale.

_____ 5. The pulse of an infant is taken on the carotid artery.

_____ 6. To prevent accidental or careless exposure, do not eat, drink, or touch your face during emergencies without first washing your hands.

_____ 7. A bolus of food is the most common object that adults choke on.

_____ 8. If direct pressure for bleeding does not stop the flow, a tourniquet must then be applied by a physician.

_____ 9. Usually an animal bite must be reported to the local animal control department.

_____ 10. In an emergency, if a person can wheeze, make a high-pitched sound, cough, or speak, do not take any action.

FILL IN THE BLANK

Using words from the list below, fill in the blanks to complete the following statements.

105° F	dressings	ligaments
advice	EMS	massage
bright red	exposure	overdose
bruising	flushing	perspire
chemical	gentle stream	poisoning
cleansed	hard	pressure
contamination	healing	rub
copious	heart	strains
darker in color	immobilize	tendons
direct pressure	infection	underlying tissues
dislocations	insidious	water
distally to proximally		

1. Arterial bleeding is usually _____, rapid, _____, and often spurts. Venous bleeding is slower, _____, and can usually be controlled by _____.

2. An individual experiencing heat stroke usually fails to _____ and has a body temperature of _____ or higher.

3. Internal bleeding may be obvious or _____. _____ or discoloration of the skin may be an indication of bleeding in the _____.

4. Open wounds must be _____, and most wounds require some type of dressing to promote _____ and prevent _____.

5. Bandages are used to anchor _____ in place, prevent _____ of a recent wound or surgical site, support and _____ injured extremities, and may be used to apply _____ to slow and/or stop bleeding.

6. If tissue has been frozen and is _____ to the touch, call _____ or the physician. Never _____, squeeze, or _____ frozen tissue.

7. Musculoskeletal injuries involve bones, muscles, _____ and _____ and include fractures, _____, sprains, and _____.

8. Poison Control Centers offer emergency _____ concerning accidental _____ and _____, this service is usually provided at no charge.

9. To help venous blood flow return to the _____, always apply bandages _____, or far to near.

10. If a liquid chemical is the cause of a burn, remove it from the skin by _____ with copious amounts of _____. If it is a dry or powdery _____, it should be carefully wiped from the victim while avoiding _____ to yourself or bystanders, then flush the area with a copious but _____ of water.

Procedure 23-1

Perform Adult Rescue Breathing and One-Rescuer CPR

Objective: The student, using the supplies and equipment listed below, will demonstrate how to administer rescue breathing for an adult and one-rescuer CPR for an adult.

Supplies: approved mannequin, gloves, ventilator mask, mouth guard

Notes to the Student:

_____

_____

_____

_____

_____

_____

Skills Assessment Requirements

Read and familiarize yourself with the procedure; complete the minimum practice requirements. Document each MPR using proper charting technique. Complete each procedure within a reasonable amount of time, with a minimum of 85% accuracy.

Name: _____

Date: _____

POINT VALUE ✦ = 3-6 points ∗ = 7-9 points		PRACTICE TRIAL	GRADED TRIAL # 1	GRADED TRIAL # 2	NOTES:
1. ✦	Assess the victim and determine if help is needed. Shout "Are you OK?" while gently shaking the victim's shoulders.				
2. ∗	If there is no response, assess the ABCs. *Airway:* Perform a head-tilt chin lift, or, if a neck injury is suspected, a jaw thrust. Look and feel for breath and chest movements. Attempt to get another person to call 911. If you are alone, begin the rescue sequence for 1 minute and then attempt to call yourself. If gloves are available, put them on. If you have a ventilator mask, place it on the victim.				
3. ✦	*Breathing:* If breathing is absent, put on a mouth guard and administer two rescue breaths. If your breaths do not cause the chest to rise, tilt the head again and make a second attempt.				
4. ∗	If the breath still does not enter the chest, proceed to the Heimlich maneuver for unconscious victims.				
5. ∗	*Circulation:* If the breaths cause the chest to rise, assess the patient's circulation by feeling for a pulse at the carotid artery. If you feel a pulse, begin rescue breathing. Administer 1 breath every 5 seconds, or 10–12 every minute. After 1 minute, reassess the victim for breathing and pulse.				

		PRACTICE TRIAL	GRADED TRIAL # 1	GRADED TRIAL # 2	NOTES:
6. ★	If you do not feel a pulse, begin chest compressions. Kneel at the victim's side. Find the sternum and place the heel of one hand 2–3 fingers' width above that space.				
7. ✦	Place your other hand on top of the first hand, making sure to lift your fingers off the chest, using only the heels of your hands to administer compressions.				
8. ✦	Keeping your shoulders directly over your hands, compress the chest 1 1/2 to 2 inches, then allow the sternum to relax. Do not lift your hands off the chest.				
9. ★	Continue to compress the chest a total of 30 times, then administer 2 breaths.				
10. ✦	Repeat this sequence for 4 total cycles. Reassess the victim.				
11. ✦	If necessary, continue CPR until pulse and breathing return or you are relieved by more advanced medical personnel.				

Name: _____

Date: _____

Document: Enter the appropriate information in the chart below.

Grading

Points Earned	_____		
Points Possible	_____	81	81
Percent Grade (Points Earned/ Points Possible)	_____		
PASS:	_____	❏ YES ❏ NO ❏ N/A	❏ YES ❏ NO ❏ N/A

Instructor Sign-Off

Instructor: _____ Date: _____

Procedure 23-2

Use of an Automated External Defibrillator (AED)

Objective: The student, using the supplies and equipment listed below, will demonstrate how to use an AED.

Supplies: AED machine, patient chart

Notes to the Student:

_____

_____

_____

_____

_____

_____

Skills Assessment Requirements

Read and familiarize yourself with the procedure; complete the minimum practice requirements. Document each MPR using proper charting technique. Complete each procedure within a reasonable amount of time, with a minimum of 85% accuracy.

Name: _____

Date: _____

POINT VALUE ✦ = 3-6 points ⋆ = 7-9 points		PRACTICE TRIAL	GRADED TRIAL # 1	GRADED TRIAL # 2	NOTES:
1. ✦	Place the AED next to the victim's left ear. This position allows the rescuers clear access to the chest and airway for continued rescue measures.				
2. ⋆	Turn the AED on and follow the voice prompts.				
3. ✦	You will be prompted to attach the electrode pads to the patient's chest, on the sternum and at the apex of the heart, following the diagram for correct placement.				
4. ✦	Next, you will be directed to allow the machine to analyze the heart rhythm to determine if it is a shockable rhythm. CPR should cease while the machine is analyzing.				
5. ✦	The machine will begin a charging sequence prior to shocking and warn rescuers to stand back. The voice prompt will then tell you to press the "shock" button to administer the electrical current to the patient.				
6. ⋆	If the machine indicates "No shock is advised," assess the patient for breathing and circulation. Continue CPR as needed until advanced medical personnel arrive.				

Name: _____

Date: _____

Document: Enter the correct information in the chart below.

Grading

Points Earned	_____		
Points Possible	_____	81	81
Percent Grade (Points Earned/ Points Possible)	_____		
PASS:	_____	❏ YES ❏ NO ❏ N/A	❏ YES ❏ NO ❏ N/A

Instructor Sign-Off

Instructor: _____ Date: _____

Procedure 23-3

Respond to an Adult with an Obstructed Airway

Objective: The student, using the supplies and equipment listed below, will demonstrate how to administer the Heimlich maneuver to an adult.

Supplies: approved mannequin, gloves, ventilation mask with one-way valve for an unconscious victim

Notes to the Student:

_____

_____

_____

_____

_____

_____

Skills Assessment Requirements

Read and familiarize yourself with the procedure; complete the minimum practice requirements. Document each MPR using proper charting technique. Complete each procedure within a reasonable amount of time, with a minimum of 85% accuracy.

POINT VALUE ✦ = 3-6 points ⋆ = 7-9 points		PRACTICE TRIAL	GRADED TRIAL # 1	GRADED TRIAL # 2	NOTES:
1. ⋆	Once it has been established that the victim is choking, with no air exchange, direct someone to call 911 and shout, "Are you choking?" or "Can you speak?" If the answer is no—as indicated by a head shake—tell the victim you are going to begin emergency treatment.				
2. ✦	Stand behind the victim with your feet slightly apart, placing one foot between the victim's feet and one to the outside. This stance will give you greater stability, and if the victim should pass out, you can safely guide them to the ground by sliding them down your thigh.				
3. ✦	Place the index finger of one hand at the person's navel or belt buckle. If the victim is a pregnant woman, place your finger above the enlarged uterus.				
4. ✦	Make a fist with your other hand and place it, thumb side to victim, above your other hand. If the person is very pregnant, the uterus is pushing the stomach and other internal organs under the rib cage and you may have to do chest compressions.				
5. ✦	Place your marking hand over your curled fist and begin to give quick inward and upward thrusts.				

	PRACTICE TRIAL	GRADED TRIAL #1	GRADED TRIAL #2	NOTES:
6. ✦ There is no set number of thrusts to give to an adult who remains conscious. Continue to give thrusts until the object is removed or the victim becomes unconscious.				
7. ✦ If the victim becomes unconscious, gently lower them to the ground.				
8. ✦ If gloves are available, put them on, open the victim's mouth, and perform a finger sweep to try to remove the foreign object.				
9. ✦ If the object cannot be removed, perform a head-tilt chin lift (in case of possible neck injury, use a jaw thrust) and administer two rescue breaths.				
10. ✦ If the air does not cause the chest to rise, tilt the head again and attempt two more breaths.				
11. ⋆ If your attempts are unsuccessful, straddle the victim's thighs and place the heel of one hand 2-3 finger widths above the navel and place your other hand on top, interlocking the fingers.				
12. ✦ Give five quick inward and upward abdominal thrusts.				

		PRACTICE TRIAL	GRADED TRIAL # 1	GRADED TRIAL # 2	NOTES:
13. ★	Move to the head of the victim and perform another finger sweep. If the object has not been expelled into the mouth, tilt the head again and attempt two more rescue breaths.				
14. ✦	Continue the cycle of five thrusts, finger sweep, and two breaths until the object is expelled or advanced medical personnel arrive to relieve you.				
15. ✦	The victim may lose the pulse, but you cannot proceed to CPR chest compressions until the foreign airway obstruction is cleared.				

Name: _____

Date: _____

Document: Enter the correct information in the chart below.

Grading

Points Earned	_____		
Points Possible	_____	99	99
Percent Grade (Points Earned/ Points Possible)	_____		
PASS:	_____	❑ YES ❑ NO ❑ N/A	❑ YES ❑ NO ❑ N/A

Instructor Sign-Off

Instructor: _____ Date: _____

Procedure 23-4

Administer Oxygen

Objective: The student, using the supplies and equipment listed below, will demonstrate how to administer oxygen therapy to an adult.

Supplies: portable oxygen tank; pressure regulator; oxygen flow meter; sterile, prepackaged, disposable nasal cannula with tubing; gloves; oximeter, patient chart

Notes to the Student:

_____

_____

_____

_____

_____

_____

Skills Assessment Requirements

Read and familiarize yourself with the procedure; complete the minimum practice requirements. Document each MPR using proper charting technique. Complete each procedure within a reasonable amount of time, with a minimum of 85% accuracy.

Name: _____

Date: _____

POINT VALUE ✦ = 3-6 points ⋆ = 7-9 points		PRACTICE TRIAL	GRADED TRIAL # 1	GRADED TRIAL # 2	NOTES:
1. ✦	Gather all needed equipment.				
2. ✦	Wash your hands.				
3. ⋆	Identify the patient and confirm the physician's order for oxygen therapy.				
4. ✦	Check the pressure reading on the oxygen tank to make sure it has enough oxygen in it.				
5. ✦	Start the flow of oxygen by opening the cylinder.				
6. ✦	Attach the cannula tubing to the flow meter. Adjust the oxygen flow to the physician's order.				
7. ✦	Hold the cannula tips over the inside of your wrist, without touching the skin, to determine if the oxygen is flowing.				
8. ✦	Don gloves, if necessary. You may prefer to wear gloves with patients who demonstrate a chronic cough, nasal drip, or other situation of potential exposure.				
9. ✦	Place the tips of the nasal cannula into the patient's nostrils. Wrap the tubing behind the patient's ears.				
10. ✦	Instruct the patient to breathe normally through the mouth and nose. Some patients instinctively hold their breath or avoid breathing through the nose when an object is placed in the nostrils.				

		PRACTICE TRIAL	GRADED TRIAL # 1	GRADED TRIAL # 2	NOTES:
11. ✦	Check the patient's oxygen level with an oximeter. Place the probe over the index finger and record the reading. If necessary, have the patient take a short walk to verify that the oxygen flow rate is sufficient for activity.				
12. ∗	Document the procedure in the patient's chart.				

Document: Enter the correct information in the chart below.

Grading

Points Earned	_____		
Points Possible	_____	78	78
Percent Grade (Points Earned/ Points Possible)	_____		
PASS:	_____	❏ YES ❏ NO ❏ N/A	❏ YES ❏ NO ❏ N/A

Instructor Sign-Off

Instructor: _____ Date: _____

Procedure 23-5

Demonstrate the Application of a Pressure Bandage

Objective: The student, using the supplies and equipment listed below, will demonstrate the application of a pressure dressing.

Supplies: dressing supplies or makeshift materials, gloves and/or other PPE available

Notes to the Student:

_____

_____

_____

_____

_____

_____

Skills Assessment Requirements

Read and familiarize yourself with the procedure; complete the minimum practice requirements. Document each MPR using proper charting technique. Complete each procedure within a reasonable amount of time, with a minimum of 85% accuracy.

POINT VALUE ✦ = 3-6 points ∗ = 7-9 points		PRACTICE TRIAL	GRADED TRIAL # 1	GRADED TRIAL # 2	NOTES:
1. ✦	Escort the patient immediately to an examination room.				
2. ✦	Wash your hands. Put on disposable gloves.				
3. ∗	Under physician's supervision, apply direct pressure with a dressing placed on the open wound. If possible, elevate the affected part.				
4. ✦	After assessment, the physician will decide if EMS should be activated.				
5. ✦	Apply additional dressings as needed. Do not remove the original dressing.				
6. ∗	Apply pressure to pressure points as necessary and with the physician's supervision.				
7. ✦	If bleeding is controlled, anchor the dressing to maintain pressure.				
8. ✦	Prepare the patient for transport to an emergency care facility.				
9. ✦	Dispose of waste in a biohazardous container.				
10. ✦	Remove your gloves and discard. Wash your hands.				
11. ∗	Document the procedure.				

Document: Enter the correct information in the chart below.

Grading

Points Earned	_____		
Points Possible	_____	75	75
Percent Grade (Points Earned/ Points Possible)	_____		
PASS:	_____	❏ YES ❏ NO ❏ N/A	❏ YES ❏ NO ❏ N/A

Instructor Sign-Off

Instructor: _____ **Date:** _____

Procedure 23-6

Demonstrate the Application of Triangular, Figure 8, and Tubular Bandages

Objective: The student, using the supplies and equipment listed below, will demonstrate how to apply triangular, figure 8, and tubular bandaging.

Supplies: elastic bandage, roller bandage, Kling™ bandage, tubular gauze and applicator, triangular bandage, tape, scissors

Notes to the Student:

_____

_____

_____

_____

_____

_____

Skills Assessment Requirements

Read and familiarize yourself with the procedure; complete the minimum practice requirements. Document each MPR using proper charting technique. Complete each procedure within a reasonable amount of time, with a minimum of 85% accuracy.

POINT VALUE ✦ = 3-6 points ⋆ = 7-9 points		PRACTICE TRIAL	GRADED TRIAL # 1	GRADED TRIAL # 2	NOTES:
1. ✦	Escort the patient immediately to an examination room. You may need to assist the patient, depending on the severity, location, and type of injury.				
2. ✦	Explain the procedure to the patient.				
3. ✦	Wash your hands.				
4. ✦	Gather necessary supplies.				
5. ⋆	**Triangular bandage:** • Keep the injured arm as immobile as possible. • Carefully slide the triangular bandage under the area to be held. The two shorter sides of the triangle should be pointing toward the elbow, and the remaining longer edge should be parallel to the opposite body side. • Bring the lowest side of the triangle up and over the arm • Tie the ends of the bandage behind and slightly to the side of the neck. • Tuck the peak of the bandage in toward the elbow point of the bandage. • The triangular bandage may also be wrapped around the head as a turban to anchor dressings onto the head.				

		PRACTICE TRIAL	GRADED TRIAL # 1	GRADED TRIAL # 2	NOTES:
6. ⋆	**Figure 8 bandage:** • Place the thumb of one hand on one end of the bandage to hold it in place. • Anchor the bandage with your other hand, then complete one circle around the extremity or body part. • Continue to alternate wrapping above and below the body joint or dressing and circling behind the joint or dressing area until the injured area is covered adequately.				
7. ⋆	**Tubular bandage:** • Choose an applicator that is larger than the extremity to be bandaged. • Cut an approximate amount of tubular gauze bandage and slide the gathered bandage onto the applicator. • Slide the applicator over the extremity. • Hold the bandage against the proximal end of the extremity and pull the applicator approximately 1 inch past the distal end. • Twist the bandage gauze one complete turn.				

		PRACTICE TRIAL	GRADED TRIAL # 1	GRADED TRIAL # 2	NOTES:
	• Next, slide the applicator toward the proximal end of the injury. • Hold the proximal end of the tubular bandage gauze in place, and pull the applicator toward the distal end. • After pulling past the distal end, complete one twist. • Slide back and forth and twist the distal end of the dressing until the injured area is adequately covered. Cut excess dressing, but remember to anchor the bandage at the proximal end. • Instruct the patient to watch for signs of circulation impairment.				
8. ✦	Wash your hands.				
9. ★	Document the procedure and patient teaching.				

Document: Enter the correct information in the chart below.

Grading

Points Earned	_____		
Points Possible	_____	66	66
Percent Grade (Points Earned/ Points Possible)	_____		
PASS:	_____	❏ YES ❏ NO ❏ N/A	❏ YES ❏ NO ❏ N/A

Instructor Sign-Off

Instructor: _____ **Date:** _____

Procedure 23-7

Demonstrate the Application of a Splint

Objective: The student, using the supplies and equipment listed below, will demonstrate how to apply a splint.

Supplies: makeshift or sterile dressing supplies, stiff or solid materials to immobilize the extremity, bandages or strips of material to secure splint materials

Notes to the Student:

_____

_____

_____

_____

_____

_____

Skills Assessment Requirements

Read and familiarize yourself with the procedure; complete the minimum practice requirements. Document each MPR using proper charting technique. Complete each procedure within a reasonable amount of time, with a minimum of 85% accuracy.

POINT VALUE ✦ = 3-6 points ✶ = 7-9 points	PRACTICE TRIAL	GRADED TRIAL #1	GRADED TRIAL #2	NOTES:
1. ✦ Identify yourself to the patient.				
2. ✦ Obtain vital signs.				
3. ✦ Ask the patient, if conscious, to speak his or her name.				
4. ✶ Ask about medical allergies and medications and whether or not the patient has a medical history.				
5. ✦ Assess the area of suspected fracture for bruising, bleeding, and open areas or protruding bones				
6. ✶ Moving the limb as little as possible and with gentle traction on the distal side, place the splint with padding under the limb or alongside the limb. You may have to ask other clinical staff for help to ensure the least amount of discomfort for the least amount of time.				
7. ✦ Place sterile dressings or clean makeshift dressings gently over open areas.				
8. ✶ Secure the splint by wrapping bandages or strips of material around the splint and the limb. The ties must be above and below the joints on both sides of the suspected fracture.				
9. ✦ Add additional ties as necessary along the length of the splint.				
10. ✦ If possible, leave an exposed area, such as toes or fingers, so that circulation can be monitored.				
11. ✶ The splint should be snug enough to immobilize the limb, but not tight.				

Name: _____

Date: _____

Document: Enter the correct information in the chart below.

Grading

Points Earned	_____		
Points Possible	_____	78	78
Percent Grade (Points Earned/ Points Possible)	_____		
PASS:	_____	❏ YES ❏ NO ❏ N/A	❏ YES ❏ NO ❏ N/A

Instructor Sign-Off

Instructor: _____ Date: _____

CHAPTER 24
Gastroenterology and Nutrition

CHAPTER OUTLINE

Review the Chapter Outline. If any content area is unclear, review that area before beginning workbook exercises.

    A. The Medical Assistant's Role in the Gastroenterology Office

    B. The Anatomy and Physiology of the Gastrointestinal System

    C. Diseases and Disorders of the GI Tract

    D. Nutrition

    E. Diagnosis and Treatment of GI Disorders

CHAPTER REVIEW

The following is a summary of the chapter. If any of this material is unclear, review it in the textbook.

The gastrointestinal system has the primary responsibility of nourishing the body; therefore, knowledge of nutrition is a major part of working in a gastroenterology office. The medical assistant will take the medical history and vital signs, record symptoms, assist the physician, arrange appointments, and provide patient instruction. To do these tasks, the MA must know the anatomy and physiology of the GI system, healthy living habits, nutrients, and weight management along with MyPyramid, and food allergies. An understanding of the diseases and conditions of this system are also vital.

LEARNING ACTIVITIES AND STUDY AIDS

Review the following study aids and/or complete the activities to ensure that you have achieved the learning objectives for this chapter.

1. Define the role of the medical assistant in the GI medical office.

    _____

    _____

    _____

    _____

    _____

    _____

    _____

    _____

2. Make a list of the anatomical parts of the GI system and include a brief explanation of the function of each part. List the accessory organs in this body system.

_____

_____

_____

_____

_____

_____

_____

3. Review Table 24-10 in the textbook. Make flash cards to study the diseases and disorders of the GI system and the accessory organs. Put the disease or disorder's name on one side of a card, and put a brief definition or description, as appropriate, on the other side. By transferring the information from the table to the cards, you will not only be reviewing the material again but you will have a quick reference as well as an excellent study tool.

_____

_____

_____

_____

_____

_____

_____

4. Write a list with the following basic food components: proteins, carbohydrates, fiber, lipids, vitamins, minerals, and water. Write a brief statement on the basic function of each.

_____

_____

_____

_____

_____

_____

_____

5. Visit the website www.MyPyramid.com as referred to in your textbook. If you have not entered information to get a pyramid specifically for *you*, then do so. It is quick and easy, and very informative since it is personal. This should enhance your understanding of MyPyramid guidelines and help you in your role of patient education and instruction. In your own words, explain how MyPyramid is used for healthy meal planning.

_____

_____

_____

_____

_____

_____

_____

6. Review the section on Nutrition and Health in your textbook. Close the book and answer the following questions from memory. Once you have written your answers, go back and check the book to ensure you included all the information.

   a. Name and define the three effects that nutritional status has on an individual's health.

   _____

   _____

   _____

   _____

   b. Why is dental health a contributing factory to nutritional status?

   _____

   _____

   _____

   _____

7. State the three factors that may affect caloric intake as discussed in the textbook. Give a one-sentence definition of each factor.

   _____

   _____

   _____

   _____

   _____

   _____

   _____

   _____

8. Explain the effects of alcohol on nutritional status.

   _____

   _____

   _____

   _____

   _____

   _____

   _____

Next, match the following parts of statements together. In the line space provided on the left, fill in the letter of the choice that completes the numbered statement.

   1. _____ Pregnant women are advised against taking *any* alcohol because of
   2. _____ Long-term alcohol use leads to other medical disorders, including malnutrition,
   3. _____ When too much alcohol is delivered to the liver,
   4. _____ The metabolism of alcohol prevents enzyme use
      a. obesity, ulcers, cancer, hypertension, and diabetes mellitus.
      b. for other necessary nutritional reactions.
      c. its devastating effects on the fetus, a condition known as fetal alcohol syndrome.

d. it accumulates as fat and may eventually cause cirrhosis.

9. Review the section in this chapter on The Effects of Aging on Nutritional Status. Close the book and make a list of all the effects you can recall. When you have completed the list, go back to the book and review the material to ensure you have included all of the effects.

_____

_____

_____

_____

_____

_____

_____

10. There are seven types of major disorders associated with altered nutritional status stated in your textbook. Review this section in your textbook, close your book, and make a list from memory of these seven items. When you have completed your list, if you have not recalled all seven, go back and review the material again.

_____

_____

_____

_____

_____

_____

_____

11. Make a list with three columns: common food allergies in adults, food allergies in children, and food intolerances in adults and children. Then in your own words, explain how food allergies are tested to arrive at a diagnosis for the patient.

_____

_____

_____

_____

_____

_____

_____

12. Review Figures 24-7 and 24-8 in your textbook. On a separate sheet of paper draw two simple torsos with the navel for a landmark. On one torso, draw lines to indicate the nine anatomical regions of the abdominopelvic cavity and label each region. One the other torso, draw lines to indicate the four clinical quadrants and label each one.

13. Make a list of the diagnostic procedures performed for GI disorders that are discussed in this chapter. For each one, indicate "yes," "no," or "possible" for whether the medical assistant would be likely to assist with or perform the procedure/test in the typical GI office.

_____

_____

_____

_____

_____

_____

_____

_____

14. (a) Make flash cards of the special and therapeutic diets that are commonly prescribed for GI patients and are often covered by the medical assistant during patient instruction. It would be helpful to have these cards for a quick reference. On one side of the card, write the name or type of special diet and write the dietary concepts on the other side.

(b) Review Table 24-12: Therapeutic Diets. Make a one-page list with two columns titled "Avoid" and "Substitute." You will prepare a handout that will be easy to read on what foods to eat and which to avoid from the Heart-Healthy Dietary Guidelines (American Heart Association). In the left column, list those things that should be avoided. In the right column, list those things that should be substituted. These lists are the type of patient education handouts that you may be asked to prepare in the workplace.

_____

_____

_____

_____

_____

_____

_____

_____

_____

MEDICAL TERMINOLOGY REVIEW

Use a dictionary and highlighted terms in the textbook to define the following terms.

Terms

absorption _____

_____

alimentary canal _____

_____

alimentation _____

_____

amino acids _____

_____

anastomosis _____

anorexia _____

anus _____

bolus _____

calorie _____

carbohydrates _____

cholesterol _____

chyme _____

colonoscopy _____

colostomy _____

complete protein _____

digestion _____

dyspepsia _____

dysphagia _____

electrolytes _____

elimination _____

emesis _____

emulsification _____

fats _____

feces _____

fiber _____

flatulence _____

gastric _____

gastroenterology _____

gastroscopy _____

hematemesis _____

hepatomegaly _____

ileostomy _____

incomplete protein _____

jaundice _____

kilocalorie _____

lipids _____

lower gastrointestinal tract _____

malnutrition _____

melena _____

metabolism _____

mineral _____

obesity _____

overweight _____

peristalsis _____

polyps _____

portal hypertension _____

proctology _____

protein _____

saturated fats _____

total parenteral nutrition _____

triglycerides _____

unsaturated fats _____

upper gastrointestinal tract _____

vitamins _____

Abbreviations

DGA _____

DHHS _____

ERCP _____

FNB _____

GI _____

HDL _____

LDL _____

LGI _____

LLQ _____

LUQ _____

RDA _____

RLQ _____

RUQ _____

TPN _____

UGI _____

USDA _____

CRITICAL THINKING

1. A patient has just been given some medication rectally and has been kept in the office for about 30 minutes. She is experiencing some sleepiness and dizziness, and her sister will be driving her home. Give her patient education of any side effects she may experience.

   _____

   _____

   _____

2. Mr. McNeill is experiencing constipation and has called in for advice on how to deal with this. Try to recall what you have read in this chapter of your textbook and use your common sense to list a few things that may help. After you have done that, check the book and review items you may have not learned yet.

   _____

   _____

   _____

3. You take a call from a patient who had a sigmoidoscopy earlier today. She is complaining of excess gas. What suggestions can you give her to give her some relief at home until she can pass the gas?

   _____

   _____

   _____

   _____

4. From your own understanding, without reviewing the textbook first, explain why HDL lipoproteins are considered the good cholesterol and LDL lipoproteins are considered the bad cholesterol.

_____

_____

_____

5. Your patient, Millie Stewart, is chatting while you are getting her ready for an exam. She tells you she has tried every kind of diet and many have worked well and rapidly, but the weight always comes back. Ms. Stewart explains that she has decided that she is just supposed to be 20 pounds overweight and she isn't going to diet any more; she is going to enjoy her food and her life. How would you respond to this? Consider that the information on Fad Diets under Tips for Success in your textbook is a resource for you to follow while working in a GI office. Plan your answer and write it out based on the information you know or deduce. You can check the book later, but respond to this using your common sense and critical thinking.

_____

_____

_____

CHAPTER REVIEW TEST

MULTIPLE CHOICE

Circle the letter of the correct answer.

1. Which of the following are not common-sense treatments of nausea as discussed in your text? (circle all that apply)
   a. Keep eyes open.
   b. Drink flat carbonated soft drinks.
   c. Drink clear liquids.
   d. Increase fiber in the diet.

2. Which of the following food choices are complex carbohydrates? (circle all that apply)
   a. fruit
   b. whole grains
   c. honey
   d. potatoes

3. Which of the following disorders may benefit from a therapeutic diet? (circle all that apply)
   a. diabetes mellitus
   b. hypercholesterolemia
   c. polyps
   d. hypertension

4. The initial mechanical breaking up of food starts in the mouth with: (circle all that apply)
   a. tongue.
   b. pharynx.
   c. salivary glands.
   d. mandible.

5. Which of the following is not a complete protein?
   a. eggs
   b. whole grains
   c. meat
   d. fish

6. Which of the following are warning signs of GI problems? (circle all that apply)
   a. melenoma
   b. hematemesis
   c. coffee-ground emesis
   d. flatulence

7. Which of the following is a layer of the alimentary canal? (circle all that apply)
   a. serosa
   b. submuscular
   c. mucosa
   d. muscularis

8. Which of the following activities burns the most calories?
   a. swimming
   b. tennis
   c. aerobics
   d. running

9. Which of the following are consequences of dehydration? (circle all that apply)
   a. increased blood volume
   b. hypotension
   c. increased urine production
   d. possibly hypovolemic shock

10. Which of the following is not located in the lower right quadrant of the abdomen?
    a. cecum
    b. appendix
    c. spleen
    d. right ureter

TRUE/FALSE

Indicate whether the statement is true (T) or false (F).

_____ 1. Energy released from the metabolism of proteins, fats, and carbohydrates is measured in units of kilograms.

_____ 2. LDLs transport fats from body cells to the liver for disposal.

_____ 3. Bright red blood in the stools is an indicator of gastric cancer.

_____ 4. A good post-op diet is the clear liquid diet.

_____ 5. Water, fluids, and electrolytes are absorbed mainly in the large intestine.

_____ 6. A person's religion can play a role in his or her nutrition.

_____ 7. In a heart-healthy diet, avoid tuna packed in oil.

_____ 8. Carbohydrates are the body's primary source of energy and are found primarily in breads, cereals, pasta products, rice, fruit, and potatoes.

_____ 9. Lipids (fats) are a primary source of energy.

_____ 10. For rapid absorption of a medication without the risk of GI upset, you must inject medication.

FILL IN THE BLANK

◪

Using words from the list below, fill in the blanks to complete the following statements.

affected length	examine	non-nutrient
ages	four clinical	nourishment
alimentation	good eating habits	resection
bleeding	immune system	stomach
cancer	IV therapy	total parenteral nutrition (TPN)
colostomy	lifestyle habits	tube feedings
efficient	liver	tumors
elimination of the waste	mental alertness	USDA
energy levels	nine anatomical	younger years

1. Good nutritional habits help the body maintain a strong _____ and maintain healthy _____ and _____.

2. The Food Guide Pyramid was an educational tool developed by the _____ to help healthy Americans maintain _____.

3. If a patient cannot take nutrients orally, the physician will prescribe _____ by _____ directly into the stomach or by _____.

4. The major functions of the GI system are digestion and _____, which provide _____ for the body, and the _____ products of digestion.

5. Alcohol is a _____, which yields 7 kcal/gram that is absorbed by the _____ and small intestine and broken down by the _____ before it is excreted from the body.

6. To correctly evaluate suspected lower GI disorders, _____, positive fecal blood tests, _____, polyps, or suspected _____, the physician must _____ the lower GI system.

7. The physiological functioning of the GI system becomes less _____ as an individual _____.

8. There are two methods for describing the location of abdominopelvic regions when the physician is trying to diagnose conditions and disorders: the _____ divisions and the _____ quadrants.

9. The nutritional status of the elderly is the result of _____ and choices made in their _____.

10. Obstructive conditions of the colon may require surgical intervention, including _____, either temporary or permanent, or _____ (surgical removal) of the _____ of the colon.

Procedure 24-1

Assist with a Colon Endoscopic/Colonoscopy Exam

Objective: The student, using the supplies and equipment listed below, will demonstrate how to set up an exam room and assist the physician with a colon endoscopic procedure.

Supplies: 2 pairs of nonsterile gloves, instrument for viewing, depending on procedure being performed, water-soluble lubricant, patient drapes and gown, sterile cotton-tipped applicators, for collection of fecal samples, suction device, sterile biopsy forceps, disposable or sterile rectal speculum, specimen containers with lab requisition form, as needed, disposable tissue, biohazard container, patient chart

Notes to the Student:

_____

_____

_____

_____

_____

_____

Skills Assessment Requirements

Read and familiarize yourself with the procedure; complete the minimum practice requirements. Document each MPR using proper charting technique. Complete each procedure within a reasonable amount of time, with a minimum of 85% accuracy.

POINT VALUE ✦ = 3-6 points ∗ = 7-9 points		PRACTICE TRIAL	GRADED TRIAL # 1	GRADED TRIAL # 2	NOTES:
1. ✦	Gather all needed supplies.				
2. ∗	Identify the patient and explain the procedure. Verify that the patient has followed pre-exam instructions regarding foods, medications, and activities to avoid, such as enemas. The patient should be asked to empty the bladder prior to the exam.				
3. ✦	Give the patient drapes and a gown and instructions on proper gown opening placement.				
4. ✦	Take the patient's vital signs.				
5. ✦	Assist the patient to the table and position him or her for the exam.				
6. ✦	Wash your hands and put on gloves.				
7. ∗	Assist the physician by handing him or her supplies as requested. To ease equipment entry into the anal canal, the physician will use an anal speculum. A suction device may be required to remove any fecal matter that obstructs the physician's view. If polyp tissue samples are needed, the physician will use sterile biopsy forceps.				
8. ✦	To ease any discomfort, instruct the patient to breathe slowly and deeply. Observe the patient for any change in vitals, increased pain level, or other undue reactions.				

		PRACTICE TRIAL	GRADED TRIAL #1	GRADED TRIAL #2	NOTES:
9. ✦	After the physician has collected the necessary samples, you will place them in sterile specimen containers.				
10. ✦	When the physician has completed the examination, cleanse the patient's anal area with tissues.				
11. ✦	Remove the gloves, wash your hands, and assist the patient into a recovery position.				
12. ⋆	While the patient is resting, recheck vital signs. Invasive procedures often cause a drop in blood pressure.				
13. ✦	Once the blood pressure is stable, allow the patient to get off the exam table and get dressed.				
14. ✦	Complete laboratory forms. Seal the specimen containers in an appropriate biohazard labeled transport bag.				
15. ✦	When the patient has been released from the room, wash your hands, put on new gloves, and disinfect the area. A disposable speculum should be discarded into a biohazardous container; a stainless steel speculum should be prepared for autoclaving				
16. ⋆	Document the procedure in the patient's chart.				

Document: Enter the correct information in the chart below.

Grading

Points Earned	_____		
Points Possible	_____	108	108
Percent Grade (Points Earned/Points Possible)	_____		
PASS:	_____	❏ YES ❏ NO ❏ N/A	❏ YES ❏ NO ❏ N/A

Instructor Sign-Off

Instructor: _____ Date: _____

Procedure 24-2

Assist with a Sigmoidoscopy

Objective: The student, using the supplies and equipment listed below, will demonstrate how to set up an exam room and assist the physician with a sigmoidoscopy procedure.

Supplies: sigmoidoscope, insufflator, water-soluble lubricant, patient drapes and gown, sterile cotton-tipped applicators, suction device, sterile biopsy forceps, as directed by physician, disposable or sterile rectal speculum, specimen containers with lab requisition form, as needed, disposable tissue, chucks pads, water basin, 500 ml of warmed water, gloves, biohazard container, patient chart

Notes to the Student:

_____

_____

_____

_____

_____

_____

Skills Assessment Requirements

Read and familiarize yourself with the procedure; complete the minimum practice requirements. Document each MPR using proper charting technique. Complete each procedure within a reasonable amount of time, with a minimum of 85% accuracy.

POINT VALUE ✦ = 3-6 points ⋆ = 7-9 points		PRACTICE TRIAL	GRADED TRIAL # 1	GRADED TRIAL # 2	NOTES:
1. ✦	Gather all needed supplies.				
2. ⋆	Identify the patient and explain the procedure. Verify that the patient has followed pre-exam instructions regarding foods, medications, and activities to avoid and performed an enema. The patient should be asked to empty the bladder prior to the exam for greater comfort.				
3. ✦	Give the patient drapes and a gown and instructions on proper gown opening placement.				
4. ✦	Take the patient's vital signs.				
5. ✦	Assist the patient to the table and position for the exam.				
6. ✦	Place a chucks pad, examination pad, or other absorbent material under the patient's perineal area.				
7. ✦	Wash your hands and put on gloves.				
8. ⋆	Assist the physician as needed.				
9. ⋆	Attach the light source and insufflator to the sigmoidoscope, but do not turn on the light until the physician is ready to use it. The light generates heat the longer it is on and can potentially burn the patient.				

		PRACTICE TRIAL	GRADED TRIAL #1	GRADED TRIAL #2	NOTES:
10. ✦	To ease the patient's discomfort, instruct him or her to breathe slowly and deeply. Observe the patient for any change in vitals, increased pain level, or other undue reactions				
11. ✦	When the physician has completed the examination, cleanse the patient's anal area with tissues.				
12. ✦	Remove the gloves, wash your hands, and assist the patient into a recovery position.				
13. ✦	While the patient is resting recheck vital signs. Invasive procedures often cause a drop in blood pressure.				
14. ✦	Once the blood pressure is stable, allow the patient to get off the exam table and get dressed.				
15. ✦	Complete the laboratory forms and send samples to be examined.				
16. ✦	When the patient has been released from the room, wash your hands, put on new gloves, and disinfect the area.				
17. ✶	Document the procedure in the patient chart.				

Document: Enter the correct information in the chart below.

Grading

Points Earned	_____		
Points Possible	_____	114	114
Percent Grade (Points Earned/Points Possible)	_____		
PASS:	_____	❏ YES ❏ NO ❏ N/A	❏ YES ❏ NO ❏ N/A

Instructor Sign-Off

Instructor: _____ Date: _____

Procedure 24-3

Insert a Rectal Suppository

Objective: The student, using the supplies and equipment listed below, will demonstrate how to administer a rectal suppository.

Supplies: physician-prescribed rectal suppository, water-soluble lubricant, tissues, biohazardous container, disposable gloves, patient instructions, patient chart

Notes to the Student:

_____

_____

_____

_____

_____

_____

Skills Assessment Requirements

Read and familiarize yourself with the procedure; complete the minimum practice requirements. Document each MPR using proper charting technique. Complete each procedure within a reasonable amount of time, with a minimum of 85% accuracy.

Name: _____

Date: _____

POINT VALUE ✦ = 3-6 points ★ = 7-9 points		PRACTICE TRIAL	GRADED TRIAL # 1	GRADED TRIAL # 2	NOTES:
1. ✦	Verify the patient's identification and check for allergies.				
2. ★	Verify the physician's medication order.				
3. ✦	Collect all necessary supplies.				
4. ✦	Explain the procedure to the patient.				
5. ✦	Wash your hands and put on gloves.				
6. ✦	Ask the patient to remove all clothing from the waist area down.				
7. ✦	Assist the patient into a Sims position and provide proper drapes.				
8. ✦	Take the protective foil wrap from the suppository and carefully smooth any rough or jagged edges. Lubricate the suppository with the water-soluble lubricant.				
9. ✦	Expose the patient's buttocks.				
10. ★	Holding the suppository in one hand, lift the upper buttock with your other hand, exposing the anus.				
11. ★	Firmly guide the suppository into the anus with your index finger, past any fecal masses and the internal sphincter. This will prevent it from being expelled.				

		PRACTICE TRIAL	GRADED TRIAL # 1	GRADED TRIAL # 2	NOTES:
12. ✦	With a tissue, apply firm pressure on the anus for 1–2 minutes to allow the medication to be retained. Discard the tissue into the biohazardous container.				
13. ✦	With another tissue, wipe away any excess lubricant or fecal matter from the anus and discard the tissue into the biohazardous container.				
14. ✦	Instruct the patient to get into a comfortable position and rest for 30 minutes as the medication is absorbed.				
15. ✦	Clean the area, providing a new drape if necessary, and dispose of all materials in the biohazardous container				
16. ✦	Remove the gloves and wash your hands.				
17. ⋆	Document the procedure in the patient chart.				

Gastroenterology and Nutrition **631**

Document: Enter the correct information in the chart below.

Grading

Points Earned	_____		
Points Possible	_____	114	114
Percent Grade (Points Earned/Points Possible)	_____		
PASS:	_____	❑ YES ❑ NO ❑ N/A	❑ YES ❑ NO ❑ N/A

Instructor Sign-Off

Instructor: _____ Date: _____

CHAPTER 25
Orthopedics and Physical Therapy

CHAPTER OUTLINE

Review the Chapter Outline. If any content area is unclear, review that area before beginning workbook exercises.

    A.   The Medical Assistant's Role in the Orthopedic Office

    B.   The Anatomy and Physiology of the Musculoskeletal System

    C.   Common Musculoskeletal Diseases and Disorders

    D.   Diagnostic Procedures

    E.   Treatment of Musculoskeletal Conditions in the Orthopedic Office

CHAPTER REVIEW

The following is a summary of the chapter. If any of this material is unclear, review it in the textbook.

Orthopedics is a specialty that sees a wide variety of patients, both in age and in types of disease or injury. The two body systems—the bones and the muscles—work together, and knowing the unique anatomy and physiology is vital for those working in an orthopedic office. A medical assistant should be familiar with musculoskeletal conditions including congenital, infectious, neoplastic (whether malignant or benign), and injuries such as fractures and dislocations. Examples of what the MA would do or assist with could include physical therapy tasks, thermodynamics (the application of heat and/or cold therapy), fitting and teaching about assistive aids for ambulation, and ROM exercises. For the health and safety of the MA and all healthcare workers, proper body mechanics should be utilized at all times.

LEARNING ACTIVITIES AND STUDY AIDS

Review the following study aids and/or complete the activities to ensure that you have achieved the learning objectives for this chapter.

1. Define the role of the medical assistant in the orthopedic office.

_____

_____

_____

_____

_____

_____

_____

_____

2. Since the medical assistant must know the anatomy and physiology of all body systems, answer the following questions regarding the skeletal and muscular systems.

   a. State the functions of the skeleton and of the muscles.

   _____

   _____

   b. Name the two parts of the skeleton with examples of the bones of each part.

   _____

   _____

   c. Define cartilage and ligament and briefly state their function(s). What do tendons connect?

   _____

   _____

   d. Where does hematopoiesis occur?

   _____

   _____

   e. Name the three major types of joints.

   _____

   _____

   f. What are the three types of muscle tissue?

   _____

   _____

   g. Explain the contraction of muscle cells.

   _____

   _____

   h. What stimulates involuntary muscle? What stimulates cardiac muscle?

   _____

   _____

3. Make a set of flash cards of the pathology of this system. On one side of the card, include each of the following classifications of conditions: congenital, degenerative, infectious, malignant, and traumatic musculoskeletal conditions and on the other side of the card, list the conditions that are discussed in the textbook.

   _____

   _____

   _____

   _____

   _____

   _____

   _____

4. Make a table with two columns of the diagnostic procedures for musculoskeletal conditions that are covered in your textbook. List the procedures on the left side and on the right side list the purpose for the procedure.

   _____

   _____

   _____

_____

_____

_____

_____

5. State in your own words what a splint is used for and what a brace is used for.

_____

_____

_____

_____

_____

_____

_____

6. Make flash cards of the different types of casts and the points of each one. Make points brief enough to fit on one side of the card for a quick reference. Be concise, and don't include words or details that you do not need in order to do the step correctly.

_____

_____

_____

_____

_____

_____

_____

7. Make a list of the major physical therapy modalities, including thermodynamics, and state for each modality the purpose only, not the description.

_____

_____

_____

_____

_____

_____

_____

8. Briefly explain why a patient would use one of the four ambulation gaits when walking with crutches. State why a patient would use a cane and why a patient would use a walker.

_____

_____

_____

_____

9. What are some prostheses used in medicine today? Give two examples of prostheses in orthopedics.

_____

_____

_____

_____

_____

_____

10. Describe the proper body mechanics for lifting a box of supplies.

_____

_____

_____

_____

_____

_____

MEDICAL TERMINOLOGY REVIEW

Use a dictionary and highlighted terms in the textbook to define the following terms.

Terms

amphiarthrosis _____

_____

arthritis _____

_____

articular _____

_____

atony _____

_____

atrophy _____

_____

axillary _____

_____

body mechanics _____

_____

bursa (plural: bursae) _____

_____

bursitis _____

_____

cartilage _____

_____

cast _____

_____

compress _____

_____

cryotherapy _____

_____

diarthrosis _____

_____

endosteum _____

_____

hematopoiesis _____

_____

ligament _____

_____

neoplasia _____

_____

orthopedics _____

_____

osteoblast _____

_____

periosteum _____

_____

prosthesis (plural: prostheses) _____

_____

range of motion _____

_____

reduction _____

_____

soak _____

_____

splint _____

_____

synarthrosis _____

_____

Orthopedics and Physical Therapy   **637**

tendon _____

_____

tetany _____

_____

thermodynamics _____

_____

thermotherapy _____

_____

Abbreviations

AKA _____

_____

BEA _____

_____

BKA _____

_____

C1 _____

_____

Ca _____

_____

DJD _____

_____

Fx _____

_____

L1 _____

_____

LLE _____

_____

LLL _____

_____

LS _____

_____

LUE _____

_____

PT _____

_____

RA _____

_____

RLE _____

_____

RLL _____

_____

ROM _____

_____

RUE _____

_____

T1 _____

_____

CRITICAL THINKING

1. Consider that you have a 7-year-old male patient with a fractured ankle. He is full of energy and seems to be the type who will be running around in his cast and be pretty hard on it. Which casting material would you choose for this child and why? (The answer is not in the book; use your reasoning or critical thinking and decide on your answer.)

_____

_____

_____

_____

2. Review the Case Study at the beginning of this chapter in the textbook. Explain why the x-ray may not show a fracture of a bone.

_____

_____

_____

_____

3. You were at the scene of an injury to a 14-year-old female who had fallen off of her bike. You can see that a portion of her flesh and a piece of bone has been torn away and is lying in the dirt at the edge of the sidewalk. Should you save that piece of tissue and if so, how would you prepare/store it until it can be given to a doctor?

_____

_____

_____

_____

4. Without looking back at the material right now, picture that you are working in an orthopedic office and a 19-year-old college football player has been brought into the clinic by his coach. He has been seen by the doctor, and x-rays have been taken and looked at by the doctor. He was diagnosed with a strain, and you are preparing him for application of a cast by the technician. The patient insists he has a sprain, not a strain, and asks that you explain to him the difference between the two. From your memory of the material, write your answer. Then go back and check the book and write a correct answer if yours differs.

_____

_____

_____

_____

5. A patient calls in and has questions after reading her cast care written instructions. She asks how she is supposed to apply ice to the injury when she has a cast on over the injury. What patient education/instruction would you give her?

_____

_____

_____

_____

CHAPTER REVIEW TEST

MULTIPLE CHOICE

Circle the letter of the correct answer.

1. Bones are classified according to structure, and four are listed in your textbook. Which of the following is not one of the four structure classifications?
   a. flat
   b. round
   c. short
   d. long

2. Your text includes five classifications of common musculoskeletal diseases and disorders. Which of the following are included in these classifications as stated in the book? (circle all that apply)
   a. congenital
   b. malignant
   c. infectious
   d. degenerative
   e. traumatic

3. Arthritis is the inflammation and degeneration of joint structures. Which of the following is not a form of arthritis?
   a. osteoarthritis
   b. rheumatoid arthritis
   c. bursitis
   d. gouty arthritis

4. Which of the following is a diagnostic procedure that could diagnose/confirm intervertebral disc disorders?
   a. electromyogram
   b. arthrogram
   c. bone scan
   d. myelogram

5. Involuntary muscles are controlled by the
   a. autonomic nervous system.
   b. peripheral nervous system.
   c. sympathetic nervous system.
   d. parasympathetic nervous system.

6. Which of the following types of fracture usually does not require surgical intervention at an emergency or urgent care center?
   a. displaced
   b. greenstick
   c. avulsed
   d. compound

7. There are three types of muscle tissue in the body. Which of the following are not one of those three types? (circle all that apply)

   a. tendon
   b. cartilage

   c. cardiac
   d. smooth

8. Trauma to the musculoskeletal system does NOT include insults in the form of:

   a. fractured bones.
   b. insults to muscles.
   c. soft-tissue insults to ligaments and tendons.

   d. arthritis.

9. A complete or partial dislocation is called a

   a. manipulation.
   b. laceration.

   c. subluxation.
   d. displacement.

10. Degeneration of the neuromuscular system is discussed briefly in your textbook under The Contraction of Muscle Cells, and three examples of diseases in this category are given. Which of the following is not one of the three?

   a. Parkinson's disease
   b. muscular dystrophy

   c. atrophy
   d. multiple sclerosis

TRUE/FALSE

Indicate whether the statement is true (T) or false (F).

_____ 1. The correction of a fracture, in which the bone fragments or parts are realigned, is called reduction.

_____ 2. Flexion increases the angle of the joint.

_____ 3. A torn meniscus (cartilage in the knees and other joints) often results from a fall, but could also result from a twisting motion or a sports injury.

_____ 4. A splint is a more permanent device than a brace.

_____ 5. The scapula is part of the axial skeleton.

_____ 6. Applying heat to an injury will help prevent inflammation.

_____ 7. Cartilaginous joints allow free movement.

_____ 8. A cast cutter is used in a procedure known as bivalving a cast.

_____ 9. A swing gait is a type of walking with crutches.

_____ 10. Calcium is important for blood clotting (coagulation).

FILL IN THE BLANK

Using words from the list below, fill in the blanks to complete the following statements.

24 hours	healing	sitting
abnormal	heard by the human ear	still attached
amount of movement	heat	straight
amputated	home	synaptic gap
articulation	inflammation	temperature
benign	malignant	thermotherapy
blood vessels	muscle	tissue construction
body mechanics	neuromuscular	tissue injury
circulation	one hour	tumors
cryotherapy	pain	walking
day-to-day	prompt a response	weight-bearing
excite	risk of injury	

1. A joint, or _____, is the point at which two bones meet. Joints are classified according to the _____ between the bones and the _____ allowed by each joint.

2. A nerve cell contacts the muscle cell at the _____ junction. Between the nerve cell and the muscle cell is a small space called a _____. A stimulus causes the release from the neuron neurotransmitters that _____ and _____ from the muscle fiber or cell.

3. Neoplasia and/or _____ musculoskeletal conditions may involve any of the structures of this system and usually take the form of _____. Not all _____ tissue growths (neoplasia) are malignant; some may be _____.

4. With a plaster cast, avoid _____ activity for _____. With a synthetic cast, avoid activity for _____.

5. Cryotherapy constricts _____; slows _____ to the affected area; reduces swelling, _____, and pain; and decreases body _____.

6. To prevent musculoskeletal injuries and maintain health and safety, healthcare team members must practice proper _____ such as keeping the back _____ when _____, standing, and _____.

7. The goal of proper patient instruction in the use of crutches is to reduce the _____ and accidents in the patient's _____ and during _____ activities.

8. Ultrasound waves, with frequencies that cannot be _____, penetrate deep into _____ tissue and are converted to _____.

9. Thermodynamics consists of heat (_____) or cold (_____) applications that promote _____ and prevent further _____ to areas affected by trauma, infections, and inflammation.

10. After an amputation, the individual may feel _____ or other sensations in the area where the _____ part had been, as if it were_____.

Name: _____

Date: _____

Procedure 25-1

Assist with Fiberglass Cast Application

Objective: The student, using the supplies and equipment listed below, will demonstrate how to assist with the application of a fiberglass cast.

Supplies: rolls of fiberglass casting material, stockinette, padding, tape, blunt/sharp nose scissors (for cutting material), warm tap water, basin (2–4 liter), bandage, gloves, stool or low chair for support (if casting a foot or lower leg), patient drapes

Notes to the Student:

_____

_____

_____

_____

_____

_____

Skills Assessment Requirements

Read and familiarize yourself with the procedure; complete the minimum practice requirements. Document each MPR using proper charting technique. Complete each procedure within a reasonable amount of time, with a minimum of 85% accuracy.

Name: _____

Date: _____

POINT VALUE ✦ = 3-6 points ⋆ = 7-9 points		PRACTICE TRIAL	GRADED TRIAL #1	GRADED TRIAL #2	NOTES:
1. ✦	Assist the patient to the exam room and into a comfortable position. Explain that the patient should be comfortable to avoid having to shift the body weight during the lengthy casting process.				
2. ⋆	Identify the patient and verify the physician's orders.				
3. ✦	Explain the procedure.				
4. ✦	Wash your hands and put on gloves.				
5. ⋆	Cleanse and inspect the area to which the cast will be applied. Note any open wounds, bruising, or excessive swelling and report these to the physician.				
6. ✦	Drape the patient to protect clothing.				
7. ✦	Open one package of fiberglass material. Do not open the other packages until they are needed, to prevent waste.				
8. ✦	Hand the physician the materials requested. If your clinic allows medical assistants to perform casting, cut the stockinette to fit the area.				

		PRACTICE TRIAL	GRADED TRIAL # 1	GRADED TRIAL # 2	NOTES:
9. ★	Cover the affected body part with the stockinette, making sure it is smooth against the patient's skin and extends 1–2 inches beyond where the cast will end. If the stockinette is allowed to wrinkle or become bulky, it may cause a pressure sore on the patient's skin.				
10. ◆	If you are casting the ankle, cut away excess wrinkled stockinette from the bend in the front of the ankle.				
11. ★	Use a spiral bandage turn to cover the casting area with padding. Apply extra padding to any bony areas.				
12. ◆	Soak the inner layer of fiberglass tape in the basin of warm water. The tape material will be activated on contact with the water, so only wet as much as you need at a time.				
13. ◆	The physician will roll and form the cast to the patient.				
14. ◆	Roll the excess stockinette over the edges of the casting material to form a smooth edge.				
15. ◆	Open the package of outer fiberglass tape for the physician.				
16. ◆	The physician will shape and smooth the cast or may direct you to do so.				
17. ◆	Clean up the work station. Remove the gloves and wash your hands.				
18. ★	Document the procedure in the patient chart.				

Name: _____

Date: _____

Document: Enter the correct information in the chart below.

Grading

Points Earned	_____		
Points Possible	_____	123	123
Percent Grade (Points Earned/ Points Possible)	_____		
PASS:	_____	❏ YES ❏ NO ❏ N/A	❏ YES ❏ NO ❏ N/A

Instructor Sign-Off

Instructor: _____ Date: _____

Name: _____

Date: _____

Procedure 25-2

Assist with Cast Removal

Objective: The student, using the supplies and equipment listed below, will demonstrate how to assist in the removal of a cast.

Supplies: cast-cutting device, cast spreader, bandage scissors, heavy-duty bag in which to discard cast materials, patient drape, 500-ml basin, 500 ml of warm water, hypoallergenic soap, towel, hypoallergenic lotion

Notes to the Student:

_____

_____

_____

_____

_____

_____

Skills Assessment Requirements

Read and familiarize yourself with the procedure; complete the minimum practice requirements. Document each MPR using proper charting technique. Complete each procedure within a reasonable amount of time, with a minimum of 85% accuracy.

POINT VALUE ✦ = 3-6 points ⋆ = 7-9 points	PRACTICE TRIAL	GRADED TRIAL #1	GRADED TRIAL #2	NOTES:
1. ✦ Gather equipment and supplies.				
2. ⋆ Greet and identify the patient. Explain the procedure				
3. ⋆ Making certain that the limb is properly supported, make two cuts along the medial and lateral side of the long axis of the cast.				
4. ✦ Pry the cast apart with a cast spreader.				
5. ✦ Carefully remove the two halves of the cast.				
6. ✦ Cut away the stockinette and padding with the large bandage scissors.				
7. ✦ Wash the previously casted area with hypoallergenic soap.				
8. ✦ Dry the skin and apply a gentle skin lotion.				
9. ⋆ Provide the patient with written and verbal instructions for care of the limb.				
10. ⋆ Document procedure in patient chart.				

Name: _____

Date: _____

Document: Enter the correct information in the chart below.

Grading

Points Earned	_____		
Points Possible	_____	72	72
Percent Grade (Points Earned/ Points Possible)	_____		
PASS:	_____	❏ YES ❏ NO ❏ N/A	❏ YES ❏ NO ❏ N/A

Instructor Sign-Off

Instructor: _____ Date: _____

Procedure 25-3

Assist the Patient with Cold Application/Cold Compress

Objective: The student, using the supplies and equipment listed below, will demonstrate how to apply a cold compress.

Supplies: water, 4 × 4 gauze pads or other absorbent material or washcloths, waterproof pad, waterproof wrap (plastic bag or plastic wrap), basin, ice cubes

Notes to the Student:

_____

_____

_____

_____

_____

_____

Skills Assessment Requirements

Read and familiarize yourself with the procedure; complete the minimum practice requirements. Document each MPR using proper charting technique. Complete each procedure within a reasonable amount of time, with a minimum of 85% accuracy.

POINT VALUE ✦ = 3-6 points ⋆ = 7-9 points		PRACTICE TRIAL	GRADED TRIAL #1	GRADED TRIAL #2	NOTES:
1. ✦	Wash your hands.				
2. ⋆	Identify the patient and verify the physician's order.				
3. ✦	Explain the procedure to the patient.				
4. ✦	Fill the basin with ice and water and soak the gauze pads or washcloths.				
5. ✦	Wring out the compress so it is damp but not dripping.				
6. ✦	Place the compress on the patient's injured body part and wrap it with plastic wrap to protect the patient's clothing.				
7. ⋆	Check the compress every 3–5 minutes, replacing it with a colder compress as needed. Remove water as necessary from the basin and add more ice to keep the water cold.				
8. ✦	After applying compresses for the time specified by the physician, remove them and dry the affected area. Call the physician if you notice increased swelling and redness, or if the pain intensifies.				
9. ✦	Launder the linens or place them in the appropriate laundry hamper, according to office protocol, and clean the room.				
10.⋆	Wash your hands and document the procedure.				

Name: _____

Date: _____

Document: Enter the correct information in the chart below.

Grading

Points Earned	_____		
Points Possible	_____	69	69
Percent Grade (Points Earned/ Points Possible)	_____		
PASS:	_____	❑ YES ❑ NO ❑ N/A	❑ YES ❑ NO ❑ N/A

Instructor Sign-Off

Instructor: _____ **Date:** _____

Procedure 25-4

Assist the Patient with Hot Moist Application/Hot Compress

Objective: The student, using the supplies and equipment listed below, will demonstrate how to apply a cold compress.

Supplies: water, digital or disposable strip thermometer, 4 × 4 gauze pads or other absorbent material or washcloths, waterproof pad, waterproof wrap (plastic bag or plastic wrap can be used), basin

Notes to the Student:

_____

_____

_____

_____

_____

_____

Skills Assessment Requirements

Read and familiarize yourself with the procedure; complete the minimum practice requirements. Document each MPR using proper charting technique. Complete each procedure within a reasonable amount of time, with a minimum of 85% accuracy.

POINT VALUE ✦ = 3-6 points ⋆ = 7-9 points		PRACTICE TRIAL	GRADED TRIAL # 1	GRADED TRIAL # 2	NOTES:
1. ✦	Wash your hands.				
2. ⋆	Identify the patient and verify the physician's order.				
3. ✦	Explain the procedure to the patient.				
4. ✦	Fill the basin with water heated to 105–110°F, as verified with the thermometer, and soak the gauze pads.				
5. ✦	Wring out the compress so it is damp but not dripping.				
6. ✦	Place the waterproof pad under the injured body part. Apply the compress to the patient's injured body part and wrap with plastic wrap to protect clothing. Ask the patient to confirm that the temperature is comfortable but not burning.				
7. ⋆	Check the compress every 3–5 minutes, replacing it with a warmer compress as needed. Call the physician if you notice increased swelling and redness, or if pain increases.				
8. ✦	After applying the compress for the time specified by the physician, remove it and dry the affected area.				
9. ✦	Launder the linens or place them in the appropriate laundry hamper, according to office protocol, and clean the room.				
10. ⋆	Wash your hands and document the procedure.				

Name: _____

Date: _____

Document: Enter the correct information in the chart below.

Grading

Points Earned	_____		
Points Possible	_____	69	69
Percent Grade (Points Earned/ Points Possible)	_____		
PASS:	_____	❏ YES ❏ NO ❏ N/A	❏ YES ❏ NO ❏ N/A

Instructor Sign-Off

Instructor: _____ **Date:** _____

Procedure 25-5

Assist with Therapeutic Ultrasonography

Objective: The student, using the supplies and equipment listed below, will demonstrate how to assist with therapeutic ultrasonography.

Supplies: ultrasound gel (coupling agent), ultrasound machine, tissue, patient chart

Notes to the Student:

_____

_____

_____

_____

_____

_____

Skills Assessment Requirements

Read and familiarize yourself with the procedure; complete the minimum practice requirements. Document each MPR using proper charting technique. Complete each procedure within a reasonable amount of time, with a minimum of 85% accuracy.

Name: _____

Date: _____

		PRACTICE TRIAL	GRADED TRIAL #1	GRADED TRIAL #2	NOTES:
	POINT VALUE ✦ = 3-6 points ✶ = 7-9 points				
1. ✶	Prepare the equipment and identify the patient.				
2. ✶	Verify the physician's orders for duration and frequency of treatment.				
3. ✦	Explain the procedure and encourage the patient to inform you of any pain or discomfort.				
4. ✦	Have the patient remove clothing from the area to be treated.				
5. ✦	Apply warmed ultrasonic gel to the area to be treated and to the applicator head.				
6. ✦	Set the machine at the lowest treatment setting and increase gradually as needed. Set the timer to the specified treatment time.				
7. ✶	Place the applicator head firmly against the patient's skin and move the applicator in a circular motion at a speed of 2 inches per second. Keep the applicator head in contact with the patient's skin and moving at all times when the machine is running.				
8. ◆	When the set time has expired, the machine will shut off automatically.				
9. ✦	Return the intensity control back to zero.				
10. ✦	Wipe the ultrasonic gel from the patient's skin and assist with dressing if necessary.				
11. ✶	Wash your hands and document the procedure in the patient's chart.				

Name: _____

Date: _____

Document: Enter the correct information in the chart below.

Grading

Points Earned	_____		
Points Possible	_____	78	78
Percent Grade (Points Earned/ Points Possible)	_____		
PASS:	_____	❏ YES ❏ NO ❏ N/A	❏ YES ❏ NO ❏ N/A

Instructor Sign-Off

Instructor: _____ Date: _____

Procedure 25-6

Demonstrate Measuring for Axillary Crutches

Objective: The student, using the supplies and equipment listed below, will demonstrate how to measure for axillary crutches.

Supplies: patient chart, order for axillary crutches, adjustable axillary crutches

Notes to the Student:

_____

_____

_____

_____

_____

_____

Skills Assessment Requirements

Read and familiarize yourself with the procedure; complete the minimum practice requirements. Document each MPR using proper charting technique. Complete each procedure within a reasonable amount of time, with a minimum of 85% accuracy.

POINT VALUE ✦ = 3-6 points ⋆ = 7-9 points	PRACTICE TRIAL	GRADED TRIAL #1	GRADED TRIAL #2	NOTES:
1. ✦ Wash your hands and gather the necessary materials.				
2. ⋆ Identify the patient and escort him or her to the treatment area.				
3. ⋆ Assist the patient, with shoes on, to a standing position. With the crutch armrests under the patient's axillae, adjust the crutches first for height and then for hand position, using the following criteria: **a.** a space of two finger widths between the axilla and the crutch armrest **b.** body weight supported by the hands on the hand grips **c.** crutch tip placement approximately 2 inches in front of the foot and 4 to 6 inches from the lateral aspect.				
4. ✦ After the crutches have been correctly measured and fitted to the patient, provide verbal and written instruction about general guidelines, crutch gait, and symptoms of improper fit.				
5. ✦ Document the procedure and prepare the treatment area for the next patient.				

Name: _____

Date: _____

Document: Enter the correct information in the chart below.

Grading

Points Earned	_____		
Points Possible	_____	36	36
Percent Grade (Points Earned/ Points Possible)	_____		
PASS:	_____	❏ YES ❏ NO ❏ N/A	❏ YES ❏ NO ❏ N/A

Instructor Sign-Off

Instructor: _____ Date: _____

Procedure 25-7

Assist a Patient with Crutch Walking

Objective: The student, using the supplies and equipment listed below, will demonstrate how to assist a patient with crutch walking.

Supplies: crutches correctly fitted to the patient

Notes to the Student:

_____

_____

_____

_____

_____

_____

Skills Assessment Requirements

Read and familiarize yourself with the procedure; complete the minimum practice requirements. Document each MPR using proper charting technique. Complete each procedure within a reasonable amount of time, with a minimum of 85% accuracy.

Name: _____

Date: _____

POINT VALUE ✦ = 3-6 points ⋆ = 7-9 points	PRACTICE TRIAL	GRADED TRIAL # 1	GRADED TRIAL # 2	NOTES:
1. ✦ Wash your hands and gather the necessary materials.				
2. ⋆ Identify the patient and escort him or her to the treatment area.				
3. ✦ Inspect the crutches for correctly fitted arm pads, tight wingnuts, and comfortable handgrips.				
4. ◆ Instruct the patient to relax the injured knee and keep it slightly bent to avoid touching the foot to the ground.				
5. ✦ Instruct the patient in the crutch-walking gait ordered by the physician.				
6. ⋆ Have the patient practice taking several steps to ensure correct technique.				
7. ⋆ Document patient education in the patient's chart.				

Name: _____

Date: _____

Document: Enter the correct information in the chart below.

Grading

Points Earned	_____		
Points Possible	_____	51	51
Percent Grade (Points Earned/ Points Possible)	_____		
PASS:	_____	❏ YES ❏ NO ❏ N/A	❏ YES ❏ NO ❏ N/A

Instructor Sign-Off

Instructor: _____   **Date:** _____

Procedure 25-8

Assist a Patient Using a Cane

Objective: The student, using the supplies and equipment listed below, will demonstrate how to instruct a patient on correct cane use.

Supplies: single-tipped cane as ordered by physician, gait belt

Notes to the Student:

_____

_____

_____

_____

_____

_____

Skills Assessment Requirements

Read and familiarize yourself with the procedure; complete the minimum practice requirements. Document each MPR using proper charting technique. Complete each procedure within a reasonable amount of time, with a minimum of 85% accuracy.

POINT VALUE ✦ = 3-6 points ⋆ = 7-9 points		PRACTICE TRIAL	GRADED TRIAL # 1	GRADED TRIAL # 2	NOTES:
1. ⋆	Identify the patient and explain why instruction in cane use is necessary.				
2. ✦	Wash your hands.				
3. ✦	Verify the type of cane the patient and physician have agreed on and assemble equipment.				
4. ✦	Make sure the suction tip on the cane is in good condition.				
5. ✦	Place the gait belt snugly around the patient's waist, tucking any excess length into the belt.				
6. ⋆	Place the cane tip 4–6 inches to the side of the patient's foot, on the patient's stronger, unaffected side. Adjust the cane so that the handle grip is level with the patient's hip and the patient's elbow is flexed at a 20- to 30-degree angle.				
7. ✦	Stand on the patient's weaker side with a firm underhand grip on the gait belt.				
8. ✦	Instruct the patient to move the injured leg and cane forward simultaneously.				
9. ✦	The patient should then advance the stronger leg and rest it slightly in front of the injured leg. Repeat this process.				
10. ✦	*Going up stairs:* Instruct the patient to use hand rails whenever possible.				

		PRACTICE TRIAL	GRADED TRIAL # 1	GRADED TRIAL # 2	NOTES:
11. ✦	The patient moves the stronger leg forward to the next step while the injured leg and cane rest on the lower step.				
12. ✦	With a firm grip on the cane and the handrail, the patient moves the injured leg up to the same step as the uninjured leg. Repeat as needed.				
13. ✦	*Going down stairs:* The patient steps down with the uninjured leg and the cane. The injured leg follows to the same step.				
14. *	Document patient education in the patient's chart.				

Name: _____

Date: _____

Document: Enter the correct information in the chart below.

Grading

Points Earned	_____		
Points Possible	_____	93	93
Percent Grade (Points Earned/ Points Possible)	_____		
PASS:	_____	❑ YES ❑ NO ❑ N/A	❑ YES ❑ NO ❑ N/A

Instructor Sign-Off

Instructor: _____ **Date:** _____

Name: _____

Date: _____

Procedure 25-9

Assist a Patient Using a Walker

Objective: The student, using the supplies and equipment listed below, will demonstrate how to teach a patient how to use a walker.

Supplies: walker, gait belt

Notes to the Student:

_____

_____

_____

_____

_____

_____

Skills Assessment Requirements

Read and familiarize yourself with the procedure; complete the minimum practice requirements. Document each MPR using proper charting technique. Complete each procedure within a reasonable amount of time, with a minimum of 85% accuracy.

POINT VALUE ✦ = 3-6 points ⋆ = 7-9 points		PRACTICE TRIAL	GRADED TRIAL # 1	GRADED TRIAL # 2	NOTES:
1. ⋆	Identify the patient and explain why instruction in walker use is necessary.				
2. ✦	Wash your hands.				
3. ✦	Place a gait belt snugly around the patient's waist. Tuck any excess belt length under the belt near the hip.				
4. ✦	Position the patient inside the walker. Adjust the height of the walker as needed. The patient's arms should be flexed at a 30-degree angle when resting on the hand grips.				
5. ✦	Stand behind and slightly to the side of the patient, with an underhand grip on the gait belt.				
6. ✦	Instruct the patient to move the walker directly ahead until the back supports of the walker are even with the patient's toes.				
7. ✦	Instruct the patient to grip the handles firmly and step toward the walker with the stronger leg first, then the other leg.				
8. ✦	Repeat: the patient moves the walker first, then moves toward the walker.				
9. ✦	Watch the patient for signs of fatigue. Some walkers are equipped with platforms on which the patient can sit to rest.				
10. ⋆	Document patient education in patient's chart.				

Document: Enter the correct information in the chart below.

Grading

Points Earned	_____		
Points Possible	_____	66	66
Percent Grade (Points Earned/ Points Possible)	_____		
PASS:	_____	❏ YES ❏ NO ❏ N/A	❏ YES ❏ NO ❏ N/A

Instructor Sign-Off

Instructor: _____ Date: _____

Procedure 25-10

Assist a Patient in a Wheelchair to and from an Exam Table

Objective: The student, using the supplies and equipment listed below, will demonstrate how to transfer a patient from a wheelchair to an examination table and from an examination table to a wheelchair.

Supplies: gait belt, long-handled stool (if exam table is not equipped with pull-out step)

Notes to the Student:

_____

_____

_____

_____

_____

_____

Skills Assessment Requirements

Read and familiarize yourself with the procedure; complete the minimum practice requirements. Document each MPR using proper charting technique. Complete each procedure within a reasonable amount of time, with a minimum of 85% accuracy.

POINT VALUE ✦ = 3-6 points ★ = 7-9 points	PRACTICE TRIAL	GRADED TRIAL #1	GRADED TRIAL #2	NOTES:
1. ★ Identify the patient and explain what you are going to do.				
2. ✦ Wash your hands.				
3. ✦ Position the wheelchair so that the patient is sitting with his or her strongest side next to the examination table.				
4. ★ Lock the wheelchair brakes.				
5. ✦ Place the gait belt snugly around the patient's waist, making certain the belt is tight enough that it will not slip and put unnecessary pressure on the ribs. Tuck any excess belt length under the belt.				
6. ✦ If the wheelchair allows, remove the foot rests. If not, move them as far out as possible to avoid hitting your shins against them during the transfer.				
7. ★ Standing directly in front of and as close to the patient as possible, grip the gait belt with both hands in an underhand grip. Bend at the knees and hips to avoid back strain.				
8. ✦ If the patient is able, have him or her grip the arm rests and push off at the same time that you lift, for added leverage. If possible, the patient can also assist by pushing upward with his or her legs.				

		PRACTICE TRIAL	GRADED TRIAL # 1	GRADED TRIAL # 2	NOTES:
9. *	With the patient now standing, have him or her place the stronger leg on the stool or exam table step, and together you will lift as the patient steps up.				
10. ✦	Have the patient place one hand on the table and guide him or her to a sitting position.				
11. ✦	Move the wheelchair out of the way.				
12. *	To transfer the patient back to the wheelchair: After identifying the patient, explaining the procedure, and washing your hands, place the stool (if the exam table does not have a step) next to the exam table.				
13. ✦	Place the wheelchair next to the exam table with the brakes locked.				
14. *	With a firm underhand grip on the gait belt, assist the patient to a standing position. If the patient is able, have him or her push off with the legs and arms. Once the patient is steady on the step or stool, have him or her step to the floor with the stronger leg.				
15. ✦	Have the patient take small steps backward until the backs of the knees touch the wheelchair.				

Orthopedics and Physical Therapy **681**

		PRACTICE TRIAL	GRADED TRIAL # 1	GRADED TRIAL # 2	NOTES:
16. ✦	Ask the patient to reach back and place the hands on the wheelchair armrests for support. Bending at the hips and knees, slowly lower the patient to the chair.				
17. ✦	Help the patient adjust to a comfortable position in the wheelchair.				
18. ✦	Replace the foot rests.				

Name: _____

Date: _____

Document: Enter the correct information in the chart below.

Grading

Points Earned	_____		
Points Possible	_____	126	126
Percent Grade (Points Earned/ Points Possible)	_____		
PASS:	_____	❏ YES ❏ NO ❏ N/A	❏ YES ❏ NO ❏ N/A

Instructor Sign-Off

Instructor: _____ Date: _____

CHAPTER 26
Obstetrics and Gynecology

CHAPTER OUTLINE

Review the Chapter Outline. If any content area is unclear, review that area before beginning workbook exercises.

    A. The Medical Assistant's Role in the OB/GYN Office

    B. The Anatomy and Physiology of the Female Reproductive System

    C. The Menstrual Cycle

    D. Contraception

    E. Pregnancy and the Birth Process

    F. Gynecological Diseases and Disorders

    G. Routine Assessment

    H. Diagnostic Procedures

    I. Treatment Modalities

CHAPTER REVIEW

The following is a summary of the chapter. If any of this material is unclear, review it in the textbook.

The specialty of OB/GYN is one of the most varied in tasks for the medical assistant as well as in the exams and procedures performed in an office. Obstetrics addresses pregnancy and childbirth while gynecology addresses the female reproductive system. The MA would do the usual patient history and vital signs, prepare and assist the physician with exams and procedures such as colposcopies and fetal ultrasounds, and often patient education, which includes teaching the patient to do a breast self-exam, nutritional requirements, labor and delivery, and breast and formula feeding, as examples. Knowledge is needed regarding hormonal changes in various life stages, menopause, disorders of the menstrual cycle, contraception, infertility, the prenatal period and visits, and diseases and disorders of the reproductive system. Understanding STDs is another aspect, as are breast health and disease, cancer, and psychological issues.

LEARNING ACTIVITIES AND STUDY AIDS

Review the following study aids and/or complete the activities to ensure that you have achieved the learning objectives for this chapter.

1. Describe the medical assistant's role in the obstetric/gynecology medical office.

_____

_____

_____

2. Make a list of the anatomical parts in the female reproductive system and the major functions of the female reproductive system.

_____

_____

_____

_____

_____

_____

3. Review the material on the menstrual cycle and menopause, then explain both in your own words. Be concise and summarize the entire detailed process in one paragraph.

_____

_____

_____

_____

_____

_____

4. Make a list of the common disorders and conditions related to the menstrual cycle. State the name and the basic issue of each.

_____

_____

_____

_____

_____

5. Review the material in your textbook on the different methods of contraception. Prepare flash cards on the various methods that are discussed in your book. Put the name of the contraceptive method on one side and how it works on the other.

_____

_____

_____

_____

_____

_____

_____

6. Review the material about infertility in the textbook and, as you do, list the causes of female infertility that are discussed.

_____

_____

_____

_____

_____

_____

7. Describe in a list format, and in your own words, the process of pregnancy and the process of childbirth. Explain each from start to finish.

_____

_____

_____

_____

_____

_____

_____

8. Review the list of important information for a complete obstetrical history. Then close your textbook and list as many of the items as you recall. Once you have finished, go back to the book and check your answers. Add items to your list that have not yet been included there.

_____

_____

_____

_____

_____

_____

9. Make a list of the common complications of pregnancy that are addressed in your textbook. Choose two of the conditions on the list, then research them both on the Internet (at a reputable site). Read the additional information there that can supplement the textbook. Print only the page at that site that states or describes what that condition/complication is and ensure the URL of the site is printed on the bottom.

_____

_____

_____

_____

_____

_____

_____

10. Make a chart of the benefits and drawbacks of breastfeeding and formula feeding.

_____

_____

_____

_____

_____

_____

_____

11. Make flash cards of the disease conditions related to the female reproductive system. Put the name on one side and the signs and symptoms on the other side.

_____

_____

_____

_____

_____

_____

12. How can vaginal bleeding be assessed?

_____

_____

_____

_____

_____

13. Make flash cards of sexually transmitted diseases affecting women. Put the name of the disease and the signs/symptoms on one side and the treatment on the other.

_____

_____

_____

_____

14. Read through the section in Chapter 26 of your textbook on Breast Disorders and Conditions. List each disorder or condition below. Then list each test or diagnostic procedure. Finally, make a list of the signs and symptoms that are mentioned.

_____

_____

_____

_____

_____

_____

_____

15. Describe what patient assessment includes in the OB/GYN office.

_____

_____

_____

_____

_____

_____

_____

_____

16. Review the information on diagnostic procedures performed in an OB/GYN clinic as discussed in the chapter. Pay attention to the name of each test and what it is for (or what it will tell the doctor). Close the book and write a list of as many of the procedures as you can recall, including a brief statement of what each is for. Go back to the book after you have completed the list from memory and fill in those that you may have left out.

_____

_____

_____

_____

_____

_____

17. The book discusses nine major treatment modalities for OB/GYN patients. Make flash cards with the name of each procedure on one side and a brief explanation on the other.

_____

_____

_____

_____

18. At times psychological interventions are needed for various OB/GYN conditions. Review the list of psychologically sensitive issues listed in the book. Close the book and list all of the examples you can think of. When you have finished, go back and locate the ones you may have forgotten and add them to your list.

_____

_____

_____

_____

_____

_____

_____

_____

MEDICAL TERMINOLOGY REVIEW

Use a dictionary and highlighted terms in the textbook to define the following terms.

Terms

amniocentesis _____

_____

cervix _____

_____

colostrum _____

_____

effacement _____

_____

embryo _____

_____

endometrium _____

_____

fetus _____

_____

fundal height _____

_____

gravida _____

_____

gynecology _____

_____

gynecologist _____

menarche _____

menopause _____

menses _____

obstetrician _____

obstetrics _____

ovum (plural: ova) _____

para _____

perineum _____

postnatal/postpartum _____

prenatal _____

zygote _____

Abbreviations

AFT _____

BSE _____

C-section _____

EDC _____

EDD _____

FHT _____

g _____

GU _____

L & D _____

LH _____

OB/GYN _____

PP _____

P _____

UCG _____

CRITICAL THINKING

1. A patient, 18-year-old Maria Riojas, has come in with a chief complaint of bleeding between periods. This will be her third GYN visit since menarche, and she is still quite apprehensive about the exams and getting undressed. She says she hopes the doctor won't have to do a pelvic exam today; she just wants a stronger or different birth control pill. Her friend told her she has break-through bleeding because she is on the wrong pill. What would you say to the patient?

   _____

   _____

   _____

   _____

2. Considering the case study in your textbook for this chapter, if the patient is encouraged by the physician to take the hormone replacement anyway but the patient refuses, does it mean she will develop a disease or problem from not taking it? What is the worst thing for the patient if she does not take treatment of any kind?

   _____

   _____

   _____

   _____

3. A patient has come in and from her patient health history, you find she has had three abortions in the past and is now pregnant for the fourth time. She is scheduled for a prenatal work-up today. Your personal morals are against abortion, but you know that abortions can be therapeutic (by choice or for medical reasons) or spontaneous (miscarriage), and you don't know which type her abortions were. What, if any, of your personal beliefs can be conveyed to the patient? Would you say anything about her OB history?

   _____

   _____

   _____

   _____

4. A patient comes in with her husband, and she asks that he be allowed to come into the exam room with her. When you ask her to disrobe, she looks hesitant then looks at her husband and doesn't move to take the gown and drape. What do you anticipate is happening? What should you do?

_____

_____

_____

_____

5. A patient who is six months pregnant calls in saying that she has been bleeding a little (just spotting) all morning and wanted to let the doctor know. She wants an appointment for Thursday and today is Monday. What would you say?

_____

_____

_____

_____

CHAPTER REVIEW TEST

MULTIPLE CHOICE

Circle the letter of the correct answer.

1. Risk factors for cervical and uterine cancer include all of the following except:
   a. frequent douching.
   b. nonsurgical menopause.
   c. frequent vaginal infections.
   d. promiscuous sexual behavior.

2. Routine prenatal visits are usually scheduled once a month until the _____ month.
   a. sixth
   b. seventh
   c. eighth
   d. ninth

3. The first step in the female reproductive process is:
   a. when the zygote is formed.
   b. when the cell begins to divide.
   c. when an ovum is released.
   d. when the ovum is fertilized by the sperm.

4. Which of the following is not a treatment modality for cervical dysplasia?
   a. chemicals
   b. electricity
   c. dilation and curettage
   d. cryocauterization

5. In the prenatal patient, a history of certain previous or current medical conditions presents a challenge to the obstetrical team. Which of the conditions below is not one of the challenges?
   a. hyperthyroidism
   b. diabetes mellitus
   c. hypertension
   d. hormonal imbalance

6. Which two of the following can be used to estimate date of delivery?

    a. Nagele's Rule
    b. lunar method

    c. fundal height method
    d. Lamaze method

7. Cryosurgery is a technique that uses liquid

    a. hydrogen.
    b. oxygen.

    c. nitrogen.
    d. nitrous oxide.

8. The _____ is/are responsible for producing some estrogen and large amounts of progesterone.

    a. graafian collicles
    b. ovarian follicles

    c. endometrium
    d. corpus luteum

9. Which of the following are methods of birth control or contraception? (circle all that apply)

    a. barrier
    b. chemical contact

    c. hormonal control
    d. surgical sterilization

10. Which of the following are among the many risk factors for breast cancer? (circle all that apply)

    a. ethnicity
    b. high alcohol intake
    c. later age at first full-term pregnancy (30 and over)

    d. early onset of menarche

TRUE/FALSE

Indicate whether the statement is true (T) or false (F).

_____ 1. In some cultures, female patients are prohibited from disrobing in view of others.

_____ 2. Cilia are responsible for the propelling movement of the ovum along the fallopian tube.

_____ 3. Many pregnancy tests are so sensitive to the hormone hCG that a pregnancy can be detected as early as five days after conception.

_____ 4. A colposcopy is a special examination of the ovaries and fallopian tubes.

_____ 5. A primary symptom of problems in the female reproductive tract is lower abdominal pain.

_____ 6. An episiotomy is an incision made in the perineum to facilitate the delivery of an infant.

_____ 7. Periodic sexual abstinence involves avoiding sexual intercourse during the probable fertile period of the menstrual cycle.

_____ 8. Glucose tolerance testing is now becoming a routine part of prenatal care.

_____ 9. Colostrum is a fluid secreted from the breast that enriches the milk.

_____ 10. Menarche signals the beginning of the female's reproductive capability.

FILL IN THE BLANK

Using words from the list below, fill in the blanks to complete the following statements.

38	contact numbers	not successful
266	contraception	permanent
after	contractions	physician
age and sex	counselors or other professionals	positive
amount lost	date of confinement	semen
blood	effacement	sensitive
blood tests	estrogen-progestin	sexually transmitted diseases
breast cancer	examinations	subsequent routine
cervix	fertilization	their families
color	gynecological	ultrasound examination
compassion	menstrual flow	vagina
conception	needs	vaginal secretions
congenital		

1. In a normal delivery, the _____, or mouth of the uterus, dilates and begins _____, and uterine _____ propel the fetus through the _____ and into the external environment.

2. When a patient reports abnormal vaginal bleeding, even an unusually heavy _____, the actual _____, as well as its _____, must be determined.

3. Both OB and GYN offices care for patients with contagious diseases that are transmitted through sexual contact, commonly referred to as _____ or venereal diseases. STDs may be experienced by either males or females and are transmitted during sex by _____, _____, and _____.

4. Many psychologically _____ issues are addressed in the OB/GYN office. It is important to listen with _____ to patients and _____ as they present with various problems.

5. The normal gestational period is _____ days, or _____ weeks, from the date of _____. The expected date of delivery is also called the estimated _____.

6. Recent studies on hormone replacement therapy (HRT) suggest that this therapy, especially the _____ combination, increases a woman's risk for _____.

7. The use of ultrasound during a pregnancy, as well as to assess _____ conditions, is becoming more common. The _____ of the fetus and possible _____ conditions are often determined during an _____.

8. Keep in mind that not every pregnancy is a planned or _____ event. Be sympathetic to the patient's _____ and have appropriate _____ available for reference to _____.

9. The first prenatal appointment takes more time than _____ visits and includes several _____, manual _____, and consultation with the _____.

10. A tubal ligation is a _____ form of _____, as it prevents the sperm from meeting the egg for _____. Reversal is generally _____, and there are recorded instances of females conceiving _____ a tubal ligation.

Procedure 26-1

Assist with a Prenatal Exam

Objective: The student, using the supplies and equipment listed below, will demonstrate how to assist with a prenatal exam.

Supplies: EDD calculator, full Pap and pelvic exam setup, gloves, patient's chart

Notes to the Student:

_____

_____

_____

_____

_____

_____

Skills Assessment Requirements

Read and familiarize yourself with the procedure; complete the minimum practice requirements. Document each MPR using proper charting technique. Complete each procedure within a reasonable amount of time, with a minimum of 85% accuracy.

POINT VALUE ✦ = 3-6 points ⋆ = 7-9 points	PRACTICE TRIAL	GRADED TRIAL # 1	GRADED TRIAL # 2	NOTES:
1. ⋆ Verify the patient's identification.				
2. ✦ Explain the tests that will be done as a baseline to compare to in the later stages of pregnancy.				
3. ✦ Measure the patient's height and weight.				
4. ⋆ Depending on your office requirements, you may be asked to take a complete physical history of the patient. Obtain her menstrual history (age of onset, duration, flow rate, and intervals) and pregnancy history (number of pregnancies, number of live births, number of miscarriages, number of abortions).				
5. ✦ Obtain a urine sample to run a UA.				
6. ✦ Assist the physician with the Pap and pelvic examination as required by office protocol.				
7. ⋆ Document required information in the patient's chart.				

Document: Enter the correct information in the chart below.

Grading

Points Earned	_____		
Points Possible	_____	51	51
Percent Grade (Points Earned/ Points Possible)	_____		
PASS:	_____	❏ YES	❏ YES
		❏ NO	❏ NO
		❏ N/A	❏ N/A

Instructor Sign-Off

Instructor: _____ **Date:** _____

Procedure 26-2

Instruct the Patient in Breast Self-Examination

Objective: The student, using the supplies and equipment listed below, will demonstrate how to instruct the patient in the performance of breast self-examination.

Supplies: patient chart, educational materials such as patient brochures or breast models

Notes to the Student:

_____

_____

_____

_____

_____

_____

Skills Assessment Requirements

Read and familiarize yourself with the procedure; complete the minimum practice requirements. Document each MPR using proper charting technique. Complete each procedure within a reasonable amount of time, with a minimum of 85% accuracy.

POINT VALUE ✦ =3-6 points ✶ = 7-9 points		PRACTICE TRIAL	GRADED TRIAL # 1	GRADED TRIAL # 2	NOTES:
1. ✦	Wash your hands and gather the necessary supplies.				
2. ✦	Escort the patient to the patient education area.				
3. ✶	Emphasize the following habits for the monthly self-exam: **a.** Premenopausal women should perform the examination about one week after the menstrual period, when the breasts are not swollen. Postmenopausal women should select a specific date of the month. **b.** Perform a visual inspection while standing in front of a mirror. With the arms hanging at the sides, above the head, or forward, away from the body, or with the hands positioned on the hips, observe for bilateral similarities or differences, for color or texture changes in the skin and nipples, and for nipple discharge. **c.** Examine each breast in side-lying and flat positions, starting with the same breast each time. For the flat position, place a pillow under the shoulder on each side.				

		PRACTICE TRIAL	GRADED TRIAL # 1	GRADED TRIAL # 2	NOTES:
	d. Palpate each breast with the fingertip pads of the opposite hand, using a dime-sized, circular motion. Use the same search pattern of vertical strip, wedge, or circle search for both breasts.				
	e. Finish the breast examination by squeezing for nipple discharge and palpating the breast into the axillary area.				
	f. Report any abnormalities or changes to the physician.				
4. ∗	Document your patient instruction in breast self-examination. Note the patient's level of understanding.				
5. ✦	Perform any necessary cleaning of teaching models and store for the next patient use.				

Document: Enter the correct information in the chart below.

Grading

Points Earned	_____		
Points Possible	_____	36	36
Percent Grade (Points Earned/ Points Possible)	_____		
PASS:	_____	❑ YES ❑ NO ❑ N/A	❑ YES ❑ NO ❑ N/A

Instructor Sign-Off

Instructor: _____ **Date:** _____

Procedure 26-3

Assist the Physician in the Performance of a Pelvic Examination and Pap Test

Objective: The student, using the supplies and equipment listed below, will demonstrate how to assist the physician during the performance a pelvic examination and Pap test.

Supplies: Patient chart; examination gloves; water-soluble lubricant; physician's gown and eye protection; vaginal speculum; gooseneck or other light source; slide container, glass slides, marker to label slides, and slide fixative for Pap smear; cervical/spatula scraper; cotton-tipped applicators; lab requisition form

Notes to the Student:

_____

_____

_____

_____

_____

_____

Skills Assessment Requirements

Read and familiarize yourself with the procedure; complete the minimum practice requirements. Document each MPR using proper charting technique. Complete each procedure within a reasonable amount of time, with a minimum of 85% accuracy.

	POINT VALUE ✦ = 3-6 points ⋆ = 7-9 points	PRACTICE TRIAL	GRADED TRIAL # 1	GRADED TRIAL # 2	NOTES:
1. ✦	Wash your hands and assemble the equipment. Label the slide containers with patient information. Label the frosted edge of each slide with patient information and the location from which the specimen was taken.				
2. ⋆	Identify the patient and escort her to the examination room. Obtain the mensuration required by the physician (usually weight, temperature, blood pressure, pulse, and respirations).				
3. ✦	Interview the patient for the following information: • chief complaint (reason for visit) • medications and known allergies • start date of last menstrual period • date of most recent Pap smear				
4. ✦	Explain the procedure to the patient.				
5. ✦	Before the procedure, assist the patient to the bathroom to void.				

		PRACTICE TRIAL	GRADED TRIAL # 1	GRADED TRIAL # 2	NOTES:
6. ★	When the patient returns to the examination room, instruct her to remove clothing from the waist down. Assist as necessary. Provide a drape for the body from the waist down. If a breast examination is also to be performed, the patient will need to completely disrobe. Provide a gown cover for the chest area as well. The patient may sit on the examination table or lie comfortably until the physician arrives.				
7. ✦	When the physician is present, assist the patient into a supine/dorsal recumbent position if a breast exam is to be performed. Slide the patient toward the stirrups and into the lithotomy position for the remainder of the pelvic examination and the Pap test.				
8. ★	Observe the patient's tolerance of the procedure and hand the slides, cervical/spatula scraper, and cotton-tipped applicators to the physician for the Pap smear. After the physician has placed the specimen on the slides, immediately spray or apply ethyl alcohol liquid fixative. Give the physician water-soluble lubricant for the pelvic examination.				

		PRACTICE TRIAL	GRADED TRIAL # 1	GRADED TRIAL # 2	NOTES:
9. ✦	When the procedure has been completed, assist the patient to a sitting position. Leave the room to allow her to dress in private, or assist if necessary.				
10. ✦	Remove the used implements to the cleaning area. Dispose of disposable and biohazardous materials in the appropriate containers. Wash your hands				
11. ✦	Transport the labeled specimen to the laboratory, or arrange for transport, with the appropriate lab requisitions. Assist the patient with the scheduling of additional procedures, if necessary.				
12. ⋆	Document the patient's response to the procedure, any future appointments, and other patient information, including prescriptions or patient instruction.				

Name: _____

Date: _____

Document: Enter the correct information in the chart below.

Grading

Points Earned	_____		
Points Possible	_____	84	84
Percent Grade (Points Earned/ Points Possible)	_____		
PASS:	_____	❏ YES ❏ NO ❏ N/A	❏ YES ❏ NO ❏ N/A

Instructor Sign-Off

Instructor: _____ Date: _____

Procedure 26-4

Perform a Urine Pregnancy Test

Objective: The student, using the supplies and equipment listed below, will demonstrate how to test a patient's urine for the presence of hCG.

Supplies: gloves, urine sample, hCG test, hCG positive urine control, hCG negative urine control, timer, disinfectant, patient chart

Notes to the Student:

_____

_____

_____

_____

_____

_____

Skills Assessment Requirements

Read and familiarize yourself with the procedure; complete the minimum practice requirements. Document each MPR using proper charting technique. Complete each procedure within a reasonable amount of time, with a minimum of 85% accuracy.

POINT VALUE ✦ = 3-6 points ⋆ = 7-9 points		PRACTICE TRIAL	GRADED TRIAL #1	GRADED TRIAL #2	NOTES:
1. ✦	Assemble all necessary equipment.				
2. ✦	Wash your hands and put on gloves.				
3. ⋆	Follow the manufacturer's directions for using the negative control serum				
4. ✦	When you are satisfied that the tests are reliable, test the patient's urine sample.				
5. ✦	Report the results to the physician.				
6. ✦	Disinfect the work area.				
7. ⋆	Document the test and results in the patient's chart.				

Name: _____

Date: _____

Document: Enter the correct information in the chart below.

Grading

Points Earned	_____		
Points Possible	_____	48	48
Percent Grade (Points Earned/ Points Possible)	_____		
PASS:	_____	❏ YES ❏ NO ❏ N/A	❏ YES ❏ NO ❏ N/A

Instructor Sign-Off

Instructor: _____ Date: _____

Procedure 26-5

Assist with Cryosurgery

Objective: The student, using the supplies and equipment listed below, will demonstrate how to assist with a cryosurgery.

Supplies: gloves, patient drapes, light source, liquid nitrogen, vaginal speculum, sterile specimen container (if needed), patient chart

Notes to the Student:

_____

_____

_____

_____

_____

_____

Skills Assessment Requirements

Read and familiarize yourself with the procedure; complete the minimum practice requirements. Document each MPR using proper charting technique. Complete each procedure within a reasonable amount of time, with a minimum of 85% accuracy.

POINT VALUE ✦ = 3-6 points ⋆ = 7-9 points		PRACTICE TRIAL	GRADED TRIAL # 1	GRADED TRIAL # 2	NOTES:
1. ⋆	Verify the patient's identification.				
2. ✦	Explain the procedure to the patient.				
3. ✦	If necessary, assist the patient in undressing from the waist down. Provide proper patient drapes.				
4. ✦	When the patient is undressed and draped, assist her into the lithotomy position.				
5. ⋆	Assist the physician as needed.				
6. ✦	Reassure the patient that as the probe moves over the affected tissue and the liquid nitrogen freezes and kills the tissue, she will feel some discomfort, similar to menstrual cramping. The discomfort should not be unbearable, however.				
7. ✦	After the procedure, assist the patient to a seated position and help her dress as needed.				
8. ✦	Clean and disinfect the room.				

Name: _____

Date: _____

Document: Enter the correct information in the chart below.

Grading

Points Earned	_____		
Points Possible	_____	54	48
Percent Grade (Points Earned/ Points Possible)	_____		
PASS:	_____	❏ YES ❏ NO ❏ N/A	❏ YES ❏ NO ❏ N/A

Instructor Sign-Off

Instructor: _____ Date: _____

CHAPTER 27
Pediatrics

CHAPTER OUTLINE

Review the Chapter Outline. If any content area is unclear, review that area before beginning workbook exercises.

- A. The Medical Assistant's Role in Pediatrics
- B. Physical, Developmental, and Emotional Growth of a Child
- C. Routine Visits (Well-Baby Checks)
- D. Common Pediatric Diseases and Conditions
- E. Diagnostic Procedures

CHAPTER REVIEW

The following is a summary of the chapter. If any of this material is unclear, review it in the textbook.

Because of the unique patient population in pediatrics and the many well- and sick-child aspects, pediatrics can be an excellent specialty for the MA who not only has the technical knowledge and skill to work with children, but who also can understand the needs and concerns of both parents and the child. Taking growth measurements of growing children is vital, as is the administration of immunizations. The variety of conditions covers a wide range from common diaper rash and ear inflammation to serious respiratory conditions including RSV and cystic fibrosis that need immediate care. Children can have blood disorders such as leukemia or anemia or congenital problems such as heart disorders. Some children may be born addicted to illegal drugs, or born with fetal alcohol syndrome. A few of the diagnostic procedures in pediatrics are strep tests, urinalysis and culture and sensitivity testing, and blood tests such as hematocrit and hemoglobin.

LEARNING ACTIVITIES AND STUDY AIDS

Review the following study aids and/or complete the activities to ensure that you have achieved the learning objectives for this chapter.

1. Explain the medical assistant's role in a pediatric specialty office.

   _____

   _____

   _____

   _____

   _____

   _____

2. Review Figures 27-1 through 27-7. This is an excellent resource for quick "at-a-glance" information on the developmental milestones that occur in the various age groups. It is worth your time to make a flash card for each stage from infant to preadolescent/teenager. State the age group on one side and list of the aspects of development on the other side.

_____

_____

_____

_____

_____

_____

_____

3. Since the medical assistant works closely in preparing for and assisting with procedures that may be performed during a well-child visit, it is important to know these well. Make a list of each procedure performed at this visit.

_____

_____

_____

_____

_____

_____

_____

4. Why is growth measurement so important in the routine or well-child visit?

_____

_____

_____

_____

_____

_____

5. Prepare a one-page reference sheet listing recommended child immunizations and the possible side effects of each.

_____

_____

_____

_____

_____

_____

6. Make flash cards of the common contagious diseases of childhood, putting the disease on one side and a brief description on the other.

_____

_____

_____

_____

_____

_____

7. Review Table 27-4: Congenital Neurological Disorders. Spinal fusion disorders are spina bifida occulta, meningocele, and myelomeningocele. Cranial fusion disorders are hydrocephalus, microencephaly, and anencephaly. Develop a list and add a brief description and the symptoms of each defect to make a table of this information.

_____

_____

_____

_____

_____

_____

_____

8. Review Table 27-5: Congenital Heart Conditions, in the textbook. In this activity, state the name of each condition, the description, the symptoms, and the treatments.

_____

_____

_____

_____

_____

_____

_____

9. List and describe the three blood disorders in Table 27-6: Blood Disorders, with more detail. Include the disorder name, the symptoms, and the treatment.

_____

_____

_____

_____

_____

10. List and describe the following pediatric diagnostic procedures that are discussed in the textbook: urinalysis, strep screen, hemoglobin, hematocrit, and culture and sensitivity. Use a medical dictionary or other chapters in your textbook to describe those procedures; be concise in one to two sentences.

_____

_____

_____

_____

_____

_____

_____

11. Describe the four techniques used to position and secure the child for an examination and/or treatment.

_____

_____

_____

_____

_____

_____

_____

12. Explain how you would collect a pediatric urine specimen in a collection bag.

_____

_____

_____

_____

_____

_____

_____

MEDICAL TERMINOLOGY REVIEW

Use a dictionary and highlighted terms in the textbook to define the following terms.

Terms

acyanotic_____

_____

cyanotic _____

_____

fontanelle _____

_____

lavage _____

_____

pediatrician _____

_____

pediatrics _____

_____

Abbreviations

FAS _____

_____

MMR _____

_____

VIS _____

_____

CRITICAL THINKING

1. If you needed to give an injection in the vastus lateralis muscle to a 9-month-old, and the child was crying and kicking, what could you do to ensure safety and proper administration? List a few ideas that would be appropriate.

_____

_____

_____

_____

2. You have an order to obtain blood for a test for a patient, who is a 4 1/2-year-old girl here with her father. She starts to get tears in her eyes when you approach, and the father tells her to quit that crying or he'll tell the MA to stick her a second time. What would you do?

_____

_____

_____

3. You have a parent of a 3-month-old baby who calls in two to three times per day, extremely anxious and worried over every little thing and leaving messages with questions for the doctor. When you get the advice from the physician and return her calls, she keeps talking in detail for long periods of time. This is her first child, and she has no family in town to help her through this time of learning how to care for an infant. Everyone in the office is aware of her neediness and many feel some annoyance at the amount of time and attention this one patient requires. How would you handle the continuing phone calls? What would you do and/or say?

_____

_____

4. The MA should document immunizations on the patient's chart and on the parent's copy of the child's immunization record. Considering other types of documentation you have learned in your program so far, think of two examples of other places that immunization documentation may be needed (depending on the type of practice and the office policies). This is not stated in this chapter, so use prior knowledge, common sense, and critical thinking to find examples.

_____

_____

_____

_____

5. A parent brings in a child and a jar with a urine specimen in it. The parent thought the urine may be needed, and explained that it is so difficult to keep her child on a urine pediatric collection bag, so she collected the specimen about three hours ago and has kept it refrigerated. Would this urine be useful? Provide your reason why or why not.

_____

_____

_____

_____

CHAPTER REVIEW TEST

MULTIPLE CHOICE

Circle the letter of the correct answer.

1. In cystic fibrosis, a thick and sticky mucus is produced by the _____ glands.

   a. endocrine
   b. exocrine
   c. sweat
   d. sebaceous

2. Which of the following choices is not a common indication of otitis media?
   a. fussiness
   b. vomiting
   c. pulling at ear
   d. holding head to one side

3. The chapter states that certain contagious diseases are common among children, particularly school-age children, and then goes on to list three more serious conditions for which treatment is required immediately. Which of the following is NOT one of the more serious conditions?
   a. congenital heart conditions
   b. neural tube defects
   c. blood disorders
   d. oral thrush

4. Which of the following ages is not an age when a well-baby check is recommended per the well-child visit schedule?
   a. 3 months
   b. 15 months
   c. 2 weeks
   d. 9 months

5. A child should be able to dress and undress him or herself by the time the child is a:
   a. toddler.
   b. preschooler.
   c. school-age child.
   d. infant.

6. Which two of the following choices are cyanotic conditions of congenital heart conditions?
   a. tetralogy of Fallot
   b. ventricular septal defect
   c. coarctation of the aorta
   d. transposition of the great arteries

7. A pediatrician treats children from birth to age
   a. 13.
   b. 16.
   c. puberty.
   d. 20.

8. A newborn's age range is from _____ to _____.
   a. birth, four weeks
   b. four weeks, six months
   c. four weeks, one year
   d. birth, three months

9. A parent or guardian should be allowed and encouraged to stay with the child unless his or her presence
   a. makes the child cry.
   b. makes the room crowded.
   c. hinders effective care.
   d. encourages the child to laugh and chatter, which makes it hard for the MA to hear the blood pressure.

10. If a child feels uncomfortable and threatened when clothing needs to be removed, (circle all that apply)
    a. provide a drape or sheet.
    b. provide a gown.
    c. leave the room and close the door until he or she has changed.
    d. ask the parent to do it.

TRUE/FALSE

Indicate whether the statement is true (T) or false (F).

_____ 1. A few days after birth, a baby with fetal alcohol syndrome will suffer from alcohol withdrawal.

_____ 2. Rubella is also known as the measles.

_____ 3. For a child under 2 years old, it is best to use an aural temperature.

_____ 4. Parasitic worms are helminthes.

_____ 5. The MA should provide the parent or guardian with a vaccine information sheet for each immunization given.

_____ 6. A diaper rash that has been nonresponsive may actually be of fungal origin.

_____ 7. If a child must be completely restrained and it is impossible for the parent to hold the child, a mummy restraint is used.

_____ 8. Congenital heart conditions are easily identified before birth by prenatal ultrasound examination.

_____ 9. The potency of vaccines depends on the proper refrigerator or freezer temperature.

_____ 10. The hepatitis B immunization was recently added to the list of routine vaccinations.

FILL IN THE BLANK

Using words from the list below, fill in the blanks to complete the following statements. Note: Some terms may be used in more than one statement.

Allen	illnesses	reactions
allergies	importance	respiratory or cardiac
CDC	important	route
circumcision	medical history	rubeola
diagnose	not routinely	side effects
E	parent or guardian	Snellen
effects	parotitis	spoons or cups
fifty	patterns	storage
first three years	PDR	surgically removed
five	pertussis	transfer
frequency	pharmacist	truthful
German measles	physical development	vaccine package insert
growth records	potentially painful	varicella
hospital		

1. Part of your patient instruction in administering liquid medications will be to stress the _____ of measuring with the _____ supplied by the _____ or the manufacturer.

2. Never tell a child "This will not hurt" when a _____ procedure is about to be done. Always be _____. Reassure the _____ about the procedure.

3. For immunizations, review the information from the _____ or from other sources, such as a _____ or the _____. Know the purpose of the mediac-tion, precautions, potential side _____ or adverse _____, correct _____ for administration, and _____ requirements.

4. Thanks to routine preventive inoculations, the common contagious diseases of childhood are far less prevalent now than they were _____ years ago. These diseases include chickenpox (_____), measles (_____), rubella (_____), mumps (_____), whooping cough (_____), polio, and diphtheria.

5. Measuring growth and keeping _____ for the pediatric patient is _____. The physician uses growth _____ to observe normal _____ or _____ diseases.

6. A procedure usually performed in the _____ shortly after birth is _____, in which the foreskin on an infant boy is _____.

7. Head circumference is measured during the _____ of life. Infant chest circumfer-ence is _____ measured, except when _____ abnormalities are suspected.

8. Immunizations have dramatically reduced the _____ of many childhood illnesses and the _____ of disease to other children and adults. But it is important to alert the _____ to potential _____.

9. When children require a vision check, you will use a/an _____ chart (when the child can recognize shapes but not directions), a/a _____ chart (when the child knows directions but not the alphabet), or a/an _____ chart (when the child knows the alphabet, around _____ years old).

10. Before any immunization, it is important to obtain the _____ from the _____. Ask about any known _____ or recent_____.

Procedure 27-1

Perform and Record Measurements of Height or Length, Weight, and Head or Chest Circumference

Objective: The student, using the supplies and equipment listed below, will demonstrate how to measure the child's length (height), weight, and head and/or chest circumference.

Supplies: plastic or paper tape measure, infant or platform scale, stadiometer, growth charts, patient chart

Notes to the Student:

_____

_____

_____

_____

_____

_____

Skills Assessment Requirements

Read and familiarize yourself with the procedure; complete the minimum practice requirements. Document each MPR using proper charting technique. Complete each procedure within a reasonable amount of time, with a minimum of 85% accuracy.

Name: _____

Date: _____

POINT VALUE ✦ = 3-6 points ⋆ = 7-9 points		PRACTICE TRIAL	GRADED TRIAL #1	GRADED TRIAL #2	NOTES:
1. ✦	Wash your hands and gather equipment and supplies.				
2. ⋆	Identify the parent or guardian with the child and guide them to the treatment area.				
3. ✦	Remove all clothing except the diaper before weighing.				
4. ✦	Weigh the child on the platform scale.				
5. ⋆	Record the weight on the growth charts and/or progress notes within the child's chart.				
6. ✦	Wash your hands.				
7. ✦	Move or ask the parent or guardian to move the child to the exam table.				
8. ✦	Measure the length of the child.				
9. ⋆	Record the height on the growth charts and/or progress notes within the child's chart.				
10. ✦	Measure the child's head circumference.				
11. ⋆	Record the head circumference on the growth charts and/or progress notes within the child's chart.				

		PRACTICE TRIAL	GRADED TRIAL # 1	GRADED TRIAL # 2	NOTES:
12. ✦	Measure the child's chest circumference, if necessary.				
13. ∗	Record the chest circumference on the growth charts and/or progress notes within the child's chart.				
14. ✦	Tell the physician that the child is ready.				
15. ✦	After the physician has examined the child, tell the parent or guardian to redress the child.				
16. ✦	Dispose of disposables.				
17. ✦	Clean the room. Wash your hands.				

Document: Enter the correct information in the chart below.

Grading

Points Earned	_____		
Points Possible	_____	117	117
Percent Grade (Points Earned/Points Possible)	_____		
PASS:	_____	❑ YES ❑ NO ❑ N/A	❑ YES ❑ NO ❑ N/A

Instructor Sign-Off

Instructor: _____ **Date:** _____

Procedure 27-2

Perform and Record Pediatric Vital Signs and Vision Screening

Objective: The student, using the supplies and equipment listed below, will demonstrate how to measure a child's temperature, pulse, respirations, and blood pressure and perform a vision screening test.

Supplies: pediatric blood pressure cuff, Snellen E chart, watch with a sweeping second hand, digital thermometer, patient chart

Notes to the Student:

_____

_____

_____

_____

_____

_____

Skills Assessment Requirements

Read and familiarize yourself with the procedure; complete the minimum practice requirements. Document each MPR using proper charting technique. Complete each procedure within a reasonable amount of time, with a minimum of 85% accuracy.

Name: _____

Date: _____

POINT VALUE ✦ = 3-6 points ⋆ = 7-9 points		PRACTICE TRIAL	GRADED TRIAL #1	GRADED TRIAL #2	NOTES:
	Pulse, Respirations, Axillary Temperature, and Blood Pressure				
1. ✦	Gather equipment and supplies. Wash your hands.				
2. ⋆	Identify the patient and explain the procedure to the parent or guardian.				
3. ✦	Have the parent disrobe the child down to the diaper.				
4. ✦	Place the child in the supine position or allow him or her to remain in the parent's lap for greater compliance.				
5. ⋆	Locate the apex of the heart by feeling for the fifth intercostal space to the left of the sternum on the midclavicular line.				
6. ✦	Make sure the stethoscope head is warmed and place it on the space, listening for the "lub-dub" of the heart. Count for 1 minute (each lub-dub equals one beat).				
7. ✦	Record the results.				
8. ✦	Place your hand on the child's chest and count inspirations and expirations for 1 minute. The rise and fall of the chest is counted as one breath.				
9. ⋆	Record the results.				
10. ✦	Take the temperature probe and apply a disposable sheath.				
11. ⋆	Place the probe in the infant's axillary space, holding the child's arm down close to his or her side.				

		PRACTICE TRIAL	GRADED TRIAL #1	GRADED TRIAL #2	NOTES:
12. ✦	Wait for the beep to indicate the reading has been completed, then dispose of the probe cover.				
13. ⋆	Record the results.				
14. ✦	If the physician orders that blood pressure be taken, follow the directions for taking an adult BP reading.				
15. ✦	Palpate the blood pressure first to avoid over-inflating the cuff. Make sure the cuff size is correct for the patient size.				
16. ⋆	Record the results.				
17. ✦	**Vision Screening** Take the child to the vision screening area, accompanied by the parent. Explain the chart and ask the child to stand at the correct distance from the chart. (Each chart indicates the recommended distance.)				
18. ⋆	Have the child cover one eye and read as many lines as possible. If the child misses two objects, directions, or letters in a single line, stop the test and record the line number. For example, if the child reads line 20/20 correctly with the left eye but misses multiple letters on line 20/15, the vision would be 20/20 in the left eye.				
19. ✦	Repeat the procedure for the other eye, then both eyes reading together.				
20. ⋆	Record the results in the patient's chart.				

Document: Enter the correct information in the chart below.

Grading

Points Earned	_____		
Points Possible	_____	144	144
Percent Grade (Points Earned/Points Possible)	_____		
PASS:	_____	❏ YES ❏ NO ❏ N/A	❏ YES ❏ NO ❏ N/A

Instructor Sign-Off

Instructor: _____   Date: _____

Procedure 27-3

Perform Documentation of Immunization, Both Stored and Administered

Objective: The student, using the supplies and equipment listed below, will demonstrate how to provide the parent or guardian instruction and give childhood immunizations.

Supplies: vaccine information sheets (VIS), vaccination dosage, sterile gloves, patient chart

Notes to the Student:

_____

_____

_____

_____

_____

_____

Skills Assessment Requirements

Read and familiarize yourself with the procedure; complete the minimum practice requirements. Document each MPR using proper charting technique. Complete each procedure within a reasonable amount of time, with a minimum of 85% accuracy.

Name: _____

Date: _____

		PRACTICE TRIAL	GRADED TRIAL #1	GRADED TRIAL #2	NOTES:
POINT VALUE ✦ = 3-6 points ∗ = 7-9 points					
1. ✦	Wash your hands. Gather the equipment and supplies.				
2. ∗	Identify the parent or guardian with the child and guide them to the treatment area.				
3. ✦	Ask the parent or guardian about the child's recent health and if there is medical history that would exclude the child temporarily or permanently from any of the immunizations.				
4. ∗	Provide vaccine information sheets for each immunization to be given.				
5. ✦	Take and record the child's vital signs.				
6. ✦	After the physician has seen the patient, wash your hands and put on sterile gloves.				
7. ✦	Administer the immunizations.				
8. ✦	Dispose of sharps or biohazardous materials in the appropriate containers.				
9. ✦	Wash your hands.				
10. ∗	Document on the child's immunization record for the parent or guardian and on the child's chart.				

Name: _____

Date: _____

Document: Enter the correct information in the chart below.

Grading

Points Earned	_____		
Points Possible	_____	69	69
Percent Grade (Points Earned/Points Possible)	_____		
PASS:	_____	❏ YES ❏ NO ❏ N/A	❏ YES ❏ NO ❏ N/A

Instructor Sign-Off

Instructor: _____ Date: _____

Procedure 27-4

Perform Urine Collection with a Pediatric Urine Collection Bag

Objective: The student, using the supplies and equipment listed below, will demonstrate how to collect a urine specimen in a urine collection bag.

Supplies: urine collection bag for newborn or pediatric patient, sterile gloves, sterile container with label, cotton balls, prepackaged sterile cleansing swabs or towelettes, laboratory requisition form, patient chart

Notes to the Student:

_____

_____

_____

_____

_____

_____

Skills Assessment Requirements

Read and familiarize yourself with the procedure; complete the minimum practice requirements. Document each MPR using proper charting technique. Complete each procedure within a reasonable amount of time, with a minimum of 85% accuracy.

Name: _____

Date: _____

POINT VALUE ✦ = 3-6 points ⋆ = 7-9 points		PRACTICE TRIAL	GRADED TRIAL # 1	GRADED TRIAL # 2	NOTES:
1. ✦	Wash your hands. Gather the equipment and supplies.				
2. ⋆	Identify the parent or guardian with the child and guide them to the treatment area. Explain the procedure to the parent or guardian.				
3. ✦	Put on sterile gloves.				
4. ✦	Remove the diaper and dispose of it in the appropriate container.				
5. ⋆	Wipe the child's genital area with sterile towelettes or cleansing swabs. For boy infants, wipe around and away from the urinary meatus. For girl infants, wipe from the clitoris toward the rectal area. Repeat the wipe with a separate towelette or cleansing swab a second and third time to cleanse the area immediately surrounding the urinary meatus, then cleanse the wider surrounding area.				
6. ✦	Dry the cleansed area with dry cotton balls.				
7. ✦	Remove the adhesive tabs of the urine collection bag and apply the bag to the genital area securely, without gaps between the tabs and the skin.				
8. ✦	Diaper the child.				
9. ✦	Remove gloves and wash your hands.				
10. ✦	Instruct the parent or guardian to encourage the infant or toddler to drink or nurse.				

		PRACTICE TRIAL	GRADED TRIAL # 1	GRADED TRIAL # 2	NOTES:
11. ✦	Recheck the diaper every 20 minutes until a specimen is obtained in the bag.				
12. ★	Wash your hands and put on sterile gloves.				
13. ✦	Remove the urine collection bag. Place the bagged urine specimen in the sterile cup and cover the container tightly.				
14. ✦	Diaper the child.				
15. ✦	Remove the gloves and wash your hands.				
16. ★	Prepare the container label and laboratory requisition. Transport or arrange for transport of the specimen to the laboratory.				
17. ★	Document the procedure in the child's chart.				
18. ✦	Dispose of biohazardous materials in the proper containers.				
19. ✦	Clean the area. Wash your hands.				

Document: Enter the correct information in the chart below.

Grading

Points Earned	_____		
Points Possible	_____	129	129
Percent Grade (Points Earned/Points Possible)	_____		
PASS:	_____	❑ YES ❑ NO ❑ N/A	❑ YES ❑ NO ❑ N/A

Instructor Sign-Off

Instructor: _____ Date: _____

CHAPTER 28
Neurology

CHAPTER OUTLINE

Review the Chapter Outline. If any content area is unclear, review that area before beginning workbook exercises.

    A. The Medical Assistant's Role in Neurology and Neurosurgery

    B. The Anatomy and Physiology of the Nervous System

    C. Assessing the Neurological System

    D. Disorders and Diseases of the Central Nervous System

    E. Diseases of the Peripheral Nervous System

CHAPTER REVIEW

The following is a summary of the chapter. If any of this material is unclear, review it in the textbook.

There are many parts and disorders of the nervous system and numerous opportunities for the MA to assist the patients and providers. The nervous system includes such divisions as the central nervous system, the peripheral nervous system, the autonomic nervous system, neurons, and the sympathetic and parasympathetic nervous systems. Examples of the diseases or injuries to the system include epilepsy, Parkinson's disease, headaches and migraines, head trauma such as concussion, spinal cord injuries, infectious diseases such as meningitis, among many others. This specialty is quite varied in the needs of the patients and the assessment and procedures required.

LEARNING ACTIVITIES AND STUDY AIDS

Review the following study aids and/or complete the activities to ensure that you have achieved the learning objectives for this chapter.

1. Describe the medical assistant's role in the neurology/neurosurgery practice.

_____

_____

_____

_____

_____

_____

_____

2. The two major parts of anatomy and physiology of the nervous system are the central nervous system and the peripheral nervous system. List the functions of the complete nervous system, then list the accessory parts, if any, or include any subdivisions under each system. Your list should also include a one-sentence description of the functions of the parts of the central and peripheral nervous systems.

_____

_____

_____

_____

_____

_____

_____

3. Name the structures that make up a neuron. Draw a basic picture to illustrate how a nerve impulse travels from one neuron's dendrite to another neuron's dendrite.

_____

_____

_____

_____

_____

_____

_____

_____

4. Make a chart of the basic functions of the various physiological divisions of the nervous system. This is different from the anatomy and physiology of the systems in question 2.

_____

_____

_____

_____

_____

_____

_____

5. Review the section in Chapter 28 of your textbook on neurological assessment, paying attention to the list of areas that are assessed and the methods used in the assessment. Then close the book and from memory list the areas assessed and the various methods used in the assessments. Once you have completed the list, go back to the book and check your answers. If you missed any, add those to your list so that you will have a one-page quick reference.

_____

_____

_____

_____

_____

_____

_____

6. In neurological assessment, how is the Glasgow Coma Scale used? What could be tested by doing a lumbar puncture?

_____

_____

_____

_____

_____

_____

_____

7. Make a set of flash cards of the following common diseases and disorders of the central nervous system: CVA, TIA, epilepsy, ALS, Parkinson's disease, multiple sclerosis, amyotrophic lateral sclerosis, headache, infectious conditions, head trauma, spinal cord injuries, and disk disorders. Put the name of the disease/disorder on one side of a card, and on the other put a brief description of what it is.

_____

_____

_____

_____

_____

_____

8. Make a set of flash cards as in question 7, this time of the common diseases and disorders of the peripheral nervous system: Bell's palsy, trigeminal neuralgia, and shingles.

_____

_____

_____

_____

_____

_____

_____

MEDICAL TERMINOLOGY REVIEW

Use a dictionary and highlighted terms in the textbook to define the following terms.

Terms

affect _____

_____

aura _____

_____

cephalgia _____

_____

clonic _____

_____

contrecoup _____

_____

decerebrate posture _____

_____

decorticate posture _____

_____

dermatome _____

_____

exacerbation _____

_____

hemiparesis _____

_____

innervate _____

_____

neuralgia _____

_____

neurology _____

_____

neuron _____

_____

neurotransmitter _____

_____

nuchal rigidity _____

_____

palsy _____

_____

paraplegia _____

_____

postictal _____

_____

prodromal _____

_____

projectile vomiting _____

_____

pyogenic _____

_____

quadriplegia _____

_____

tonic _____

_____

Abbreviations

ALS _____

_____

CNS _____

_____

EEG _____

_____

LP _____

_____

PNS _____

_____

CRITICAL THINKING

1. A patient, a 57-year-old female named Katie Gilpatrick, has come in following an ER visit where she was diagnosed with a cerebrovascular accident. What are the three things that could have caused this stroke in the patient? Explain why a stroke only affects one side of the body.

   _____

   _____

   _____

2. A fellow healthcare worker comes to work and states she cannot do very much because she has a "migraine." She was out late last night at a party and states that the headache is not because she had some drinks. She hopes you will help her through the day by rooming some of her patients. She is incorrect in diagnosing herself with a migraine because it is a specific type of headache, and she

has not been diagnosed with migraines by a physician. Explain why it is unlikely someone with a true migraine would be able to come to work and function even at a slow pace.

_____

_____

_____

_____

3. In the case study in this chapter, imagine that Milo does not have any blisters or lesions. Knowing that Milo had recently had varicella, what infectious condition of the central nervous system could Milo have? The medical assistant does not diagnose, but you should have knowledge of the signs and symptoms of various nervous system problems; use this knowledge to answer the question.

_____

_____

_____

4. A patient, Janis McCarty, presents with headache, fever, dizziness, blurred vision, and motor problems. When the physician examines her, she is unable to bend her head forward to touch her chin to her chest (nuchal rigidity). What condition might the physician diagnose? What would likely be done for this patient if she does, in fact, have the condition that you suspect? (Medical assistants never make a diagnosis; this is a question of your knowledge of the signs and symptoms of various conditions.)

_____

_____

_____

5. A patient, a 28-year-old male who has paraplegia, has come in to the office for an exam. The physician needs the patient on the table to do a thorough exam. How will you get the patient on to the exam table, since he cannot stand or use the bottom half of his body at all? Explain possible transfers from his wheelchair to the table.

_____

_____

_____

CHAPTER REVIEW TEST

MULTIPLE CHOICE

Circle the letter of the correct answer.

1. There are three vascular conditions in the brain that can cause a cerebrovascular accident. Which of the following is not a cause of CVA?
   a. thrombus
   b. vessel rupture
   c. seizure
   d. embolus

2. Which two of the following would complete this statement: The _____, height, _____, and rate of brain waves on an EEG are unique to each person, like a brain "fingerprint."
   a. length
   b. rhythm
   c. strength
   d. pattern

3. Sciatica is also called
   a. a spinal cord injury.
   b. Bell's palsy.
   c. spinal stenosis.
   d. paraplegia.

4. Which of the following are disease(s) whose cause is unknown? (circle all that apply)
   a. Parkinson's disease
   b. TIA
   c. trigeminal neuralgia
   d. multiple sclerosis

5. A patient must follow certain pretesting instructions prior to having an EEG. Which of the following is not part of the patient instructions?
   a. eliminate caffeine
   b. avoid smoking
   c. discontinue certain medications
   d. have a well-balanced dinner the night before the test then nothing by mouth

6. Which of the following are the two anatomical divisions of the nervous system?
   a. central nervous system
   b. autonomic nervous system
   c. peripheral nervous system
   d. brain and spinal cord

7. An epidural hematoma is
   a. above the dura mater.
   b. below the dura mater.
   c. under the arachnoid meninges.
   d. a concussion.

8. Which two of the following are not used in diagnosing epilepsy?
   a. MRI
   b. biopsy
   c. CSF studies
   d. recurrent seizure activity

9. Which of the following is not one of the common bacterial agents listed in your textbook as being a cause of meningitis?
   a. *Hemophilus influenzae type B*
   b. *Streptococcus pneumoniae*
   c. *Neisseria meningitis*
   d. *Staphlyococcus aureus*

10. Which of the following shows the correct conduction path of a nervous system impulse?
    a. dendrite, through nerve cell body, along axon, crosses synaptic gap, next dendrite
    b. dendrite, through axon, through nerve cell body, crosses synaptic gap, next dendrite
    c. dendrite, through nerve cell body, along axon, through nerve cell body, crosses synaptic gap, next dendrite
    d. dendrite, through axon, through nerve cell body, crosses synaptic gap, through the axon, next dendrite

TRUE/FALSE

Indicate whether the statement is true (T) or false (F).

_____ 1. The functional unit of the nervous system is the nerve cell nucleus.

_____ 2. Quadriplegia is caused by an insult to the spinal cord in the cervical area.

_____ 3. The medical term for a headache is cephalitis.

_____ 4. Projectile vomiting is a symptom of a head injury.

_____ 5. Most incidences of shingles are unilateral and do not cross the midline.

_____ 6. One form of encephalitis is caused by infection with the herpes simplex virus and has the lowest mortality rate when left untreated.

_____ 7. Pressure is measured with a manometer.

_____ 8. Parkinson's disease has a deficiency in the production of the neurotransmitter dopamine.

_____ 9. There are 23 pairs of spinal nerves.

_____ 10. Brain tumors can be benign or malignant.

FILL IN THE BLANK

Using words from the list below, fill in the blanks to complete the following statements.

abscess	functioning	palsy
atherosclerosis	homeostatic	peripheral
autonomic nervous system	hormonal and chemical	peristalsis
brain and spinal cord	infection and trauma	pressure
canal	infections	progressive
cerebrospinal	internal and external	respiration and heart rate
chronic	microorganisms	speech
cranial and spinal	midbrain	spinal
dementia	motor	subarachnoid
diagnostic	myelin	ventricles
emotional	neuralgia	vital
encapsulated	nonprogressive	white matter
evaluations	oxygen	

1. Cerebrovascular disease is usually a result of _____ of the cerebral arteries, which deprives the brain of _____ and is one cause of _____.

2. Infectious microorganisms that migrate to the brain from other _____ in the body may cause a brain _____. These pyogenic _____ may be in _____ or free form in the brain tissue.

3. Cerebrospinal fluid supports and cushions the _____ and protects them from _____. It is produced within the _____ and circulates through the brain and spinal cord and into the _____ space.

4. Peripheral nervous system disorders include Bell's _____, trigeminal _____, and shingles. These acute, _____ conditions affect the _____ nerves.

5. The brainstem, consisting of the _____, pons, and medulla oblongata, is composed mainly of _____ and is responsible for regulating _____ body functions such as _____.

6. A healthy nervous system coordinates the _____ reactions of body systems to _____ stimuli.

7. Multiple sclerosis is a _____ disorder that is characterized by the progressive destruction of the _____ sheath of the nerve and _____ disability.

8. The sympathetic and parasympathetic nerves comprise the _____, which is part of the _____ nervous system. These nerves regulate all involuntary _____ functions and responses, including _____, breathing, blinking, and _____ activities.

9. Assessment of the central nervous system involves different _____ to locate a deficit in the system. Areas that are assessed are mental status and _____, mood or _____ state, cognitive _____, level of consciousness, and sensory and _____ functions involving the cranial, _____, and peripheral nerves.

10. Lumbar punctures are performed as a _____ procedure to evaluate the status of the _____ fluid and to measure the _____ within the cerebrospinal _____.

Procedure 28-1

Assist in a Neurological Exam

Objective: The student, using the supplies and equipment listed below, will demonstrate how to assist with a neurological exam.

Supplies: reflex hammers; penlight; pinwheel; tongue blade; tuning fork; ophthalmoscope; cold object, as determined by physician; warm object, as determined by physician; scent object (coffee grounds, for example), as determined by physician; patient drapes as determined by office protocol; patient chart

Notes to the Student:

_____

_____

_____

_____

_____

_____

Skills Assessment Requirements

Read and familiarize yourself with the procedure; complete the minimum practice requirements. Document each MPR using proper charting technique. Complete each procedure within a reasonable amount of time, with a minimum of 85% accuracy.

POINT VALUE ✦ = 3-6 points ⋆ = 7-9 points		PRACTICE TRIAL	GRADED TRIAL # 1	GRADED TRIAL # 2	NOTES:
1. ✦	Wash your hands and gather equipment and supplies.				
2. ⋆	Greet and identify patient. Escort patient to examination room.				
3. ✦	Interview the patient according to office protocol. Ask standard questions such as: • What is your full name? • Who is the current president of the United States? • What is the date, including the month and year?				
4. ✦	If your office protocol requires patients to change into cotton shorts and a tank top shirt, assist the patient as necessary.				
5. ✦	Provide patient drapes as needed.				
6. ⋆	Follow office protocol for assisting the patient into the required positions. If the physician tests reflexes with a hammer first, assist the patient into a seated position on the exam table. Have the patient remove socks and shoes in preparation for testing the Babinski reflex.				
7. ✦	After the physician has finished reflex testing, assist the patient to dress, as needed. Escort the patient to the gait-and-movement testing area.				
8. ⋆	Document any changes in the patient chart.				

Name: _____

Date: _____

Document: Enter the correct information in the chart below.

Grading

Points Earned	_____		
Points Possible	_____	57	57
Percent Grade (Points Earned/ Points Possible)	_____		
PASS:	_____	❏ YES ❏ NO ❏ N/A	❏ YES ❏ NO ❏ N/A

Instructor Sign-Off

Instructor: _____ **Date:** _____

Procedure 28-2

Assist with a Lumbar Puncture

Objective: The student, using the supplies and equipment listed below, will demonstrate how to assist the physician with a lumbar puncture to obtain CSF.

Supplies: Lumbar puncture kit: iodine antiseptic, iodine applicator, adhesive bandages, spinal puncture needle, 4 testing tubes; patient drape; BP cuff, sized appropriately for the patient; manometer; Xylocaine 1 or 2%; syringe and needle for anesthetic; sterile gloves; gauze sponges; fenestrated drape

Notes to the Student:

_____

_____

_____

_____

_____

_____

Skills Assessment Requirements

Read and familiarize yourself with the procedure; complete the minimum practice requirements. Document each MPR using proper charting technique. Complete each procedure within a reasonable amount of time, with a minimum of 85% accuracy.

POINT VALUE ✦ = 3-6 points ⋆ = 7-9 points		PRACTICE TRIAL	GRADED TRIAL # 1	GRADED TRIAL # 2	NOTES:
1. ✦	Identify the patient and explain the procedure. Reinforce the need for postoperative care.				
2. ⋆	Verify that the patient has signed a consent form and that it has been filed in the chart.				
3. ✦	Have the patient empty his or her bowel or bladder.				
4. ✦	Obtain the patient's vital signs.				
5. ✦	Wash your hands, put on gloves, and set up a tray using sterile technique.				
6. ⋆	With the iodine in the kit, disinfect the puncture site (L3 and L4).				
7. ✦	Have the patient lie on his or her left side and curl into the fetal position. Provide drapes for patient comfort.				
8. ⋆	Assist the physician as necessary in swabbing the patient with antiseptic and placing a fenestrated drape.				
9. ✦	Assist the physician in aspirating the xylocaine.				
10. ✦	To avoid potential trauma to the spinal cord, assist the patient in maintaining the fetal position.				
11. ✦	While the physician is taking a pressure reading, remind the patient to breathe evenly and avoid talking. If the physician requests assist the patient in straightening his or her legs to get a true pressure reading.				

		PRACTICE TRIAL	GRADED TRIAL # 1	GRADED TRIAL # 2	NOTES:
12. ✦	Place a gauze pad with firm pressure over the puncture site to absorb any bleeding.				
13. ⋆	After the fluid has been collected, tighten the sample tubes and fill out a lab order form. Correctly label the samples for analysis.				
14. ✦	Move the patient to the recovery area.				
15. ✦	Clean and disinfect the treatment area.				
16. ✦	Remove the gloves and wash your hands.				
17. ⋆	Document the procedure in the patient's chart.				

Document: Enter the correct information in the chart below.

Grading

Points Earned	_____		
Points Possible	_____	114	114
Percent Grade (Points Earned/ Points Possible)	_____		
PASS:	_____	❏ YES ❏ NO ❏ N/A	❏ YES ❏ NO ❏ N/A

Instructor Sign-Off

Instructor: _____ Date: _____

Procedure 28-3

Prepare a Patient for an Electroencephalogram

Objective: The student, using the supplies and equipment listed below, will demonstrate how to assist the physician with an EEG.

Supplies: EEG machine, electrodes, approved EEG electrode adhesive

Notes to the Student:

_____

_____

_____

_____

_____

_____

Skills Assessment Requirements

Read and familiarize yourself with the procedure; complete the minimum practice requirements. Document each MPR using proper charting technique. Complete each procedure within a reasonable amount of time, with a minimum of 85% accuracy.

POINT VALUE ✦ = 3-6 points ⋆ = 7-9 points		PRACTICE TRIAL	GRADED TRIAL # 1	GRADED TRIAL # 2	NOTES:
1. ⋆	Identify the patient. Explain the procedure and why the physician has ordered it. Try to allay any anxiety the patient might be feeling.				
2. ✦	Verify that the patient has followed pre-testing procedures—avoiding caffeine and other stimulants and eating a well-balanced diet to avoid hypoglycemia.				
3. ✦	Instruct the patient to remain absolutely motionless during the baseline reading. Even tongue or eyelid movements will alter the baseline.				
4. ⋆	Connect the electrodes to the patient's scalp with the appropriate adhesive.				
5. ✦	If a sleep EEG has been ordered, the patient should not alter his or her sleeping patterns and avoid using sleep aids.				
6. ✦	The patient will be shown flickering lights to stimulate the brain. This activity will be recorded by the technician.				
7. ✦	Remove the electrodes from the patient's scalp. If the patient has been lying supine for the exam, help him or her to a sitting position. The patient should remain seated for a minimum of 1 minute to avoid dizziness caused by orthostatic hypotension.				
8. ⋆	Document the procedure in the patient's chart.				

Document: Enter the correct information in the chart below.

Grading

Points Earned	_____		
Points Possible	_____	57	57
Percent Grade (Points Earned/ Points Possible)	_____		
PASS:	_____	❑ YES ❑ NO ❑ N/A	❑ YES ❑ NO ❑ N/A

Instructor Sign-Off

Instructor: _____ Date: _____

CHAPTER 29
Mental Health

CHAPTER OUTLINE

Review the Chapter Outline. If any content area is unclear, review that area before beginning workbook exercises.

    A. The Medical Assistant's Role in the Mental Health Field

    B. The Anatomy and Physiology of Cognitive Functioning

    C. Mental Wellness

    D. General Mental Disorders

    E. Assessment and Diagnosis

    G. Standard Treatments for Mental Disorders

CHAPTER REVIEW

The following is a summary of the chapter. If any of this material is unclear, review it in the textbook.

In a mental health facility or clinic, the psychologist and the psychiatrist are usually the primary providers. Others may also be involved in a patient's care, including social workers, family counselors, and substance abuse counselors, to name a few. Certain areas of specialty knowledge are vital when working in mental health, such as cognitive brain functions, neuron physiology, and the concept of mental wellness. An understanding of pathology, symptoms, and treatments in a variety of disorders is also basic to be effective working with the patients and providers. These include schizophrenia, mood and personality disorders, anxiety, somatoform disorders, and gender identity. Some mental conditions/disorders are caused by a lack of oxygen to the brain, often prior to, during, or soon after birth. Injuries to the skull and brain can lead to mental disorders. Additionally, Alzheimer's disease, vascular dementia, mental disorders occurring in childhood, and substance abuse–related disorders are also treated in mental health.

LEARNING ACTIVITIES AND STUDY AIDS

Review the following study aids and/or complete the activities to ensure that you have achieved the learning objectives for this chapter.

1. Identify the medical assistant's role in the mental health field.

_____

_____

_____

_____

_____

2. What is meant by cognitive function? Write a brief explanation (one to two sentences) of how the brain maintains the body's homeostasis and clarify how that process relates to cognitive functioning.

_____

_____

_____

_____

_____

_____

3. After reading Chapter 29 in your textbook, explain in your own words the concept of mental wellness.

_____

_____

_____

_____

_____

_____

_____

4. Make a list of the symptoms of schizophrenia. State the treatment for this disorder.

_____

_____

_____

_____

_____

_____

5. Make two flash cards for the mood disorders of major depressive disorder and bipolar disorder. Put the name and symptoms on one side and the treatments on the other.

_____

_____

_____

_____

_____

_____

_____

6. Make ten flash cards for the personality disorders discussed in the textbook in Table 29-5: Classifications and Symptoms of Personality Disorders. Put the name on one side and the symptoms on the other. In the corner on either side of the card, put an A or B or C to indicate which cluster that disorder is in.

_____

_____

_____

_____

_____

_____

_____

_____

7. Make flash cards for each of the four anxiety disorders that are presented in the textbook. Put the name and a one- to two-sentence statement of what the disorder is on one side and put the symptoms and treatment on the other side.

_____

_____

_____

_____

_____

_____

_____

_____

8. Make flash cards for each of the four somatoform disorders as stated in this chapter of your book. Put the name and a one- to two-sentence statement of what the disorder is on one side and put the symptoms and treatment on the other side.

_____

_____

_____

_____

_____

_____

_____

_____

9. Express in your own words what having a gender identity disorder means.

_____

_____

_____

_____

_____

_____

_____

_____

10. What is mental retardation? Name the symptoms. What are the treatments?

_____

_____

_____

_____

_____

_____

_____

11. The following are types of dementia: Alzheimer's disease, vascular dementia, and dementia due to head trauma. For each of these three, describe the form, state the symptoms, and outline the treatment.

_____

_____

_____

_____

_____

_____

_____

_____

12. Name the four mental disorders that originate in childhood. Provide the symptoms for each.

_____

_____

_____

_____

_____

_____

_____

13. Furnish the medical terms for three possible end results of abuse. Give the three types of substance abuse disorders with examples provided for each type.

_____

_____

_____

_____

_____

_____

_____

14. Review the information on Assessment and Diagnosis in the textbook. Close the book and state the aspects of assessment in mental disorders. Additionally, from memory, make a one-sentence statement on how mental disorders are diagnosed.

_____

_____

_____

_____

_____

_____

_____

15. Reread the information on Standard Treatments for Mental Disorders in Chapter 29. Close the book and from recall, list the two major categories of treatment and then as many of the various types of one category (it is obvious by reading which one has variations stated in the textbook).

_____

_____

_____

_____

_____

_____

_____

_____

_____

MEDICAL TERMINOLOGY REVIEW

Use a dictionary and highlighted terms in the textbook to define the following terms.

Terms

addiction _____

_____

antidepressant _____

_____

antipsychotic _____

_____

comorbid _____

_____

dementia _____

_____

dependence _____

_____

phobia _____

_____

psychiatrist _____

_____

psychiatry _____

_____

psychologist _____

_____

psychology _____

_____

psychosis _____

_____

psychotherapeutic _____

_____

psychotherapy _____

_____

psychotropic _____

_____

tolerance _____

_____

Abbreviations

ADHD _____

_____

DSM-IV _____

_____

MAO _____

_____

OCD _____

_____

ODD _____

_____

PD _____

_____

PTSD _____

_____

SAD _____

_____

SSRI _____

_____

CRITICAL THINKING

1. Explain why the *Diagnostic and Statistical Manual of Mental Disorders IV* is used to diagnose patients with mental disorders. This is not stated in the book, but common sense and critical thinking skills should give you ideas.

   _____

   _____

   _____

   _____

2. Referring to the case study in the textbook, what are some of the possible sources of assistance this family could benefit from if Yolanda were willing? The answer is not in the book. Read the case study carefully to determine their problems and needs. Then list what you feel would be potential resources and what they may offer. There is a wide range of appropriate things, so list as many as you can.

   _____

   _____

   _____

   _____

3. Can you think of someone you know or have met or that you know of whom you consider to be "mentally well"? Consider this carefully and decide on someone as your example. Don't state names or identifying personal information, but write a paragraph on why you feel this person is mentally well. (What are the traits or characteristics or actions, etc., that give you the impression of mental wellness?)

   _____

   _____

   _____

   _____

4. If a patient mentions to you that she was thinking about suicide recently and asks you not to tell the doctor because she would "never really do it," what would you say or do? The answer is not in the book, but use knowledge from what you have learned in your program so far and your thoughts to formulate a few sentences for your answer.

   _____

   _____

   _____

   _____

5. You have a patient who is a 4-month-old female infant, and the mother has come in today for test results on the child. The infant was diagnosed with mental retardation, and the mother was told by the physician that there is no treatment that will help the child. The mother is upset and wants to know why there is no treatment available when modern medicine can transplant hearts and do brain surgery. What will you tell her?

   _____

   _____

   _____

   _____

CHAPTER REVIEW TEST

MULTIPLE CHOICE

Circle the letter of the correct answer.

1. The two major types of treatment of mental disorders today are: (circle two)
   a. stress reduction therapy.
   b. medication.
   c. supportive care.
   d. therapy.

2. Symptoms of vascular dementia include all of the following except:
   a. memory lapses.
   b. irritability.
   c. loss of intellectual faculties.
   d. personality changes.

3. The two cerebral hemispheres contain four lobes. Which of the choices below are lobes?
   a. thalamus
   b. cerebral cortical area
   c. occipital
   d. parietal

4. Schizophrenia is treated with _____ medications such as phenothiazines.
   a. anti-anxiety
   b. antipsychotic
   c. sedative
   d. mood stabilizer

5. Personality disorders are divided into three classifications or clusters. One cluster is referred to as the Odd Cluster and includes the paranoid personality. Which cluster is this?
   a. Cluster A
   b. Cluster B
   c. Cluster C

6. Which of the following choices is *not* an end result of substance abuse?
   a. dependence.
   b. tolerance.
   c. altered
   d. addiction.

7. A person's wakefulness or sleepiness, motivation, and attention span are determined by: (circle the two correct answer choices)
   a. purines.
   b. monoamines.
   c. acetylcholine.
   d. glutamate.

8. Iatrophobia is a fear of
   a. physicians.
   b. snakes.
   c. thunder and lightning.
   d. darkness.

9. Which of the following choices are part of the assessment and diagnosis? (circle all that apply)
   a. mental status examination
   b. treatment plan
   c. mental health intake questionnaire
   d. physical exam

10. Information regarding the patient's thoughts, plans, or history of suicidal thoughts or attempts would be included in which one of the items of assessment and diagnosis?
    a. mental status examination
    b. treatment plan
    c. mental health intake questionnaire
    d. physical exam

TRUE/FALSE

Indicate whether the statement is true (T) or false (F).

_____ 1. Some alcohol addicts have been known to go so far as to drink after-shave lotion.

_____ 2. Stuttering is a physical problem instead of a learning disorder.

_____ 3. A person with panic disorder often expresses the fear that he or she is dying.

_____ 4. Malingering is faking or exaggeration of symptoms and complaints.

_____ 5. Analgesics are over-the-counter drugs that are subject to abuse.

_____ 6. Psychology deals with diagnosis, treatment, and prevention of mental disorders.

_____ 7. Caffeine and nicotine are legal substances that can be abused.

_____ 8. Many mental disorders are caused by a chemical balance in the brain.

_____ 9. Mental retardation occurs as the result of an interruption in the intellectual growth of the child, either during prenatal development or the birth process or after birth.

_____ 10. The patient should be included in or give input into the treatment plan.

FILL IN THE BLANK

Using words from the list below, fill in the blanks to complete the following statements. Note: Some terms may be used more than once.

absence	diagnose	psychological
affect	educational	psychosis
anger	emotions and thoughts	reference
behavior	ethnic	relationships
brain	frequent phenomenon	repaired
capacity to cope	homeostasis	safety
childbirth	impending	schizophrenia
compromised brain cells	implemented	social
concurrent	insidious	society
constructive	judgment	state of being
crying spells	medical	*Statistical*
daily living	mental and physical	substance
degenerative	*Mental Disorders*	visual or auditory
deteriorate		

1. Patients going through _____ withdrawal and others with _____ problems may experience periods of _____ and angry behavior. Healthcare providers must be alert to _____ anger and use _____ approaches to help manage that anger and provide _____ for themselves, the patient, and others.

2. Substance abuse occurs among people from every _____, professional, _____, racial, and _____ background. The economic cost to _____ is immeasurable.

3. Disordered or disorganized thinking, inappropriate _____, unpredictable _____, and _____ hallucinations are all symptoms of _____.

4. Substances that have the capacity to alter _____, impair _____, and create _____ problems. Social and family _____ suffer and may _____.

5. The brain maintains the body's _____ by reacting to sensory inputs, including _____, with processing and interpretation.

6. The *Diagnostic and* _____ *Manual of* _____ IV (DSM-IV) is the _____ manual used by mental health providers to _____ a wide range of mental disorders.

7. Alzheimer's disease usually has an _____ onset, is a progressive _____ disease of the _____, and _____ functioning is reduced.

8. Mental wellness is a _____. It is not necessarily a/an _____ of mental problems but rather a _____ in healthy ways with the pressures of _____.

9. There is no cure or drug therapy for mental retardation, as the _____ cannot be replaced or _____. Any _____ mental disorders should be addressed and treatment options explored and _____.

10. Postpartum depression is a _____ in the first few days or weeks after _____. It ranges in severity from _____ or "new baby blues" through sadness and despair to _____, with potentially devastating outcomes.

CHAPTER 30
Oncology

CHAPTER OUTLINE

Review the Chapter Outline. If any content area is unclear, review that area before beginning workbook exercises.

    A. The Medical Assistant's Role in the Oncology Practice

    B. The Classification and Physiology of Cancers

    C. Diagnostic Procedures

    D. Cancer Treatment

    E. Hospice and Emotional Support

    F. The Cancer Prevention Lifestyle

CHAPTER REVIEW

The following is a summary of the chapter. If any of this material is unclear, review it in the textbook.

Being a medical assistant in an oncology practice requires special knowledge of this specialty including the possible causes of cancer; the detection, diagnosis, and the treatment of cancer, including radiation, chemotherapy, surgery, hormone treatment, and immunotherapy; and tumor markers, as well as the staging and grading of cancerous tumors. Knowledge of hospice and an understanding of promoting a cancer prevention lifestyle are also needed in this particular specialty. The typical duties of the MA are the same as in other specialties—taking the medical history and vital signs, preparing patient for examinations and procedures, providing patient education and community resources, scheduling appointments, and collecting specimens. A special understanding of the special effects of cancer on people's lives and emotions is important in the oncology practice.

LEARNING ACTIVITIES AND STUDY AIDS

Review the following study aids and/or complete the activities to ensure that you have achieved the learning objectives for this chapter.

1. Identify the typical duties of a medical assistant's role in the oncology office.

    _____

    _____

    _____

    _____

    _____

    _____

2. Describe the different types of malignant neoplasms in a table with two columns containing the type of malignancy or neoplasm and two examples of each one. You do not have to list more than two, even though many of the neoplasms have more. If a neoplasm only has one example, just list that one.

_____
_____
_____
_____
_____
_____
_____

3. Review the various routine cancer screening tests that are listed in your textbook and make a brief list here; you do not have to include an explanation of each.

_____
_____
_____
_____
_____
_____
_____
_____

4. What is a tumor marker and explain how it is used in cancer diagnosis?

_____
_____
_____
_____
_____
_____
_____

5. Review the staging and grading of malignancies by providing purpose and/or definition of staging, TNM, and grading. Provide a fairly thorough answer.

a. staging: _____
_____
_____

b. T: _____
_____
_____

c. N: _____

_____

_____

d. M: _____

_____

_____

e. grading: _____

_____

_____

6. Review the material on chemotherapy in this chapter to formulate a statement of one or two sentences in your own words of its role in cancer treatment.

_____

_____

_____

_____

_____

_____

_____

7. Review the material on radiation in this chapter to formulate a statement of one or two sentences in your own words of its role in cancer treatment.

_____

_____

_____

_____

_____

_____

_____

8. Describe surgical intervention in cancer treatment. Explain the importance of having clear or negative margins of tissue removed.

_____

_____

_____

_____

_____

_____

_____

9. Both hormone therapy and immunotherapy are also used as cancer treatments in addition to the options of radiation, chemotherapy, and surgery. State what each one does to treat cancer.

_____

_____

_____

_____

_____

_____

_____

10. Review the chapter's section on Side Effects of Cancer Treatment, which includes side effects from chemotherapy, radiation, and surgery as well as hormone therapy and immunotherapy. Close the book and list as many of the side effects as you can from memory. Go back to the textbook to check your answers and fill in any that you missed.

_____

_____

_____

_____

_____

_____

_____

11. Describe some recent advances in cancer research that are discussed in your textbook.

_____

_____

_____

_____

_____

_____

_____

12. Explain in your own words the philosophy of hospice care for terminally ill patients.

_____

_____

_____

_____

_____

_____

_____

13. State in your own words the cancer prevention lifestyle.

_____

_____

_____

_____

_____

_____

_____

MEDICAL TERMINOLOGY REVIEW

Use a dictionary and highlighted terms in the textbook to define the following terms.

Terms

benign _____

_____

cancer _____

_____

chemotherapy _____

_____

malignant _____

_____

metastasis _____

_____

neoplasm _____

_____

oncology _____

_____

remission _____

_____

tumor _____

_____

tumor marker _____

_____

CRITICAL THINKING

1. Your patient, Sharyn Holliker (a 44-year-old female), was told today by the doctor the results of a biopsy performed three days ago. She has a benign tumor, and the doctor recommended removal to prevent it from pushing on surrounding tissues if/when it grows. The patient was fine when talking with the doctor, but a little later when you meet with her to arrange the surgery, she starts crying and states that she "doesn't think it is benign or else the doctor wouldn't want to remove it." She feels sure she really has cancer but that the doctor won't tell her the truth. What would you say or do? The answer is not specifically in your textbook; this will be your opinion and should be based on the knowledge you have gained in your studies so far.

   _____

   _____

   _____

   _____

2. In the case study in this chapter of the textbook, what would you say to the patient, Ruth Dillan, if she asked you to explain how cancer runs in families? This answer is not specifically in the textbook so use your critical thinking skills and current knowledge to determine the most appropriate answer.

   _____

   _____

   _____

   _____

3. A patient named Claire has come in today for her annual checkup; she has been cancer free for six years now. A melanoma on her shoulder was removed with clear margins. She states she has no complaints, although you notice an open sore on her ankle. You casually ask her how long she has had it, as you put on the blood pressure cuff. She tells you she has had it for "weeks, I keep putting antibiotic ointment on it but it just doesn't go away." She confides she thinks it isn't healing because she keeps using some self-tanning cream even though it irritates the sore for a few minutes after she puts it on every day. What red flag would this raise to you? What would you say or do?

   _____

   _____

   _____

   _____

4. Explain, as if giving patient education, what remission is in oncology. You may need to do research on the Internet or in other texts to complete your answer.

   _____

   _____

   _____

   _____

5. The following is a hypothetical situation involving a patient who is a smoker with lung cancer. There is not a particular right or wrong answer, but it is meant to help the student recognize his or her own feelings, which are usually not expressed in the office. You should picture yourself in this situation as realistically as you can, and then state what you would say or do using critical thinking and common sense.

   Scenario: The patient is a 68-year-old male who was diagnosed two weeks ago with lung cancer caused by smoking. The patient is in the office today to discuss which treatment he has chosen from those offered last week by the physician. The patient, Mr. Holman, has been smoking since he was

14 years old and drinks about six beers per day. His wife passed away a few years ago, and he has no children. He tells you that he wants chemo but no radiation and that he won't quit smoking. He says that he has nothing left in life, and if drinking and smoking help him get through each day, he is too old to change it now. He thinks if cuts down, at least the chemo will still be able to kill the cancer.

Write a paragraph on what you would likely say to this patient. Then, consider how you would feel personally about this particular scenario. Even though you cannot convey your personal morals and opinions to the patient, it is important that you acknowledge your true biases. Write a paragraph about how you feel about this situation (which you would hide from the patient for professionalism). What would you be thinking about this patient's choice? Would you feel differently if he had a different type of cancer? Would you feel differently if the patient had lung cancer, had never smoked, but was a heavy drinker and he refused to stop drinking?

_____

_____

CHAPTER REVIEW TEST

MULTIPLE CHOICE

Circle the letter of the correct answer.

1. The term for cancer appearing in a secondary site elsewhere in the body is called:

   a. spreading.
   b. metastasis.
   c. malignant.
   d. eradication.

2. Carcinoma originates in _____ tissue.

   a. lymphoid
   b. stem cells
   c. basal
   d. epithelial

3. The "A" in the ABCDs of abnormalities in warts and moles stands for:

   a. asymmetry.
   b. assimilation.
   c. atrophy.
   d. alimentary.

4. There are three major methods of cancer treatment. Which of the following is NOT one of the three?

   a. chemotherapy
   b. staging and grading
   c. surgery
   d. radiation

5. The two goals of surgery for cancer as a treatment modality are: (circle both)

   a. palliative
   b. to avoid radiation and chemotherapy
   c. cure
   d. avoid the negative margins

6. Two ways to screen for prostate cancer include: (circle the two that are correct)

   a. barium enema
   b. PSA blood test
   c. digital rectal examination
   d. colonoscopy

7. Which of the following are a part of a healthy lifestyle to try to prevent cancer? (circle all that apply)
   a. Reduce intake of animal fat.
   b. Get an EKG.
   c. Apply sunscreen prior to sun exposure.
   d. Have your eyes checked.

8. Which of the following are early warning signs of breast cancer? (circle all that apply)
   a. positive occult blood test
   b. a depression or dimpling in the skin
   c. bloody or spontaneous discharge from the nipple
   d. swelling of the lymph nodes in the armpit

9. The "N" in malignancy staging by the TNM system stands for
   a. note size, depth, and location
   b. nodal involvement
   c. normal
   d. neurological involvement

10. Overexposure to the sun's UV rays raises the risk of three types of cancer. Which of the following is not one of the three types?
    a. squamous
    b. basal
    c. lymphoma
    d. melanoma

TRUE/FALSE

Indicate whether the statement is true (T) or false (F).

_____ 1. Chemotherapy is only toxic to cancer cells.

_____ 2. The human papillomavirus is a possible precursor to ovarian cancer.

_____ 3. Radiation use in an oncology office can be both diagnostic and therapeutic.

_____ 4. Leukemia is a type of cancer.

_____ 5. Mammograms are usually prescribed yearly after the age of 65.

_____ 6. Hormone therapy can be effective in all types of cancer.

_____ 7. Malignant tumor recurrence is rare after a surgical excision.

_____ 8. Benign tumor cells are differentiated; that is, they resemble the tissue of origin.

_____ 9. Chemotherapeutic cancer treatment is a challenge as the drugs may cause uncomfortable and undesirable side effects.

_____ 10. Radiation disrupts RNA replication.

FILL IN THE BLANK

Using words from the list below, fill in the blanks to complete the following statements.

1.3	life cycle	rectal
500,000	lower GI	recurrence
angiogenesis	metastasized	removed
attack	metastatic	screening
cancer	negative margins	screening tools
degree	new blood vessels	shrink
different stages	normal tissue	staged and graded
drug therapy	Pap	starving
entire tumor	prognosis	tissue
final phase	progress	treatment
genetic	prolonging	tumors
holistic care	quality of life	twenty-five
hormones	quality palliative care	

1. Every year _____ million Americans are diagnosed with cancer. _____ percent of U.S. deaths (_____) are caused by cancer.

2. Tumor markers, also referred to as _____ markers, are proteins, _____, and other substances produced by _____ and released into the blood. They are used as _____ to determine the _____ of cancer treatment or the _____ of a tumor.

3. Cancer takes on many forms and has variable outcomes, depending on the _____ or area of the body involved and the _____ to which the cancer has _____ at the time of diagnosis.

4. Routine diagnostic screening for cancer includes: colorectal _____; barium enema or _____; mammogram screening; _____ smear and pelvic examination, PSA screening, and digital _____ examination.

5. Hospice is the _____ of terminally ill patients in a home or homelike setting. The philosophy of hospice is to provide _____to patients during the _____ of life.

6. Malignancies are _____ to determine the _____ and optimum course of _____ for each patient.

7. Single or combination chemotherapy, in conjunction with other _____, is used effectively to _____ the malignancy at _____ of the cancer cell _____.

8. There is no cure for many _____ diseases, but the same treatment modalities may be useful in _____ or improving the _____.

9. When surgery is employed as a curative measure, the surgeon tries to achieve the _____ around the tumor, meaning that a certain amount of _____ is removed along with the tumor to ensure the _____ is _____.

10. Recent cancer research has explored the areas of _____ inhibitors and _____ causes. One new approach is based on "_____" the tumor by inhibiting the growth of _____ (angiogenesis) that feed the tumor, causing the tumor to _____.

CHAPTER 31
Geriatrics

CHAPTER OUTLINE

Review the Chapter Outline. If any content area is unclear, review that area before beginning workbook exercises.

    A. The Medical Assistant's Role in the Geriatric Office

    B. The Aging Process

    C. Cultural Views of Aging

    D. Promoting Health Among the Elderly

CHAPTER REVIEW

The following is a summary of the chapter. If any of this material is unclear, review it in the textbook.

Geriatrics is as unique as pediatrics in that it specializes in a certain age group or stage of life. The aging process of these patients includes physical, social, and psychosocial changes and consideration of all the various aspects of aging is needed to provide total patient care. Nutrition is important in geriatric patients, and the MA should be aware of this patient population's needs. Cultural views on aging also play a role and all healthcare workers should be aware of these various views. Often elderly patients need special assistance with health insurance, finances, or community resources for assistance. The promotion of healthy habits in the older patient is important in improving their quality of life.

LEARNING ACTIVITIES AND STUDY AIDS

Review the following study aids and/or complete the activities to ensure that you have achieved the learning objectives for this chapter.

1. Explain the medical assistant's role in a geriatric medical office.

    _____

    _____

    _____

    _____

    _____

    _____

    _____

    _____

2. Make one card and concisely list only the physical changes that take place during aging. The material does not have to be presented on the card as a term on one side and a definition on the

other. Then make a set of cards that lists a body system on one side and on the other side, list examples of common geriatric conditions for that system.

_____

_____

_____

_____

_____

_____

_____

3. Review in the textbook the psychological aspects of aging. Write a paragraph that explains your understanding of this.

_____

_____

_____

_____

_____

_____

_____

_____

4. Write a paragraph on the various changes that can happen to the aging person's social life.

_____

_____

_____

_____

_____

_____

_____

5. Review material in your book about the nutritional needs and the nutritional problems of the aging person. Make a list with two columns, one for the needs and the other for the problems in nutrition in the elderly.

_____

_____

_____

_____

_____

_____

_____

6. Explain in your own words the economic impact of aging.

_____

_____

_____

_____

_____

_____

_____

7. Review the material on the various cultural views on the place of the elderly in society. Close the book and from memory, make a list of the different views you can recall. After you have completed your list, check the textbook, and any items you may have left out should be added to your list.

_____

_____

_____

_____

_____

_____

_____

_____

8. What are some things you can do to promote health in geriatric patients?

_____

_____

_____

_____

_____

_____

_____

MEDICAL TERMINOLOGY REVIEW

Use a dictionary and highlighted terms in the textbook to define the following terms.

Terms

assisted living facility _____

_____

extended care facility _____

_____

geriatrics _____

_____

hemiplegia _____

_____

Medicare _____

_____

Medigap insurance _____

_____

orthostatic hypotension _____

_____

paraplegia _____

_____

presbycusis _____

_____

presbyopia _____

_____

short-term memory _____

_____

Abbreviations

LRI _____

_____

URI _____

_____

CRITICAL THINKING

1. Your patient is an 82-year-old woman who is in fairly good health, but she is worried about money. She states that Medicare doesn't pay for enough things, and she wonders if you know of any other resources for her. What can you suggest to this patient regarding medical costs?

   _____

   _____

   _____

2. Because your patient, Mr. Bjorklund, has a diminished short-term memory, what can you do to ensure that any patient education you deliver will not be ignored because the patient forgot?

   _____

   _____

   _____

3. Mr. and Mrs. Holman, a married couple in their 70s, are both patients at your clinic and they are both in for their annual physicals today. The woman tells you in the hallway that her husband's driving is becoming a problem. She states he has bumped into a few planters and fences when parking and that he drifts out of his lane when driving. She asks that you not tell the doctor because it would be difficult if they did not have a car. What would you do?

_____

_____

_____

_____

4. A 68-year-old patient named Mrs. Royer has come in today because she is depressed. She says she used to have lots of friends and family but now she is alone. Make a list of possible reasons that this patient feels so isolated.

_____

_____

_____

_____

5. After you have practiced Procedure 31-1: Role-Play Sensorimotor Changes of the Elderly, write at least two paragraphs on how you felt, or what it was like, or even a list of the things you didn't realize before trying this. You can choose to write a paragraph each on two of the various aging conditions (loss of vision, paralysis, etc.), or you can write two paragraphs on the overall experience. There are no right or wrong answers in this critical thinking question. This is for you to explore and consider how your patients feel and what they have to deal with. This is a valuable experience.

_____

_____

_____

_____

CHAPTER REVIEW TEST

MULTIPLE CHOICE

Circle the letter of the correct answer.

1. The typical length of time between visits by a doctor to a patient at an extended care facility is:
   a. daily.
   b. weekly.
   c. monthly.
   d. semi-monthly.

2. Which of the following is not an assistive device to aid older individuals?
   a. handrails and grab bars
   b. throw rugs
   c. bathtub seat
   d. Velcro fasteners

3. In which of the following cultures is it considered shameful not to care for elderly parents?
   a. Chinese
   b. Indian
   c. Latino
   d. Korean

4. All older patients should be encouraged to document their wishes regarding

   a. which community resources to refer them to.

   b. the extent of medical intervention they want when they cannot speak for themselves.

   c. arrangements for transportation to doctor appointments and shopping.

   d. submitting their information to the Local Councils on Aging.

5. Changes in metabolic rate are a condition of which system?

   a. endocrine

   b. cardiac

   c. integumentary

   d. gastrointestinal

6. Normal wear and tear and natural deterioration take their toll on spinal disks, and the individual may: (circle all that apply)

   a. cause orthostatic hypotension.

   b. stoop.

   c. lose muscle tone.

   d. become shorter.

7. Which of the following are true statements? (circle all that apply)

   a. The process of aging has physiological aspects.

   b. The loss of hearing, taste, smell, and mobility can lead to depression.

   c. Changes in sensorimotor abilities improve how the elderly interact with their environment.

   d. The elderly undergo changes in their physical appearance.

8. Which of the following is not listed in your textbook as one of the three examples of factors that accelerate the aging process?

   a. disease

   b. stress

   c. depression

   d. lack of social interaction

9. Seborrheic keratosis is a condition of what system?

   a. endocrine

   b. cardiac

   c. integumentary

   d. gastrointestinal

10. Three changes to hearing (related to the nervous system) are listed in the textbook. Which of the following is not one of those three?

   a. delayed auditory response

   b. damage to ossicles

   c. sensoneural damage to auditory nerve

   d. decreased equilibrium

TRUE/FALSE

Indicate whether the statement is true (T) or false (F).

_____ 1. Solitude during mealtimes is one of the nutritional aspects of aging.

_____ 2. An extended care facility is also called a nursing home.

_____ 3. Hemiplegia is paralysis of the lower half of the body.

_____ 4. An aging circulatory system prevents orthostatic hypotension.

_____ 5. High blood pressure can affect the kidneys.

_____ 6. Short-term memory loss usually happens over a short period of time.

_____ 7. The aging process becomes more intense during middle age.

_____ 8. Circulatory problems that change the blood supply to the brain may lead to improved mental functioning.

_____ 9. Cumulative trauma to all body tissues causes aches and pains, accompanied by reduced range of motion and activity occurs.

_____ 10. Only geriatric specialists will see elderly patients.

FILL IN THE BLANK

Using words from the list below, fill in the blanks to complete the following statements.

65	feel	quality of life
76 years	healthcare	residence
activity	heating pad	resources
address or cope	home upkeep	retirement
average	identify	senile
diminished	medical intervention	speak for themselves
discussion	medication	specialize
economic	nutritional	susceptible
elderly	physical	unsafe situation
exacerbate		

1. Our culture has set the age of _____ as a rite of passage from _____ and regular employment to _____.

2. Elderly persons who have symptoms as a result of a medical condition, a _____ deficit, or noncompliance with _____ administration are sometimes labeled "_____."

3. Life expectancies of different population groups vary, depending on social, _____, environmental, _____, and genetic factors. The _____ expectancy in the United States is _____.

4. As the immune system declines, the body is more _____ to disease conditions that _____ the aging process.

5. As part of total patient care, you will help older patients _____ these changes and how to _____ with them in order to improve their overall _____.

6. Changes in financial _____ and an inability to cope with the physical demands of _____ often lead to a change in _____.

7. All patients should be encouraged to document their wishes regarding the extent of _____ they desire when they are no longer able to _____.

8. Sensation may be _____, which can present certain hazards. For example, an older individual is less able to _____ the burning of an overly hot _____.

9. As the size of the aging population grows, the need for _____ will grow as well. There will be greater need for healthcare professionals who _____ in diseases and disorders of the _____.

10. It is important for the medical assistant to document any _____ with the patient concerning a potentially _____.

Name: _____

Date: _____

Procedure 31-1

Role-Play Sensorimotor Changes of the Elderly

Objective: The student, using the supplies and equipment listed below, will demonstrate how to understand the changes that aging patients undergo.

Supplies: 2 pairs of laboratory goggles, yellow tissue paper (such as gift wrap), pastel-colored candy, Vaseline, earmuffs, black construction paper, swimming goggles with one lens blacked out, heavy dishwashing gloves, long (50" or more) belt, walker, tongue depressors, ace bandages, regular print newspaper, coins (pennies and dimes), button-front shirts, textbook, tape, gallon jug of water

Notes to the Student:

_____

_____

_____

_____

_____

_____

Skills Assessment Requirements

Read and familiarize yourself with the procedure; complete the minimum practice requirements. Document each MPR using proper charting technique. Complete each procedure within a reasonable amount of time, with a minimum of 85% accuracy.

POINT VALUE ✦ = 3-6 points ∗ = 7-9 points	PRACTICE TRIAL	GRADED TRIAL # 1	GRADED TRIAL # 2	NOTES:
1. ✦ **Vision loss:** **a.** Put on the swimming goggles and wait for your partner's directions. **b.** Have your partner stand out of the line of vision and give directions to cross the room and pick up a specific textbook.				
2. ✦ **Vision loss accompanied by hearing loss:** **a.** Continue to wear the swimming goggles and put on the earmuffs. **b.** Have your partner stand out of the line of sight and tell you to retrieve a different textbook.				
3. ✦ **Difficulty distinguishing colors:** **a.** Remove the goggles and earmuffs. Put on the laboratory goggles, which should be covered with yellow paper to simulate yellowing of the lens. **b.** Have your partner spread the pastel candy on a table and give you directions to pick up specific colors and quantities of each color.				
4. ✦ **Difficulty focusing:** **a.** Put on a set of lab goggles that have been smeared with Vaseline. **b.** Without speaking, your partner must get you to walk a specific distance using hand signals.				

	PRACTICE TRIAL	GRADED TRIAL # 1	GRADED TRIAL # 2	NOTES:
5. ✦	***Loss of peripheral vision:*** **a.** While wearing goggles with black construction paper taped to the sides, have your partner stand out of your line of vision and give you directions to follow. **b.** Have your partner lead you through several turns and doors if possible.			
6. ✦	***Aphasia and partial paralysis:*** **a.** Bend one arm at the elbow, with your fingertips touching your shoulder. Have another student wrap the ace bandage around your arm, securing it in this position. Bend one leg at the knee with your foot near your buttocks. Have another student secure your leg in place with the belt. Finally, have someone tape your mouth shut. **b.** Your partner should stand several feet away. Communicate to your partner that you need to go to the bathroom.			

	PRACTICE TRIAL	GRADED TRIAL #1	GRADED TRIAL #2	NOTES:
7. ✦ **Loss of dexterity:** **a.** Put on the dishwashing gloves and try to button a shirt, tie your shoes, and pick up the coins off a flat surface.				
8. ✦ **Problems with mobility:** **a.** Use a walker to move across the room. **b.** When you have traveled 2 feet, have your partner hand you a gallon of water to carry.				

Name: _____

Date: _____

Document: Enter the correct information in the chart below.

Grading

Points Earned	_____		
Points Possible	_____	48	48
Percent Grade (Points Earned/ Points Possible)	_____		
PASS:	_____	❑ YES ❑ NO ❑ N/A	❑ YES ❑ NO ❑ N/A

Instructor Sign-Off

Instructor: _____ Date: _____

CHAPTER 32
Alternative Medicine

CHAPTER OUTLINE

Review the Chapter Outline. If any content area is unclear, review that area before beginning workbook exercises.

    A. Complementary and Alternative Medical Systems

    B. Alternative Medicine

    C. Mind–Body Interventions

    D. Biologically Based Therapy

    E. Manipulative and Body-Based Methods

    F. Energy Therapies

CHAPTER REVIEW

The following is a summary of the chapter. If any of this material is unclear, review it in the textbook.

The medical assistant in an alternative medical office should be familiar with all of the various therapies under the heading of alternative and complementary medicine. Integrative medicine combines conventional medicine with alternative and complementary therapies. Each category has many specialties under it. It is significant to note that not all insurance plans will cover alternative and complementary methods of treatment since they are not tested, proven, and approved, so assisting the patients with this will be one of the medical assistant's tasks.

LEARNING ACTIVITIES AND STUDY AIDS

Review the following study aids and/or complete the activities to ensure that you have achieved the learning objectives for this chapter.

1. List the five NCCAM classifications of complementary and alternative medicine and include at least two examples of each class.

_____

_____

_____

_____

_____

_____

_____

_____

2. Give a brief description in your own words of the following types of alternative medicine: Ayurveda, homeopathy, naturopathy, and acupuncture.

_____

_____

_____

_____

_____

_____

3. State the basic principle of biofeedback. Then check the Internet for more information on biofeedback and list any additional reasons for biofeedback that are not included in the textbook.

_____

_____

_____

_____

_____

_____

_____

4. Briefly describe how aromatherapy and herbal medicine are used.

_____

_____

_____

_____

_____

_____

5. Write a description of the following types of manipulative and body-based therapies: hydrotherapy, acupressure, chiropractic, CranioSacral Therapy, exercise, reflexology, and massage.

_____

_____

_____

_____

_____

_____

_____

6. What is the main principle behind energy therapies?

_____
_____
_____
_____
_____
_____
_____
_____

MEDICAL TERMINOLOGY REVIEW

Use a dictionary and highlighted terms in the textbook to define the following terms

Terms

alternative medicine _____
_____

complementary medicine _____
_____

essential oils _____
_____

integrative medicine _____
_____

Abbreviations

CAM _____
_____

CRITICAL THINKING

1. As you take the patient history of a 22-year-old female patient, you ask her if she has been taking any herbal supplements or other natural remedies or receiving any alternative treatments. She looks very surprised and asks why you want to know that. She states that since her "herbal supplements are natural," they wouldn't interfere with any medications she is taking. You know this is a false statement, so explain to the patient why this information is important to the physician.

_____
_____
_____
_____

2. A patient has come in today who would like to try Ayurvedic treatment, but she wants to know how to tell if it is worthwhile. She has researched on the Internet and cannot find the accrediting board(s) for the practice of Ayurveda medicine. What would you tell her?

_____

_____

_____

_____

3. Today Mr. Arnold has an appointment. As you are noting his chief complaint, he mentions that he wants to know which herbs should be used to relieve anxiety. Which herbs would you recommend to him?

_____

_____

_____

_____

4. Your patient, a widowed 59-year-old female named Marie DuLac, has been prescribed lymphatic massage. Although she said nothing to the physician, she now admits to you that she is very worried about having it. She is concerned that it will be painful or that it is dangerous compared to traditional massage. Write out the response/patient education you would give orally to her in the office during a visit.

_____

_____

_____

_____

5. A father comes in with the patient, Paul, his 14-year-old son, who is joining a school sports team for the first time this year. Since Paul has weak knees and ankles, the provider has recommended sports massage, but the father is skeptical and feels this won't be beneficial to his son as much as aerobic or strength-building exercise. Educate the father on the benefits of sports massage.

_____

_____

_____

_____

CHAPTER REVIEW TEST

MULTIPLE CHOICE

Circle the letter of the correct answer.

1. Which two of the following are the main reasons for homeopathic treatment as listed in your text?
   a. stimulate the immune system
   b. maintain a balance of three doshas
   c. treat psychological factors
   d. strengthen the body's healing processes

2. The three major areas of care under alternative medicine are: (circle all three)
   a. integrative
   b. naturopathic
   c. alternative
   d. complementary

3. Mind-body interventions use techniques that enhance the mind's ability to influence body function and symptoms. For example, positive thinking, laughter, and personal contact help to release _____, which are natural anti-pain mediators.
   a. hormones
   b. endorphins
   c. potassium and sodium
   d. enzymes

4. Which of the following is *not* a form of hydrotherapy?
   a. hot tub
   b. moist heat pack
   c. sauna
   d. all of the above are forms of hydrotherapy

5. Which of the following types of therapies does not use conventional medicine at all?
   a. integrative
   b. complementary
   c. alternative
   d. all of the above

6. Which herb has an anti-inflammatory property?
   a. ginseng
   b. ginkgo
   c. garlic
   d. goldenseal

7. Which of the following is not considered a natural substance that can be used as the basis for biologically based therapies?
   a. hormones
   b. essential oils
   c. vitamins
   d. herbs

8. Biofeedback includes three areas in which the patient is trained. Which of the following is not one of the three areas?
   a. relaxation
   b. meditation
   c. massage
   d. visualization

9. Homeopathic treatment involves the use of natural remedies made from:
   a. plant, animal, or mineral substances.
   b. chemicals made from natural sources.
   c. natural hormones.
   d. regular household items such as vinegar and baking soda.

10. Traditional Chinese medicine is listed under which of the categories of complementary and alternative methods?
    a. mind-body interventions
    b. energy therapies
    c. biologically based therapies
    d. alternative medicine

TRUE/FALSE

Indicate whether the statement is true (T) or false (F).

_____ 1. Reflexology uses specific reflex points in the back, arms, legs, feet, and hands.

_____ 2. Harmful interactions may result when conventional and alternative medicine are used simultaneously.

_____ 3. Swedish massage uses four main strokes.

_____ 4. Leeches can be used to eat dead tissue and clean wounds.

_____ 5. There are some conditions that massage is not appropriate for.

_____ 6. There is only one licensing/accrediting board for the practice of Ayurveda in the United States.

_____ 7. Energy therapies work with electromagnetic fields that are believed to surround the human body, called biofields.

_____ 8. Accupressure is also called shiatsu.

_____ 9. Aromatherapy, reflexology, and integrative medicine used together in one session is considered an example of complementary medicine.

_____ 10. Therapeutic touch is an invasive, holistic approach to healing that attempts to stimulate the receiver's own powers of recuperation.

FILL IN THE BLANK

Using words from the list below, fill in the blanks to complete the following statements.

acupuncture	heal itself	popular
blood chemistry	healing process	practices
blood pressure	health	properties
concepts	herbs	psychological
conventional medicine	holistic	relaxation
disease process	India	safety and effectiveness
energy flow	knowledge of life	spiritual
flexibility and strength	mental	traditional exercise
hands-on manipulation	physiological health	very thin needles

1. Ayurveda is an ancient healing practice that originated in _____. It means "_____."

2. Alternative medicine has become so _____, and in many instances so promising, that the government has created the National Center for Complementary and Alternative Medicine (NCCAM) to focus on the _____ of alternative therapies.

3. Bodywork is a broad term referring to the _____ of the musculoskeletal system to promote healing, _____, pain reduction, _____, and improved _____.

4. The focus of mind-body medicine is the ways in which a person's _____, emotional, social, and _____ health directly affect his or her _____.

5. Asian medical tradition has contributed several important _____ in alternative medicine, such as _____, acupressure, and the use of _____.

6. Herbs are chosen according to their _____ and are usually used in combination with other _____ treatments.

7. "Complementary and alternative medicine," as defined by NCCAM, "is a group of diverse medical and health care systems, _____, and products that are not presently considered to be a part of _____."

8. Naturopathy is an eclectic approach that helps the body _____ by treating _____, physical, and genetic factors in addition to the _____.

9. Acupuncture involves the insertion of _____ into predetermined sites to stimulate changes in heart rate, _____, brain activity, _____, and the immune and endocrine systems.

10. Hydrotherapy increases _____ and accelerates the _____. It can be used with individuals who cannot withstand the rigors of _____ programs.